DOCTORS AT WAR

CONTRIBUTORS

GEORGE B. DARLING, M.D., Vice-Chairman of the Division of Medical Sciences, National Research Council.

HAROLD S. DIEHL, M.D., Member of the Directing Board, Procurement and Assignment Service, and Dean of the School of Medicine, University of Minnesota.

MAJOR GENERAL DAVID N. W. GRANT, The Air Surgeon.

CHARLES M. GRIFFITH, M.D., Medical Director, Veterans Administration.

MAJOR GENERAL PAUL R. HAWLEY, Chief Surgeon, ETO.

MAJOR GENERAL NORMAN T. KIRK, The Surgeon General, United States Army.

MAJOR GENERAL GEORGE F. LULL, Deputy Surgeon General.

VICE ADMIRAL ROSS T. MCINTIRE, The Surgeon General, United States Navy.

CAPTAIN FRENCH R. MOORE, Medical Corps, United States Navy.

THOMAS PARRAN, M.D., The Surgeon General, United States Public Health Service.

BRIGADIER GENERAL FRED W. RANKIN, Chief Consulting Surgeon, United States Army.

G. CANBY ROBINSON, M.D., LL.D., SC.D., National Director of the Red Cross Blood Donor Service.

COLONEL LEONARD G. ROWNTREE, Chief of the Medical Division, Selective Service System.

COLONEL HOWARD A. RUSK, Chief of the Convalescent Training Division, Army Air Forces.

BRIGADIER GENERAL JAMES STEVENS SIMMONS, M.D., Ph.D., D.P.H., Sc.D. (Hon.), Chief of the Preventive Medicine Service, United States Army.

DOCTORS AT WAR

EDITED BY

MORRIS FISHBEIN, M.D.

EDITOR OF THE *Journal of the American Medical Association*
AND OF *Hygeia,* THE HEALTH MAGAZINE

CHIEF EDITOR OF *War Medicine*

CHAIRMAN OF THE COMMITTEE ON INFORMATION
OF THE DIVISION OF MEDICAL SCIENCES
OF THE NATIONAL RESEARCH COUNCIL

*ILLUSTRATED
WITH PHOTOGRAPHS
AND CHARTS*

Essay Index Reprint Series

BOOKS FOR LIBRARIES PRESS
FREEPORT, NEW YORK

Library of Congress Cataloging in Publication Data

Fishbein, Morris, 1889-   ed.
    Doctors at war.

    (Essay index reprint series)
    1. World War, 1939-1945--Medical and sanitary
affairs. 2. Medicine, Military. I. Title.
D806.F5 1972   940.54'7573   72-4477
ISBN 0-8369-2943-8

Dedicated to the

ONE HUNDRED AND EIGHTY-SIX THOUSAND
PHYSICIANS OF OUR COUNTRY

who, in the armed forces, in industry
and in civilian life,
maintained us in health
during the war years

CONTENTS

LIST OF ILLUSTRATIONS

PREFACE

THIS BOOK *makes available the personal accounts of many of the medical leaders who directed the work of vital military and civilian agencies during the war years. These accounts provide inspiring documentary proof that the nation's doctors served nobly in every capacity to which they were called.*

Several medical histories of the Second World War have been projected, including a great work in fourteen volumes to be published under the auspices of the Division of Medical Sciences of the National Research Council. There will also be specialized histories dealing largely with administration of the medical departments of the Army and Navy. These works, scheduled to appear in the postwar period, will be surveys of what has been accomplished and of what has been learned. This book, however, is the record of doctors in action during the war years, written by the leaders themselves, and as such, it is my hope that the volume will occupy a unique place in the medical documentation of the war.

As editor, I would tender my special appreciation to the contributors, who have prepared their chapters under the stress of wartime work. Especially would I tender my appreciation to Mr. John Tebbel, Associate Editor of E. P. Dutton and Company, who has been helpful particularly in editing much of this material for the general reader, and in planning the entire work.

MORRIS FISHBEIN, M.D.

Chicago

DOCTORS AT WAR

CHAPTER I

DOCTORS AT WAR

By
MORRIS FISHBEIN, M.D.

*Editor, Journal of American Medical Association, War
Medicine and Hygeia, the Health Magazine; Chairman,
Committee on Information, Division of Medical Sciences,
National Research Council*

I

MILITARY PHILOSOPHERS SAY there could never be wars if there
were no doctors. No doubt they are right. The anguish and destruction of the human body in war with modern weapons would
be impossible to contemplate without the healing ministrations,
the pain-obliterating anesthesia, the body-restoring plastic surgery,
the successful combat of epidemics and insect pests that modern
medicine provides.

War medicine is no new experience to the American physician.
In great numbers he volunteered for many a previous war. His
record in those wars, with the knowledge he had at hand, was
good. But his record in World War II, where he could be found
at the fighting front in the mountain fastnesses of New Guinea,
in the mud of France, in the desert of North Africa, on the
sea and in the air, is amazing to contemplate. Never before in the
history of mankind have the statisticians been able to record such
magnificent results. Brigadier General Hugh Morgan is authority
for these comparative figures:

	World War I	*World War II*
Death rate in wounded	8.1%	3.3%
Meningitis mortality	38.0%	4.0%
Pneumonia mortality	28.0%	0.7%
Dysentery mortality	1.6%	0.05%

Annual death rate per 1,000 for all diseases in the Army, excluding surgical conditions	*World War I*	*World War II*
	15.6%	0.6%

The people of the United States who remained at home, giving their utmost in industry, on the farm, in the shops, in transport and in all the other activities of the war years, have been healthy beyond any morbidity and mortality rates achieved by even our own nation in times of peace. The death rate, exclusive of enemy action, for the people of the United States during the first six months of 1944 was the lowest for the like period of any year except the record health years of 1941 and 1942. This means that all our services for maintaining sanitary conditions, controlling infectious diseases and taking care of the sick were still operating efficiently after three years of war. Despite shortages in trained personnel, medicine has been able to carry on for our civilian population at the same highly efficient level as that established for the armed forces.

Suppose you were a doctor in the United States in June, 1940, and that you were attending the annual meeting of the American Medical Association, which was held that year in New York. About 13,000 doctors attended. In the House of Delegates rose Colonel George Dunham, now a brigadier general in charge of all medical aspects of the work of the Coordinator of Inter-American Affairs. He spoke as a representative of the Surgeon General of the United States Army, and warned the delegates that they should be getting ready to play their part in any military activities into which the United States might be drawn. The House of Delegates of the American Medical Association immediately developed a special committee on medical preparedness, charged with developing the necessary personnel for military activities.

The doctor was needed from the day when registrants first appeared before Selective Service boards. Great numbers of specialists were needed for appeal boards. The Army and the Navy had their own induction boards in the camps and in the cantonments. Doctors were needed in the field and in the base hospitals. They were responsible for sanitation. They were concerned with men on the march, with their physiology and with their hygiene. Doctors carried on research dealing with new methods of treatment. They acted as executives in large hospitals and in headquarters units where only medical knowledge makes it possible for an executive to be efficient.

Although the American Medical Association had in its headquarters office the only complete record of doctors available in the United States, appropriations were made by the Board of Trustees of the American Medical Association to improve the system of recording and classifying doctors. A questionnaire was sent to every doctor licensed to practise in the United States, asking him to supply the necessary information which would enable those responsible to determine his availability for military service. As the information was received, it was transferred to a punch-card system as rapidly as possible. The county and State medical societies of the United States were mobilized to bring in the completely filled-out questionnaires. In many a county, committees of doctors called personally on others who, because they were too busy or perhaps slightly neglectful, had failed to return the questionnaires.

At the meeting of the American Medical Association in Cleveland in 1941, when war was even more imminent, a motion was passed by the House of Delegates and forwarded to the President of the United States, the Secretary of War, the Secretary of the Navy and the Surgeons General of the Army, Navy and Public Health Service, advising the establishment of an agency for the procurement and assignment of medical personnel for the various departments of the government related to the war. This agency, appointed by the President, was functioning by the end of 1941. Its services have been instrumental in maintaining a minimum of one doctor for every 1,500 people for most of the United States, in maintaining physicians in the medical schools, in research institutions, in hospitals and all the various medical agencies that have functioned so efficiently during the war. The story of the Procurement and Assignment Service is told fully in this book by Dr. Harold S. Diehl, who has been a member of its directing board since its organization.

Simultaneously with the organization of personnel came the organization of research and standardization of services. These were the tasks of the Office of Scientific Research and Development and the Division of Medical Sciences of the National Research Council. Dr. George B. Darling, in the last chapter of this book, outlines fully the immense contributions that they have made. The high quality of the service rendered our troops in wartime owes much to the distinguished specialists in every field of medical science who throughout the war years have gone week after week, month after month, to Washington to contribute of their knowledge and of their experience to the standardization of medical procedures for the Army and the Navy. Out of the research carried on under their direction, and independently by the various branches of the Army and Navy, have come many discoveries which will be carried over to civilian practice for the benefit of mankind throughout the world in the postwar years.

The education of an American physician yields a product about as well trained and efficient as can be found in any human activity. A young man who wants to study medicine must finish a high school course; he must have two, three, or better, four years of premedical education in a university; he must have four years of medical education in a medical school standardized as to curriculum, quality of teaching and content; he must then have a year or two years of internship and, if he wants to specialize, about three years of residency in some hospital. The demands of war have done strange things to medical education. The curriculum has been condensed, speeded up, accelerated. Americans speak of the wartime medical curriculum as an accelerated curriculum; the British call it a contracted curriculum. Perhaps that is symbolic of the way in which the people of the two nations confront war. The American speeds up and drives forward. The British tighten their belts and doggedly carry on.

Medical schools with diminished faculties admitted 10 per cent more students during the war years, gave them four years of medical education in two and one-half years of continuous study, and speeded their premedical course into one and one-half years. The internship was shortened to nine months, and the residency was shortened to nine months for most young men and to eighteen for a few. At the war's end, it was estimated about 20,000 young men would have had that kind of medical education, together with some war service, to substitute for the kind of medical education that prevailed before the war. American medicine has been taking the necessary steps to make certain that these young men, when they come out of the Army and Navy, will have an opportunity to equip themselves further to meet the demands of the American people for a physician as fully trained as they have had in the past.

The doctors in the medical schools have had many a special burden placed on them in the war period. They have had to double their teaching, do without their vacations, attend the sick in the teaching hospitals, participate in the activities of the National Research Council and the Office of Scientific Research and Development, give graduate courses in hospitals and schools in camps throughout the nation, participate in medical meetings and conferences so that civilian physicians might be kept abreast of wartime medicine. They will need plenty of help in the postwar years. Late in 1944 an appeal was made to Federal agencies, urging that among the first of the physicians to be released in the postwar period be those who held positions as teachers before they joined the Army or the Navy.

Out of 1,000 military physicians who were asked what they wanted most in the immediate postwar years, 796 said they wanted additional postwar training. Nearly 46 per cent requested further work in hospitals for periods of six months to three or more years. Those medical officers whose education was interrupted or diminished by the war merit special consideration in order that they may equip themselves to practise on an equal basis with those who did not participate in military service.

The doctor's contribution to the Selective Service System is well and fully told by Colonel Leonard G. Rowntree in his chapter in this book. More than 33,000 doctors volunteered their time, their knowledge and their skill for this essential war service. They have worked to meet demands that taxed the resources of manpower in the nation. While they were working, even in late 1944, bitter controversies were raging as to just how good a people we are from the point of view of our physical fitness.

Are we, or are we not, a nation of physical weaklings? Is the American recruit of today as good a man physically as were his father, grandfather and great-grandfather in previous wars? Is it true that one-third of our prospective soldiers had to be rejected because of defects in nutrition? How does the American recruit compare with the fighters of our allies and the soldiers of the Axis? If every nation measured its fighters with the same yardstick, the comparisons would be simple. Actually, however, no two nations measure their soldiers by the same standards. We do not

measure the soldiers of World War II as we measured those of
World War I and of the Civil War.

A few simple measurements are obviously the same under all
standards. Thus, we know that the average height of the American
soldier in the Civil War and in World War I and World War II
was 5 feet 7½ inches. His weight, however, differed. In the Civil
War, he weighed 136 pounds; in World War I, he weighed 142
pounds; the soldier of 1944 averaged 150 pounds in weight. The
average height and weight of the class 1A group of selectees in
World War II was 68.1 inches and 152 pounds, while the average
height of men actually inducted into the Army was 68.23 inches,
and the average weight 150 pounds. In Canada the average height
of registrants was 66.6 inches; the average weight 144.6 pounds.

The proponents of new schemes for improving physical fitness
tell us that GI Joe was a flabby soldier. They insist that the coming
of the machine age, with the motor car, the elevator, the tractor,
the crane and all the other machines that substitute steam, air,
gas or electric power for muscle, has given us an individual in-
capable of withstanding the rigors of war. Yet, by every possible
functional test of endurance, the boys of today stand up as well
as did those of previous generations.

After the Selective Service Act was passed, committees of medical experts met with military authorities to establish the standards
by which young men were to be accepted by the local draft boards
or rejected. The Army induction boards rejected young men after
they had been passed by the local board examiners. The difference was in the approach to the problem. The local board examiner wanted to pass every man he could pass as suitable for
military service. He had to make certain that no likely man was
denied the privilege of appearing before an induction board. The
specialists who did the examining for the induction boards put
their emphasis on the need for the protection of the armed forces
against men who were likely to break down in service. That
meant future protection of the taxpayers against the expense involved in carrying such men all the subsequent years of their lives.

Out of the first 2,000,000 men examined, about 1,000,000 were
rejected. Out of the 1,000,000 rejectees, 900,000 were rejected
because of physical defects and 100,000 were rejected because of
illiteracy. Illiteracy, it must be remembered, by Army standards
means that the man concerned has not achieved an education

equivalent to the fourth grade in our public schools. This perhaps is more shameful for the nation than any number of physical defects. Of the 900,000 men who were rejected because of physical defects, 188,000, or 20.9 per cent, were rejected because of dental defects. This was the first war in the history of the United States in which a definite standard prevailed in regard to teeth. No other army in the world ever had such a standard. We demanded at least six good teeth in the upper jaw, including three incisors and three molars, opposite six others in the lower jaw.

In the German army the following conditions prevailed, according to Dr. Hans Müller: "In estimating fitness, we can only assume the stand that a man subject to military service, who is in good general condition and is not dependent on a special diet, is capable of complying with his service duty in either the work service or the armed forces. . . . In case of artificial teeth, it is to be stressed that well-fitting artificial teeth are to be estimated like the natural teeth. In case of removable dentures, the most important factor is not the number of missing and artificially replaced teeth but rather the efficiency of the artificial denture."

After more than a year of experience with our own standards, the Selective Service System announced that a standard similar to that of the German army would thereafter prevail in examining our own recruits. Incidentally, the British said that "partial or total absence of teeth will not constitute grounds for rejection." The Japanese considered rejection because of teeth only when the loss was detrimental to mastication or to speech. The Russians simply said that their teeth were good. They attributed the quality of their teeth, incidentally, to the fact that the Russian diet contains large quantities of black bread.

From the point of view of height, the French soldiers averaged 5 feet 5 inches, the Russians 5 feet 6 inches, the Japanese a little over 5 feet. We insisted in the American Army on a height of at least 5 feet 2 inches, but the British would accept a man only 5 feet tall. Our average weight was 150 pounds. The Japanese would take a man weighing as little as 106 pounds, and the British would take one weighing as little as 113 pounds.

I have endeavored from all the available sources to determine the main causes for rejections of recruits in the other armies of the world. For the Russian army, exact figures are apparently not available, but most authorities estimate that the reasons for rejection were tuberculosis, syphilis, defects of the eyes, rickets and ruptures. The data for the Japanese indicated that trachoma, venereal disease, and difficulties of vision were the main causes for rejection. Among the British, the chief causes included ruptures, difficulties with the eyes, diseases affecting the lungs, defects of hearing, and body deformities. Rejections from the French army were associated with defects of body structure, difficulties in vision and with hearing, and undernourishment. German rejects were refused because of difficulties of vision, total disability due to diseases of the heart and blood vessels, musculoskeletal defects, and venereal and genitourinary diseases.

Through the well-designed plans of the Selective Service System, the Army and Navy medical departments and the scientifically organized services for standardizing nutrition and medical care, men of the highest possible quality of physical fitness have been chosen for service in the armed forces, and every possible means necessary to maintain that kind of physical fitness has been provided.

The great victories won by American troops all over the world were not won by weaklings. The American soldier proved himself to be a competent fighter. He represented a selection of the best physical specimens that our nation had developed. To a group of men chosen by Selective Service and then re-examined by the physicians of the Army and Navy medical departments, there have been applied technics for physical and military training that the years have proved to be efficient.

The 4,000,000 men rejected by Selective Service because they could not meet physical or mental standards are in need of what medicine and physical training have to offer. Many of the registrants were found to be pampered and soft and in need of conditioning. It would be folly for a nation as wealthy and as efficient as ours to fail to give to these people the most that medicine and physical training can give in order to make them effective.

Modern medicine knows that not every person who is mentally or physically unfit can be benefited. Many defects are not preventable with the knowledge that medicine now has to offer. Numerous defects cannot be corrected. Perhaps 1,500,000 of the 4,000,000 referred to would be in this category. Nevertheless, that would leave 2,500,000 men who could be benefited by the application of proper medical treatment and modern physical conditioning. Many of these men could be made to meet the needs of the armed forces. Most of them could be made much more effective in the occupations which they fill in civilian life.

The doctors of the United States have joined with the National Committee on Physical Fitness in the development of a Joint Committee aiming to emphasize physical fitness as a special job during 1945. The knowledge that medicine has gained about life and health, and the program that has been established by experts in the field of physical education and recreation, will be combined to overcome as many as possible of the preventable and correctible defects that were responsible for the rejection of two-thirds of the men summoned to the armed forces. The physicians have the responsibility of keeping records, before and after the establishment of the physical fitness program, to determine the nature of the difficulties to be overcome, and then to determine how well the results have been accomplished.

Even ordinary physical fitness requires development. Physical fitness is a bodily state in which the tissues have power and efficiency. The basic material of the American body is sound; it needs training.

The purpose of the campaign is not the development of big muscles. Physical fitness implies that the heart, lungs, teeth, eyes and other organs are physically sound and capable of working efficiency. Physical fitness implies specific fitness or skill in certain performances. Physical fitness is needed not only by high school and college students and by the armed forces, but by every man and woman in this country. Especially is physical fitness needed in industry, where the fitness of every worker must be geared to his job. The Council on Industrial Health of the American Medical Association, working with representatives of management and labor, is concerning itself particularly with determining the physical condition of workers and with maintaining continuous records of the workers' health and fitness.

Physical fitness includes the practice of good personal hygiene and the application of established knowledge to improve the health and fitness of the human body. It includes enough sleep, the right kind of ventilation and continuous emphasis on cleanliness. It demands proper nutrition, good posture, controlled exercise and rest periods. It embraces mental hygiene and a program of recreation. The new joint campaign for better physical fitness initiated by this conference may well prove to be one of the greatest possible significance for the health and happiness of the American people.

II

Many a story of bravery beyond anything that routine demands has gradually filtered to the public from the records of the armed forces in this war. Especially conspicuous have been the achievements of the Air Forces.

There is, for instance, the story of Second Lieutenant Robert Wesselhoeft, Jr., 27 years old, who was stricken with infantile paralysis in a mountainous region of Western China. For fourteen days he was kept alive by artificial respiration, and then he was evacuated by air to a hospital in Calcutta, India, more than 1,000 miles away, where an artificial respirator—an iron lung—was available. In order to get Lieutenant Wesselhoeft to the hospital plane, he was flown on a three-and-one-half-hour flight in a small plane through weather that had grounded other planes. His pilot flew the small plane with one hand while with the other he pumped a lever to operate an improvised artificial respirator. The village at which Lieutenant Wesselhoeft was stricken was more than 100 miles from a landing field. Major Morris Kaplan, commanding officer of an Air Evacuation Unit, flew from India and, with Lieutenant Colonel John K. Burns, a Fourteenth Air Force medical officer, made the last part of the trip in a combined jeep and mule trek. The details of the story of the flight of the hospital plane and the care of this paralyzed man make one of the most dramatic stories of the war.

Sick and wounded soldiers of the United States and Allied air forces were flown 250,000 times by American military aircraft in the period between Pearl Harbor and D-Day. Almost 7,500 wounded were transported by air from Normandy to the United Kingdom in the 21 days from D-Day until July 1. All over the world, American planes have carried a thousand patients a day. One of the most amazing performances was the flying of sick and wounded from Burma in jeep planes. At first, according to Major General David N. W. Grant, our troop and cargo carriers transported up to 24 patients. During flight, medical care was provided by flight nurses, working in medical air evacuation squadrons under the supervision of flight surgeons. By 1944, planes carried even more than 24 patients at a time, and the jeep planes carried one or two patients in an emergency. From Pearl Harbor up to mid-1944, the Army Transport Command had flown more than 9,000 patients from the theaters of operations into the United States for hospitalization, and during 1944, patients arrived by plane at the rate of approximately 100 every day. This in itself is one of the major accomplishments of medicine in the war because the speed of evacuation of the wounded has been a fundamental factor in the magnificent record of recovery.

In a late report, Major General Paul R. Hawley, who describes preparations for D-Day later in this volume, said that the condition of the casualties on arrival in the United Kingdom was surprisingly fine. Fractures had been well splinted. Shock had been treated on the landing ships (tanks) and hospital carriers, so that it was a rare patient who arrived at the hospital in shock. Indeed, General Hawley asserted, there were many American soldiers who owed their lives to the surgeons aboard the LSTs, who gave immediate emergency care to casualties evacuated from the fighting. An experienced surgeon was placed on every LST, and in addition there were two young medical officers of the Navy and about twenty hospital corpsmen on D-Day and during the early operations. Especially remarkable has been the wonderful cooperation between the Army and Navy medical departments, characterized as a "model of complete cooperation."

People often wonder why the Army and Navy have to have so many doctors. We began with about 8 doctors to 1,000 men. That dropped to 6.5, and more recently to about 5.5 for the Army, and as low as 4 doctors for 1,000 men in the Navy. People should not wonder any more when they read of the importance of having a surgeon on every LST, and two naval medical officers on every small boat that transports wounded. The immediate presence of doctors in the fighting at the front must be classified as one of the major factors in saving the lives of our wounded.

Often the violent demands of military life speed the development of new methods and new technics which prove themselves so well that they become routine when peace returns. Every war in the history of mankind has brought with it new inventions and devices that modified the lives of people. Those phases of war which are concerned with the study of injuries and disease are susceptible of great advancement because the control of injuries and disease may well mean the difference between victory and defeat.

Before the beginning of World War II, medical research had begun to advance prominently along three main lines—chemotherapy, nutrition and glandular therapy. Outstanding, however, among the medical accomplishments of World War II have been those relating to chemotherapy and the control of infectious disease.

Early in the present century, medicine began to turn to chemotherapy when Paul Ehrlich made his announcement of the discovery of salvarsan, or 606, for syphilis. Ehrlich may well be called the father of modern chemotherapy. Out of his discovery came the sulfonamides. New inventions or discoveries in the field of medicine promptly stimulated great numbers of investigators to undertake work along similar lines. The technic that yielded salvarsan gave us sulfanilamide. Today the original sulfanilamide has been expanded to a wide variety of sulfonamide drugs, including sulfapyridine, sulfathiazole, sulfaguanidine, sulfadiazine, sulfasuxidine, promin and many others. Each of these is beginning to be considered especially efficient against infections of a certain type. For instance, sulfathiazole is used against infections with the gonococcus, sulfaguanidine against the intestinal infections, and promin—at least in experimental animals—against tuberculosis. Sulfadiazine is considered, in general, a less toxic, all-purpose sulfa drug, and more recently sulfamerazine has been launched for a similar purpose. In the laboratories of innumerable investigators, hundreds if not thousands of modifications of the sulfonamides are still being studied—first, isolated by the chemist; second, tested as to their virtues and toxicity by the pharmacologist; and third, applied in the clinic to the treatment of disease.

Still more amazing, perhaps, among the discoveries of World War II have been the so-called antibiotic agents, including gramicidin and tyrothricin, but even more remarkable is penicillin. This, indeed, is one of the great romances of medical science. Almost fifteen years have passed since the British bacteriologist Fleming observed in his laboratory the fact that the common mold *penicillium notatum* would prevent the growth of germs. It required the impetus of war to cause Florey to make the actual tests of the product on animals, and later on men, which gave the world this greatest of all boons for the conquest of infectious disease. It required the stimulus of war to bring about the vast production of the product in a short time, so that in 1944 American industry was producing more penicillin than was available in all the rest of the world. It required the urge and conditions of war to permit the testing of penicillin by a variety of technics on meningitis so that one naval officer was able to report 75 consecutive cases of meningitis of all types cured by this remedy.

The menace of venereal disease in wartime led to the development of special venereal disease hospitals and venereal disease centers in which new methods of treatment could be tried. Today we know that penicillin can cure gonorrhea in 24 hours and in all likelihood eliminate the menace of syphilis from the human body in five days. Indeed, late reports indicate that this drug can stop the ravages of general paresis—syphilis of the nervous system and locomotor ataxia.

In his article describing the work of the American Red Cross, Dr. G. Canby Robinson tells the amazing story of blood plasma. For many years blood transfusion had been practised, beginning with the actual tying of the blood vessel of a donor to a vein of the recipient. Then came the transfer of whole blood from one person to another with a syringe. A Russian doctor named Yudin first suggested that the blood of people who died while in good health should be taken from the bodies and preserved for transfer to the living sick who might require it. From this came the suggestion for blood banks to contain liquid blood plasma. Finally came technics for drying and preserving blood plasma, thus making it available for shipment over thousands of miles for use directly on the battlefield.

This tremendous achievement was in turn the stimulus for research studies which have led to the purification of the proteins of the blood for direct administration to the sick. Gelatin, acacia and similar chemical substances are being tested as substitutes for blood plasma. Perhaps the ultimate development will be the securing of some material in pure form from the blood of cattle or of other animals so modified that it may be given to a human being. Until that time comes, the blood donor centers of the Red Cross serve as veritable life-saving stations, not only for men in battle but for the sufferers from injuries and burns in great holocausts like the Boston and Hartford fires, in railroad wrecks, and in the other casualties of civilian life.

Outstanding also among the scientific contributions that have aided the winning of the war has been the development of the drug called atabrine as a substitute for quinine in the control of malaria. In 1940, Surgeon General Thomas Parran of the United States Public Health Service pointed out the necessity for developing as rapidly as possible a supply of quinine and of narcotics for which we looked to the Orient—a supply sufficient to last for three to five years.

When the Japanese struck at Pearl Harbor, and then swiftly at the East Indies, our supplies were shut off. More than a year before Pearl Harbor, however, the need for a drug to take the place of quinine for a war against malaria had been recognized. In the history of mankind, malaria has played a tremendous part in determining the fates of nations. In North Africa, in the South Pacific and in the Caucasus, even in France and Italy, malaria might disable, if not destroy, an army more certainly than it could be destroyed by warfare. In this country the manufacture of atabrine had been conducted on an extremely small scale, most of the product coming from abroad. When the time came to manufacture the product, it was discovered that the basic materials were lacking, the processes not clearly understood, even the necessary chemists and other personnel not yet properly trained.

Today, however, the manufacturers of the product supply more than two billion tablets of the drug, sufficient to meet not only our own needs but also those of our British, Russian and Chinese allies. Malaria and dengue fever are the principal health problems in the Solomon Islands, and there atabrine is taken routinely by the men for the control of malaria. Obviously, at the end of this war vast supplies of these and many other drugs developed for war needs will become far more widely available, and at prices much lower than now prevail, and thus will be within the reach of millions of people who might not otherwise be able to secure them.

Step by step, improvement has taken place in the manufacture of anesthetics, particularly those administered under the skin or by injection elsewhere in the body as a substitute for the anesthetics that were inhaled. In some forms of anesthesia, the barbituric acid derivatives are injected directly into the blood. In other forms, derivatives of the cocaine group are injected into the spinal fluid and act directly on the spinal cord. Most recent is the designing of a technic in which a derivative of cocaine, called metycaine, or others, such as procaine, may be injected directly into the area around the nerve roots at the base of the spinal column in the so-called sacral area, thus blocking entirely pain from all the areas served by the nerve roots which come out of the spinal cord in this region. Since the nerves of the uterus and the birth tract in women come from this area, physicians have been able to devise a means for completely painless childbirth, a goal long sought in the history of medical science.

When the forces of the United Nations entered Naples, they were confronted with the possibility of an epidemic of typhus. To their aid came a new discovery developed by the research divisions of our war effort: DDT, the miracle insecticide and repellent of World War II. No one now knows exactly what the ultimate uses of this product will be. Its presence in the seams of clothing will repel body lice. DDT is given most of the credit for stopping the outbreak of typhus in Naples. Reports say it will destroy a housefly on a wall as late as two months after the product has been put there, that it is fatal to moths, and that mosquitoes (including the malaria-bearing mosquito) cannot survive its distribution in the vicinity where they develop.

New technics for distributing insecticides have also come from this war's needs. Perhaps the freon bomb alone may, in the years to come, more than repay the costs of World War II. The Westinghouse Company, for instance, by 1944 had produced more than 10,000,000 insect bombs, each containing enough spray to remove the bugs from 150 Army pup tents or 50 giant bombers.

The National Research Council sponsored extensive studies in various clinics on the treatment of burns. Probably no other phase of medical treatment received so much attention as did the treatment of burns. Burns constituted almost 30 per cent of the injuries to men in the Navy. In all, about 80 different methods for the treatment of burns had been published up to 1944. The methods of treatment included pressure bandages, painting with paraffin films containing sulfa drugs, the giving of great amounts of blood plasma internally, and many other technics. The vast experience of this war will eventually yield standardization in a field where it might have been long postponed had it not been for the immense number of cases made available in the war effort.

These major fields of medical research are supplemented by studies of the tropical diseases which menace our men on many a foreign front, and by new technics in surgery, including particularly peripheral nerve surgery and orthopedic surgery. More than one-half of the wounds affecting our soldiers are wounds of the arms and legs, fracturing bones, cutting nerves, injuring muscles. Again and again I have seen in our hospitals most amazing reconstructive efforts involving the use of transplants of bone, wiring with tantalum wire, the use of bone screws and metal plates, and all sorts of similar technics which have been successful. Much of the success of this new surgery depends on the ability to keep the wounds free from infection by the use of penicillin. Tantalum, a new substance, is used both as a suture material and as a foil for filling defects of bone, as an intervening substance to prevent scarring around nerves, and in many other ways to help war surgery.

Interesting also in nerve surgery has been the development of the substance called fibrin foam, composed of substances taken from the by-products of blood plasma production. This fibrin foam serves to clot blood and acts as a framework for the growth of nerves. Another product of the blood plasma program has been the concentrated red blood cell solution, which, when used as such or in the form of a paste, has been found to be efficient in the healing of wounds.

The most frequent cause of discharge from the armed forces has been what is commonly called the "NP" case—the neuropsychiatric disturbance. These represent as high as 45 per cent of all cases of disability. To their study and control a variety of new technics have been applied, including the use of barbituric acid derivatives to produce a state of narcosis and thus enable the doctor to study the basic difficulties. Hypnosis has been combined with this procedure in many cases. The newer advances of psychosomatic medicine have been applied. By all these technics, great numbers of men were returned to service who might otherwise have been discharged. The neuropsychiatric casualties in civilian life are also greater because of the stresses of war, and the worker who breaks down in industry gets the benefit of these methods.

The advances that have been mentioned are but an indication of the many hundreds of technics in medicine improved by the stimulus of war and made applicable by better technics of distribution and mass production to the needs of more and more people.

New methods of overcoming contagious diseases have been developed under the Army's board for the investigation and control of infectious and other epidemic diseases. A method of oiling floors and blankets to trap the germs of air-borne infections became common practice and was instrumental in lowering the number of such infections among troops in barracks. A by-product of the blood plasma program has been the discovery that a protein of the blood called gamma globin contains the antibodies which are capable of combating measles. Through the cooperation of the Red Cross with the great industries that have been providing the necessary drugs for our armed forces, this anti-measles preparation is now being made available at cost to State health departments so that they may, in turn, provide it for the people of the individual States.

When meningitis breaks out in any Army camp, the routine taking of sulfadiazine has been found to be efficient in preventing spread of the disease.

During World War I, influenza was probably responsible for more deaths than any other single cause; indeed, the epidemic of 1918 took its toll of countless victims all over the world. Since that time, viruses known to be responsible for the development of influenza have been isolated and it has been shown that it is the combination of the streptococcus infection with a virus infection that produces the deadly epidemic. Now the streptococcus is kept under control by the sulfonamide drugs and penicillin, and vaccines have been developed which are effective against influenza A and B viruses. The organization of the Bureau of Preventive Medicine in the Army medical department includes commissions of some of the greatest experts in American medicine, who deal with acute respiratory diseases, air-borne infections, epidemics, streptococcal infections, influenza, measles, mumps, meningitis, virus diseases, pneumonia and tropical diseases. Especially dramatic was the work of the commission concerned with sandfly fever. Fourteen soldiers volunteered, as did the soldiers of the Spanish-American War, to be inoculated with this disease. In that war, under the Reed-Gorgas Commission, men volunteered to be infected with yellow fever.

Our soldiers in the tropics suffered severely with sandfly fever, also called phlebotomus fever. This fever is caused by the bite at night of a sandfly which carries the disease. The sandfly is about one-eighth of an inch long and it is only the female that bites. The fever is not contagious. The disease can be transmitted only by the bite of the sandfly which has previously bitten a person who had the fever. Experiments made by a special group of investigators showed that the virus which causes the fever in the Middle East is the same as that which caused sandfly fever in our soldiers in Sicily. All these men who volunteered for the experiments were given the Legion of Merit medals by the United States Army in recognition of their contribution to the winning of the war.

In a further experiment, it was found that two chemical insect repellents, DDT, also known as dimethyl phthalate, and a vanishing cream that was rich in pyrethrum would prevent the bite of the sandfly.

Also serious for men in the tropics has been filariasis, caused by a parasite known as the *Wuchereria bancrofti*, which is transmitted by several types of mosquitoes. This is the parasite that causes men to have elephantiasis if the disease continues for long without control. In August, 1944, 522 servicemen with filariasis came back to the United States, where they were sent at once to a special hospital for the study and control of that disease.

Outstanding among the studies of the Bureau of Preventive Medicine was the preparation of a survey of every area in the world which our soldiers were likely to invade. Thus, it became possible, when our troops were about to invade Guam, to warn servicemen that all water on Guam, regardless of its source, must be regarded as unsafe until proved otherwise, and to tell them that fly control measures should be instituted immediately on arrival because of the importance of flies in the spread of dysentery, yaws and various diseases of the skin. Complete instructions were given for the protection of soldiers from insects, and a technic of sewage disposal had to be worked out. Of necessity, many of the sewers were below sea level. The warning went forth that camps should be far from places frequented by natives and that natives should not, except under extraordinary circumstances, enter a camp area. This was done to cut down the chance of the soldiers getting hookworm, with which 25 per cent of the natives of Guam are infected. The medical services must be given much of the credit for the exceedingly low rate of disease among our troops in every invaded area.

III

Major General Paul Hawley later in this book tells of the preparations of our Army for the invasion of France. The Navy too—and indeed every branch of our armed services—had long been planning for this day, which meant the beginning of the end of the war. By August, 1941, the Navy had set up a special naval dispensary in London with a senior medical officer whose duties covered all of England. A supply and repair base had been set up at Londonderry in Ireland late in 1942 with bed facilities for 300 patients. Storehouses for medical supplies had been established in Brooklyn, in San Francisco and, still farther out, in the Pacific and in North Africa. Now it became necessary to establish such a warehouse in Great Britain.

A stock of approximately 2,000 different items is maintained in each warehouse for replenishment of drugs and dressings. The medical department of the Navy, for instance, requires 160,000 blankets every six months as replacements and 24,000 chemical heating pads with three times that number of refills for each pad. Other replenishments to be shipped twice a year include 7,200 surgical knife blades, 32,800 assorted hypodermic needles, 18,600 surgical needles, 136,000 surgical sutures, 144,000 dental burrs, 370,000 yards of gauze for dressings, 4 tons of absorbent cotton, 518,000 bandages of assorted sizes, and 179,000 battle dressings. And if these figures give you a headache, just think over the fact that the Navy uses for each storehouse 700,000 aspirin tablets every six months.

Preliminary to the invasion, hundreds of young physicians trained in Solomons Island, Maryland; San Diego, California; Great Lakes, Illinois, and Fort Pierce, Florida. Since the invasion was a cooperative effort, a procedure was planned to utilize men from both the Army and Navy. This was the planned procedure:

At 20 or 30 minutes past the hour of attack, the Army sends ashore a Battalion Landing Team of two medical officers and 32 enlisted men. They tag the wounded (men of the first waves will have been given aid by their own comrades) and mark their positions for later collectors. The Navy unit, a Medical Section Shore Party, consists of one medical officer and eight hospital corpsmen. They set up a beach evacuation station, receive the cases sent or brought to them by the Army's collecting teams, give additional first aid treatment, and prepare the casualties for evacuation.

Later Army units land with jeeps and light trucks, in which they help to gather up the litters and take them along the beach to the evacuation point. Jeeps are fitted with special racks, front and back, to carry a total of four stretchers. DUKWs, also under Army control, are a most useful member of the evacuation team. As much at home at sea as on land, they can take a load of eight or ten litters along the beach, put out to sea, and drive up the bow-ramp of a waiting ship.

The Navy medical officer, through the Beachmaster, will have secured small craft for the removal of the casualties from the evacuation station. Another essential job that must be done at this point is to keep the "running records" by which cases passing through this clearing house are identified and described.

As the position on shore becomes more firmly established, more and larger Army units go ashore and leap-frog inland as far as they may, setting up a well-defined chain of evacuation of which the Navy links are those concerned with transportation afloat. The Navy supervises the embarkation and provides boats and crews.

Before that process of evacuation is examined more closely, the question of medical supplies for the early shore parties might be noted. Since in this phase only emergency aid can be given, only the simplest equipment need be on hand. Light and easily handled waterproof packs, preferably shoulder packs, are used, permitting freedom of action on difficult terrain and under fire. Not only has the content of the pack been carefully studied, but the type of pack itself, down to such details as its compartmentation and the use of snap-fasteners. ("Zippers foul up when wet or with blood on them, therefore impractical.")

Experience in the Pacific showed that basic items that could be brought ashore in shoulder packs might soon be exhausted, since casualties tend to be greater in the early phases. Loss or premature departure of the supporting ships sometimes deprived the medical shore party of renewals. To bridge this gap, a "Medical Resupply Unit" was devised. Two waterproof bags, contained in a larger canvas bag, are packed with bandages, dressings, plasma, sulfa tablets, morphine syrettes, splints and diagnosis tags. Such a unit is placed in each of the landing boats assigned to the later assault waves, and the boat crew is made responsible for landing the unit on the beach. It weighs only 32 pounds and can readily be thrown toward the high water mark. Shore parties are then under instructions to collect these units and stack them in the medical dump. This simple expedient assures adequate material for use until the Army's larger medical units can establish themselves.

Provision is also made for an automatic exchange of certain items to keep a constant flow of indispensable medical material going forward. As a casualty arrives at an aid station, his bearers deposit him and take in return another litter and blanket, plus battle dressings and splints. This process is repeated as the various stages back to the beach are reached. Not only is item exchanged for item, but in addition spare material may be sent forward on demand.

The officer in charge of the Navy medical shore party, immediately upon landing, selects his evacuation point. It must not be too exposed, yet it must be accessible to litter-bearers and to the walking wounded. It must be centrally located, both as regards land and sea, but should not be near ammunition or fuel dumps, which also must be centrally located. The station must be easy to move, for it must follow the ebb and flow of battle if it is to serve its purpose. While some of his men are putting up this hasty shelter, others, along with the Army personnel, are scouting about the area, giving first aid, directing those who can walk to the clearing station, transporting those who cannot.

Injuries are there diagnosed and, where possible, given initial treatment. The more gravely injured are given morphine, but must await treatment later in the schedule. All patients are tagged with essential information as to what has been done for them to avoid duplication or disagreement in handling. Then, as circumstances permit, they are taken in small groups to the evacuation center next to the water line, whence they may be loaded into small boats for removal.

All this seaward movement is the Navy's responsibility. It is the Navy medical officer who supervises and integrates its factors. Army first aid units, pushing farther inland as military progress allows, send their casualties back to this waterside clearing station through the regular chain of evacuation. The casualties may be Army or Navy, American or Allied, or they may be prisoners of war, who are accorded the same expert treatment.

The next step in the process of evacuation is perhaps the most difficult. Helpless men must be taken from the beach, by way of small boats, to the larger ships which will carry them back to a friendly shore. This must be done in the heat of battle, and perhaps in rough weather. And it must be done against a heavy and urgent flow of traffic. Men and materials are being poured on to the beach with all possible speed. Against that excited, eager tide of troops and boat crews, the casualties must make their way.

Any boat used in landing operations may be utilized for embarking casualties at the beach.

Methods had, therefore, to be devised and procedures rehearsed for the most effective utilization of each of several types of boat. Take, for example, a 36-foot LCVP, a landing craft for vehicles. She will chug up to the beach, lowering her ramp as the water becomes shallower. Down will swarm men, jeeps and light trucks. A crewman will toss ashore the medical resupply unit in its canvas bag. Litters will have been waiting at the landing point, and as soon as traffic can move that way, Army litter-bearers will take the wounded aboard the LCVP. Theoretically, eight litters can be accommodated on deck, and cables rigged from side to side can make room for a second layer of six. But there are also an indefinite number of non-stretcher wounded to transport, and there may be a certain impatience to shove off and return to the parent ship. Therefore, the full stretcher load may not always be aboard.

All the many types of small landing craft are prepared to do this service, each according to its design and its capacity. Each carries first aid material in addition to that needed for its own crew.

The roomy, sea-going LSTs—landing ships for tanks—have been found the most efficient craft for the next stage of the journey. Their design adapts them for the double duty, and they are sure to be present in numbers at any scene of amphibious operation. They are, therefore, stocked with all the medical supplies and surgical equipment that may be needed. Medical officers and corpsmen are stationed aboard for these shuttle operations, and they may have the assistance of a team of Army surgeons. LST crews are specifically trained to do their share in embarking the wounded. Hands are detailed to man the hoists and to serve as litter-bearers aboard.

As fighting men and fighting materials go shoreward by way of the LST's bow-ramp, the small boats, with their helpless passengers collected at the evacuation clearing stations back on the beach, nose alongside. Casualties may then be put aboard at the rate of one per minute per lift, plus those who are driven right aboard on Army-manned DUKWs. Slings of various types are lowered overside and litters, one or two at a lift, are hoisted aboard. The less gravely wounded are also eased on deck by slings, either singly or, sitting snugly on a platform, six or eight at a time. The casualties are all on board by the time the warlike cargo has been unloaded, and the ship can then get under way for safer waters.

When a soldier has been wounded or when he breaks down from the mental stresses of war, he must be made fit again for either military service or civilian life. Colonel Howard Rusk has described the technic used by the Army Air Forces, much of it developed under his direction. The Army itself also has a large reconditioning program, including physical reconditioning, occupational, educational and recreational treatment. Although the boys who break down from either mental or physical causes are under military discipline, they are permitted latitude to follow interests which will be useful to them in later life. Army experience has shown that the majority of boys with mental or emotional upsets are benefited by being given immediately a planned program to prevent apathy, morbid introspection and manifestation of emotional disturbances. In every service command of the Army, a center for reconditioning neuropsychiatric patients has been established, and when the boys come back from overseas and are interviewed by the psychiatrists at the debarkation hospitals, they are sent, unless the condition requires immediate hospitalization, to one of these reconditioning centers.

The physical activities of men who have been wounded or who

have broken down under the strain of war are definitely related to the needs of the individual patient. While some of the exercises are general, others are designed to strengthen particular weaknesses. The men have a program which includes calisthenics, gymnastics, swimming and water-resistant exercises. Individual and group recreation includes movies, shows, dances and games, which are furnished by the American Red Cross. To a reconditioning officer of the Army medical department is assigned the special task of applying all that medicine knows to make the wounded or convalescent soldier fit for civilian or military life.

The problem of keeping men at work at machines and physically fit in wartime is just as important as the maintenance of men in the armed forces. In the United States one of our greatest problems has been the building of industrial medicine so that it might keep the health of workers at its peak. In our country, before the war, 85 to 90 per cent of industrial medicine had been carried on by general practitioners who gave part of their time to the aid of workers in industrial plants. In many a large industry the care of the workers was in the hands of specialists in the field of industrial medicine.

As a result of experience in World War II, industrial medicine has come to mean examination of the worker prior to employment, a study of his nutrition and his habits of life, control of exposure in the plant to gases and to flying particles, protection of the worker's eyes, protection against dust and protection against accidents. Industrial medicine extends into the home of the worker.

As great numbers of women came into our expanding industries, the problem of the woman in industry had to be given special consideration. Far too many of them were trying to do two jobs—one in the home and one in the factory. Special committees rendered reports on the protection of women in industry. The combined efforts of the medical profession and of various governmental agencies resulted in protection that is reflected in the sickness and death rates of our women workers.

Stimulated by the war, American medicine today is undertaking a program of education to expand the 1,500 qualified specialists in industrial medicine to at least 10,000 doctors capable of giving attention to the care of the worker in industry.

For forty years, at least, we in the United States have had more doctors proportionately to the population than any other country in the world. Our people have had, in the past two generations, the highest quality of medical service anywhere available. More and better hospitals have become easily accessible because of good roads, motor cars and telephones.

But war does things to the availability of hospitals. When a munitions plant is built forty miles out in the country and some thousands of employees congregate around it, the hospital which formerly served a community of a few hundred cannot take care of them. Doctors have to be taken to such communities; x-ray and laboratory equipment must be supplied. Many a board and many a committee has been working on this problem of the allocation of doctors.

"Dislocating" a doctor in the United States is more difficult than it might at first seem to be. Every one of our States has its own laws regulating medical licensure. In the simplest form of medical practice a doctor, finding a community in another State which requires his services, goes to that community, takes out a license to practise, opens an office, and begins taking care of the sick for whatever they can pay him. That method, which worked well under most circumstances in prewar life, is fraught with difficulties in time of war. The need for doctors becomes so great that physicians do not have to submit themselves to any risk. The lack of suitable facilities, such as hospitals, x-ray equipment and laboratories, is such a handicap to good medical practice that modern young doctors will not go into a community where those facilities are not available.

During the war, the health center movement gained speed, and some hundreds of health centers were set up by Federal funds contributed to the individual States, with a view to making good medical service more accessible to great numbers of people. New technics were developed to enable one doctor or groups of doctors to supply more and more people with needed medical care.

By such methods the medical needs of America at war have been met. By similar technics more and more medical service is likely to become available in the postwar period.

Never before in the history of the United States has it been necessary to select from the available manpower of the nation more than 10,000,000 men fit to fight. First to be called into this service were the physicians of America, because every draft board had a doctor and there were boards of consultants to give opinions in special cases. A technic of examination had to be developed and modified from time to time to meet changing needs and standards.

At first a medical officer of the regular Army, Lieutenant Colonel Charles B. Spruit, was assigned to aid in the medical aspects of the Selective Service System, but then he was called to work with the General Staff, and Colonel Leonard G. Rowntree, for many years professor of medicine at the University of Minnesota and chief of the medical division of the Mayo Foundation, was appointed to this task.

During World War I, he had served in France as an executive officer of the Air Service Research Laboratories. More recently Colonel Rowntree was appointed vice-chairman of the National Committee on Physical Fitness of the Federal Security Agency. In this capacity he has devoted himself now, and will no doubt devote himself largely in the future, to the problem of building men for America better fit to undertake the service of the nation in peace and in war.

Colonel Rowntree's contribution to this volume explains the methods by which the Army was built and the failings in our physical and mental qualifications to meet the needs, and he points the way to future progress in overcoming these defects.

CHAPTER II

FIT TO FIGHT: THE MEDICAL SIDE OF SELECTIVE SERVICE

By
Colonel Leonard G. Rowntree
Chief of the Medical Division, Selective Service System

I

The doctor's selective service work was one of the fundamental services needed in the whole program of war manpower mobilization; it was a job done quietly and effectively. The spirit of service and sacrifice was evident in the thousands of examining physicians, members of medical advisory boards, and examining dentists who participated in the work in every State and in every community.

Recorded herewith, in general outline, is the work of the medical and dental professions as examining physicians, as members of medical advisory boards, and as workers at induction centers.

The story begins with the passage of the Selective Training and Service Act of 1940, a peacetime measure enacted in the shadow of war. Originally it was designed to provide authority for the leisurely procurement of an army for national defense. As amended later, the Act provided for the wartime control of manpower allocation for both military and civilian needs: On the one hand, to obtain through selection the maximum number of qualified men needed by all the branches of the armed forces for the successful prosecution of the war; and on the other hand, to provide for war production through selective deferment of sufficient numbers of essential skilled workers in industry and agriculture.

This dual function imposed on Selective Service the need for frequent changes in policy to meet the constantly shifting demands for troops, and for manpower to produce food and armaments.

Regulations had to be amended from time to time to meet changes in policy.

In the beginning, the pool of manpower appeared so enormous as to be inexhaustible. But as the various and expanding demands were met, it became apparent that only through the wisest allocation of manpower could the national objective be fulfilled. Major adjustments became imperative in matters of marriage, fatherhood, dependency, agriculture, essential occupations, etc. Through it all, the Selective Service System strove to maintain an optimum balance in supplying all the needs defined by national objectives.

The Selective Service Act was signed by the President on September 16, 1940, and, immediately after, the Selective Service System was organized on a national basis under the guidance of Lewis B. Hershey, then a Lieutenant Colonel. Subsequently, on October 15, 1940, Dr. Clarence A. Dykstra was appointed Director, in which capacity he served until July, 1941. On December 29, 1940, the President proclaimed that this country was to become "the arsenal of democracy." Mr. Dykstra resigned on March 21, 1941, and his duties were assumed by Brigadier General Hershey, who was appointed Director on July 31, 1941. Selective Service has been fortunate, indeed, in his wise guidance.

The Act to be administered by General Hershey authorized the induction into the Army of 900,000 men a year, over a period of five years, and their retention in the Reserve thereafter for ten years. These men were selected indiscriminately from all walks of life, except those specifically exempted by the Act.

The first step was the registration of men within certain age limits. When the President signed the Selective Service Act, he issued a proclamation fixing October 16, 1940, as the first day of registration for all male citizens between 21 and 36 years of age who were residing in the United States.

The order of reporting for induction was determined by lottery. Orders for induction were issued by local boards, according to calls from military authorities to National Headquarters, thence to State Headquarters and to the local boards. The first order of business by the local board was classification in accordance with the Regulations. All registrants placed in classification 1-A were subjected to physical examination in accordance with the Standards of Physical Examination during Mobilization (MR 1-9) prescribed by the military establishment.

A second registration occurred on July 1, 1941, this one for young men who had reached the age of 21 in the interim. On February 16, 1942, came a third registration, for men who would be 21 years of age by July 1, 1942; and on April 27, 1942, there was a fourth registration, for all men between the ages of 45 and 65. The fifth registration was held on July 30, 1942, when all men born on or after January 1, 1922, or on or before June 30, 1942, were required to register. Thus all the nation's males between the ages of 18 and 65 were registered.

On October 17, 1940, the President gave the Director of the Selective Service System authority to perform the duties and functions established under the Selective Training and Service Act. These were set forth in the Regulations, which consisted of six volumes: Volume One, Organization and Administration; Volume Two, Registration; Volume Three, Classification and Selection; Volume Four, Delivery and Induction; Volume Five, Finance; and Volume Six, Physical Standards.

Selective Service authority was decentralized, with each State responsible for its quota and for the administration of the Selective Service Law, its rules and regulations. The organization included National Headquarters in Washington; 54 State and District Headquarters; 6,403 local boards (since expanded to 6,441), and 660 medical advisory boards (now numbering 812). In all, the Selective Service personnel comprised some 200,000 lay and professional workers, including some 33,000 physicians and 8,000 dentists, all serving on a voluntary basis.

National Headquarters was located in Washington, D.C. The System was under general supervision of the Director, who had as chief aides a Deputy Director, two Assistant Directors, thirteen Chiefs of Division, and eleven Assistant Executives.

The Medical Division advised and cooperated with the Director and with the State Medical Officers, and assisted in formulating policies of a medical nature. This division was staffed by a Chief and several specialized assistants. Associated with the Medical Division, there were set up a number of Advisory Committees. Such committees were appointed in the fields of psychiatry, general medicine, dentistry and statistics. Another committee, composed of deans of medical schools, advised Headquarters on problems of medical education. Additional committees were appointed to aid in the operation of the Medical Survey Program. These committees all met on call for discussion of medical problems, and submitted their recommendations. They were all purely advisory in nature and had no administrative function.

In each State there was a State Director and one or more State medical officers who were, as a rule, Medical Reserve officers placed on active duty by their respective services. The State Medical Officer was responsible to the State Director and the Governor of the State. His duties consisted of coordinating the work and cooperating with the local boards. He was the chief medical liaison officer between National and State Headquarters.

The local board was the real functioning unit of Selective Service. In it were centered the authority and responsibility for classification of all registrants. Crucial decisions, as they affected registrants, were made by the local boards.

Among the important provisions of the Act, relating to local boards, were:

1. There shall be at least one local board in each county, or political subdivision, corresponding thereto in each State, Territory, and the District of Columbia. 2. The local board shall consist of three or more members to be appointed by the President from recommendations made by the respective Governors, or other comparable executive, State or Territorial officials. 3. The boards shall have power within their jurisdiction to hear and determine all questions or claims with respect to inclusion for and exemption or deferment from training and service under the Act, of all individuals within the jurisdiction of such local boards.

(a) These determinations shall be subject to the right of appeal to the appeal boards authorized under the Act.

(b) Decisions of local boards are final, except where an appeal is authorized.

Attached to each local board were one or more examining physicians who took responsibility for all the medical phases involved. The examining physicians of the local boards carried on most of the medical function. In the beginning, they numbered some 17,000, which was later increased to 33,000. From 8,000 to 10,000 dentists also served. Originally, medical examinations were conducted in the offices of the physicians and consisted in taking medical histories and giving complete physical examinations, which included urinalysis, taking blood for serological tests, and in the majority of instances, blood pressure studies. This individual examination continued in effect in most rural communities, and proved very effective.

It is evident, from the above analysis, that the medical function has been exercised at community, State and national levels.

Physical examinations were conducted by the examining physicians, one or more of whom were attached to each local board. It was their function to procure all the information available from the family physicians, social agencies, etc.; to conduct a complete physical examination in accordance with regulations; to collect blood for serological examination; to recommend the classification in 1-A of such men as appeared satisfactory for general military service; in 1-B, of men capable of limited military service; and in IV-F, of those men who were disqualified for admission by the prevailing standards. Furthermore, the local board physicians were urged to accept or reject the registrants only if definitely certain of their grounds, otherwise to forward them to the medical advisory board for expert medical judgment and advice prior to taking action.

The medical advisory board, or any of its members, was to conduct, on request, a complete and thorough physical examination, using certain designated laboratory tests, if indicated, in order to establish the actual diagnoses. Subsequent to the examination, the registrant, the record, the diagnoses, and the opinion of the medical advisory board or board members were returned to the local board for disposition.

Registrants classified as 1-A by the local board were sent forward to the armed forces induction stations, where they were subjected to a thorough physical re-examination and either inducted or rejected. If rejected, they were returned to the local board. The board, if satisfied with the rejection, classified the registrant as IV-F; if dissatisfied, it could call for a re-examination by the medical advisory board, and on their advice resubmit the registrant to the induction station for individual versus group examinations (re-examination and reconsideration).

As time passed, a constantly growing tendency developed for the physical examination of registrants to be carried on by groups of physicians working in teams and at hospitals, rather than as individual doctors working in their own offices. While the office examination usually took from 40 to 50 minutes per man, it was found that the work could be more effectively handled by groups, cutting down the time required for each registrant, and at the same time improving the quality of the examination. The medical functions of Selective Service came to be centered in hospitals to a very great extent, in large and medium size cities. In this development, not only doctors and dentists participated, but also considerable numbers of volunteer workers, including nurses, interns, medical students, Legionnaires, etc. Selective Service benefited immeasurably by this assistance.

The groups of registrants examined varied greatly in size, according to the number of local boards concerned and the quarters, facilities and personnel available. They involved, in some instances, small numbers of 20 to 30 registrants and two to four medical examiners, and in others, large groups of 100 to 200 men with ten to twenty physicians. Many of these group examinations were efficiently organized, and furnished unusually expert medical judgment. Under such conditions the medical personnel was uncommonly enthusiastic. However, throughout the nation, individual examinations also went forward, with faithful service from thousands of examining physicians scattered over the States.

With the passage of time, and with an increasing demand for fighting men and an increasing shortage of physicians, some important experiments were carried out in various States to determine certain potentialities relative to different types of examination.

The Pennsylvania Plan provided for a continued examination by Selective Service as in the past, but combined with a preinduction examination of registrants; that is, the examination and acceptance of the selectee one month in advance of actual induction into the Army. It eliminated the injustice of late acceptance by Selective Service and the winding up of the registrant's personal affairs only to be followed later by rejection at the armed forces induction board. This plan was considered a complete success and later played an important role in wartime selection.

The Ohio Plan combined the preinduction feature with the abolition of physical examination by the medical examiners of Selective Service. The screening in this procedure was made by lay members of the local boards. Likely registrants were submitted directly to the armed forces induction boards, composed in large part of men selected from among the Selective Service medical examiners. This plan apparently failed to cover medical needs.

The Indiana Plan provided for the preinduction feature of the Pennsylvania Plan, plus a coarse screening by Selective Service examining physicians involving a careful, minute inspection of the registrant in the nude and in action, for the purpose of determining the existence of manifestly disqualifying defects. This plan met with strong approval from the Director, but not with immediate or universal acceptance by all the physicians of Selective Service. Subsequently, however, it was adopted on a national basis in wartime selection, thus replacing the complete physical examination utilized during peacetime.

As had been anticipated, the greatest difficulty in the medical phase of selection occurred in the field of nervous and mental diseases. Prior to the enactment of the Selective Service Act, Dr. Winfred Overholser, a national figure in neuropsychiatry, wrote to the President, outlining the difficulties as he envisaged them and calling Mr. Roosevelt's attention to possible future hospital needs for veterans, especially for patients suffering from nervous and mental diseases. In consequence, the Psychiatric Advisory Committee to Selective Service was appointed early in the System's history, and Dr. Harry Stack Sullivan was designated as Adviser on Psychiatry to the Director. Under his leadership, psychiatric indoctrination of all physicians participating in the examination of registrants was attempted. Medical Circular No. 1, dealing with psychiatric examinations, was provided and placed in general circulation among the examining physicians of Selective Service and armed forces induction stations.

Despite these timely efforts, it soon became apparent that selection in the field of psychiatry was poor, that men were being inducted who should have been rejected, and that perhaps many men were being rejected who could have served to advantage in the armed forces. Innumerable systems were suggested by different psychiatrists. Guidance was requested from the National Research Council, and eventually a program was forthcoming.

The rate of rejections for dental defects had been very high and was on the increase. Because of this high rate of rejections, a Dental Advisory Board was established at National Headquarters under the leadership of Dr. C. Willard Camalier and Commander (now Captain) C. Raymond Wells, DC-USNR, the latter becoming Chief Dental Officer of the Medical Division and President of the American Dental Association. This group outlined the needs of the examination, provided both personnel and facilities for local boards throughout the nation, and issued Medical Circular No. 2 (dental). As a result of their efforts, some eight to ten thousand examining dentists were added to the uncompensated personnel of Selective Service.

The rejection rate, however, continued high, so high that subsequently it became necessary for the armed forces virtually to abolish dental standards and accept men with dental defects, to rehabilitate them within the military services. Nothing could have been more satisfactory than the work of the dentists; their cooperation was splendid.

Because of the limited number of professional men, it became necessary to allocate doctors, dentists and veterinary surgeons for professional service in their respective fields. These inherent difficulties made it necessary to create a special organization for this purpose. Hence, from the Office of Defense Health and Welfare Services came the suggestion and plan for the creation and organization of the Procurement and Assignment Service. It dealt with the problem nationally and on State and local levels.

The Procurement and Assignment Service, after investigation, was to determine the essentiality of the physician in the community as against his availability for military service. This organization proved of great national value and throughout its function had the hearty support of the Selective Service System.

Because of the national shortage of physicians, and in order to meet future Army and civilian needs, it became apparent early in 1941 that the flow of medical students should be maintained at the highest possible level. Consequently, Selective Service was forced to devise a plan providing for cooperation in the matter of deferment between the schools and hospitals of the country and the local boards of Selective Service. The local boards were to be advised about supply and demand for physicians, and told of the havoc which would result from failure to keep the number of doctors at the maximum level. Deans of medical schools agreed to furnish local boards with certificates for every medical student, indicating whether or not he was satisfactory in his work.

As a result of this cooperation, it can be stated that the deferment of medical students and first-year interns was handled to the complete satisfaction of the Army, the medical schools of the country, and the majority of students concerned, as well as the general public. Subsequently, the Army and Navy both took action and set up the necessary protection.

To determine the best policy for handling second-year interns and house officers, and those men preparing themselves in various specialties, the deans of medical schools and hospital representatives were called into conference with Selective Service, along with representatives of the Surgeon General's Office.

Here again it was decided that those matters should be handled locally as far as possible, leaving any positive action by Selective Service to be taken only when necessary. To provide the requisite machinery, it was decided that one representative of the medical schools and of the hospitals should be appointed in each Corps Area to confer with the Corps Area Surgeons and with the Surgeon General to determine which men should be kept as civilians, and which should serve with the Army. It is our understanding that the Surgeons General requested the appointment of such representatives and that the plan met with their approval and that of the Army, medical schools and hospitals. This mechanism provided a plan for procurement and assignment for medical men coming within the draft age. It was adopted officially by the Association of Medical Colleges.

The rate of deferment and rejection was so high among the older registrants that it seemed to be the part of wisdom to lower the upper age limit to 28. It was found, for instance, that the rate of rejection rose rapidly with age. From 21 to 25 years, it was 30 per cent; from 26 to 30, 40 per cent; and it rose to 56 per cent from 31 to 36. In addition, military experience proved the wisdom of accepting only younger men, who as a rule make better soldiers. Hence, induction was restricted to men under the age of 28 years at that time.

The effect of this age reduction on the Army Medical Corps was considerable and certainly unexpected. In consequence, Selective Service was informed by the Surgeon General's Office that many of the medical students and interns who had been deferred according to agreement were failing to apply for or to accept commissions on establishing eligibility in the Medical Corps. A meeting was called by the Medical Division of Selective Service of all those concerned—the Army, Navy and deans of medical schools. It was decided that for the time being, at least, the problem should be handled locally by the medical colleges themselves, but that in the event of failure, Selective Service would be called upon for additional action by withholding deferment, thereby forcing the individual concerned to apply for a commission or else be inducted into the ranks.

Finally, the policy relating to medical students and first-year interns provided: Those enrolled in medical schools and listed as members of the first and second-year classes would be deferred by Selective Service; junior and senior medical students and first-year interns would be advised to apply for admission to the Medical Administrative Corps Reserve, or the Ensign Reserve, from which they would pass automatically into the Medical Reserve Corps when eligible.

Through the wisdom and cooperation of Dr. Thomas Parran, Surgeon General, the United States Public Health Service had made serological tests on all registrants at the time this was written. This procedure served a most useful purpose in identifying those men afflicted with syphilis and disclosing to the nation the magnitude of the venereal disease problem. Statistical analyses showed that positive and doubtful serology was encountered in 47 men out of every 1,000 examined among the first two million registrants. The numerical importance of venereal disease and the failure on the part of society to rehabilitate syphilitics made their induction imperative, and they were taken into the service as rapidly as facilities for their treatment would permit.

II

The subject of medical statistics has been given a great deal of careful study, attention and research, both by the Research and Statistics and by the medical divisions of Selective Service. Reports have been published from time to time both in the professional and in the lay press. Peacetime data have been adequately covered in Selective Service Medical Statistics Bulletins Nos. 1 and 2, the former published in November, 1942, the latter in August, 1943.

The significant data of the first survey are presented in Table 1. Of the first 2,000,000 men examined, 1,000,000, or 50 per cent, were rejected. This included 100,000 illiterates. The causes, numbers and percentages of the rejections for physical and mental disorders are indicated in the accompanying table.

TABLE 1. ESTIMATED NUMBER OF REGISTRANTS UNQUALIFIED FOR GENERAL MILITARY SERVICE BECAUSE OF PHYSICAL AND MENTAL REASONS

| Major Defect or Disease | Unqualified for general military service by Selective Service*a* | | | Unqualified for general service by the Army*b* | Total unqualified for general military service | Percentage of estimated total unqualified for general military service |
	Qualified for limited military service	Disqualified for any military service	Total			
Teeth	100,000	53,000	153,000	35,000	188,000	20.9
Eyes	72,000	28,000	100,000	23,000	123,000	13.7
Cardiovascular system	17,000	67,000	84,000	12,000	96,000	10.3
Musculoskeletal	27,000	25,000	52,000	9,000	61,000	6.8
Venereal	35,000	14,000	49,000	8,000	57,000	6.3
Mental and nervous	8,000	30,000	38,000	19,000	57,000	6.3
Hernia	35,000	11,000	46,000	10,000	56,000	6.2
Ears	7,000	18,000	25,000	16,000	41,000	4.6
Feet	21,000	9,000	30,000	6,000	36,000	4.0
Lungs (including tuberculosis)	6,000	11,000	17,000	9,000	26,000	2.9
Miscellaneous*c*	72,000	54,000	126,000	33,000	159,000	17.7
Total	400,000	320,000	720,000	180,000	900,000	100.0

a These estimates are based on classification reports from local boards as to the number qualified for limited military service, the number disqualified for any military service, and the rate of rejections by groups of defects or diseases by availability for military service as revealed in an analysis of 19,923 reports of physical examination. The major defect or disease for each registrant was determined by the principal cause of rejection.

b These estimates are based on the classification reports from local boards as to the total number found unqualified for general military service at the Army induction station, and the rate of rejections by groups of defects or diseases as revealed in an analysis of 123,000 reports of physical examination at the Army induction station as released by the War Department. The major defect or disease for each registrant was determined by the principal cause of rejection.

c Including diseases and defects of the mouth and gums, nose, throat, kidneys and urinary system, abdomen, genitalia, and skin; also hemorrhoids, varicose veins, tumors and infectious and parasitic diseases.

A somewhat finer breakdown, including some thirty categories, was published in Medical Statistics Bulletin No. 2. It represents a more extensive study and analysis involving 121,000 records and including twenty-one representative States. The results are presented in Table No. 2.

TABLE 2. LOCAL BOARD REJECTION RATES, BY CAUSE AND BY RACE,
NOVEMBER, 1940, THROUGH SEPTEMBER, 1941
REJECTIONS PER 1,000 REGISTRANTS EXAMINED

Principal Cause of Rejection	White and Negro			White[1]			Negro		
	All rejections	Disqualified	Limited service	All rejections	Disqualified	Limited service	All rejections	Disqualified	Limited service
All defects	437.7	221.9	215.8	433.2	221.9	211.3	472.0	222.1	249.9
Eyes	53.3	15.9	37.4	56.9	16.8	40.1	26.0	9.2	16.8
Ears	15.3	11.2	4.1	16.8	12.3	4.5	3.6	2.4	1.2
Teeth	77.5	25.0	52.5	84.1	27.2	56.9	26.8	8.4	18.4
Mouth and gums.	4.2	2.1	2.1	4.2	2.1	2.1	4.3	1.9	2.4
Nose	6.0	1.6	4.4	6.7	1.8	4.9	.8	.2	.6
Throat	1.4	.4	1.0	1.4	.4	1.0	1.4	.3	1.1
Lungs	5.4	3.1	2.3	5.7	3.3	2.4	3.0	1.6	1.4
Tuberculosis	7.4	6.9	.5	7.8	7.3	.5	3.8	3.6	.2
Cardiovascular ..	43.6	36.7	6.9	44.1	37.2	6.9	39.6	32.7	6.9
Blood and blood-forming .	.4	.3	.1	.4	.3	.1	.1	.1	0
Hernia	26.4	5.9	20.5	26.8	6.0	20.8	23.0	4.5	18.5
Kidney and urinary	4.5	3.1	1.4	4.7	3.3	1.4	3.6	2.0	1.6
Abdominal viscera	4.7	3.1	1.6	5.2	3.5	1.7	.9	.3	.6
Genitalia	6.7	1.4	5.3	6.4	1.4	5.0	9.6	1.9	7.7
Syphilis	23.1	3.8	19.3	7.5	2.0	5.5	142.3	17.7	124.6
Gonorrhea and other venereal .	3.9	.6	3.3	1.7	.4	1.3	21.1	2.4	18.7
Skin	2.7	1.1	1.6	2.8	1.2	1.6	2.0	.6	1.4
Hemorrhoids ...	2.3	.7	1.6	2.3	.7	1.6	2.4	.8	1.6
Varicose veins ..	4.8	2.7	2.1	5.0	2.8	2.2	3.7	2.1	1.6
Educational deficiency	18.6	18.4	.2	10.4	10.3	.1	81.5	81.1	.4
Mental deficiency.	9.7	9.1	.6	10.0	9.4	.6	7.7	7.1	.6
Mental disease ..	10.7	8.7	2.0	11.6	9.4	2.2	3.7	3.0	.7
Neurological	16.5	14.8	1.7	17.7	15.9	1.8	7.3	6.4	.9
Musculoskeletal..	40.6	24.1	16.5	42.2	24.5	17.7	28.5	20.8	7.7
Feet	13.7	4.5	9.2	14.2	4.6	9.6	9.8	3.1	6.7
Endocrine	6.0	4.9	1.1	6.5	5.3	1.2	1.8	1.6	.2
Neoplasms	1.7	.8	.9	1.9	.9	1.0	.9	.4	.5
Infectious and parasitic	.1	*	.1	.1	*	.1	0	0	0
Underweight, overweight and other	26.1	10.7	15.4	27.8	11.3	16.5	12.4	5.7	6.7
Non-medical reasons	.4	.3	.1	.3	.3	*	.4	.2	.2
Number rejected.	53,265	27,005	26,260	46,616	23,876	22,740	6,649	3,129	3,520

[1] Includes all races other than Negro.
* Less than 0.1 per 1,000 examined.

The influence of race on the rejection rates at local boards and induction stations is shown in Table No. 3. The influence of age is indicated in Figure 1.

The most outstanding data as to heights and weights are presented in the following tables, charts and graphs. The average age

TABLE 3. REJECTION RATES AT LOCAL BOARD AND INDUCTION STATION, BY RACE, NOVEMBER, 1940, THROUGH SEPTEMBER, 1941

| | Rejections per 100 registrants examined | | |
Racial Group	Local board[1]	Induction station[1]	Local board and induction station
White and Negro combined	43.8	16.0	52.8
White[2]	43.3	15.1	51.9
Negro	47.2	23.1	59.4

[1] Rejected registrants include men classified as available for limited service (I-B) and men disqualified for any military service (IV-F).
[2] Includes all races other than Negro.

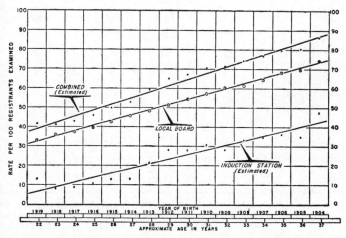

FIGURE 1. Rejection rates per 100 registrants physically examined at local boards and induction stations by year of birth, November, 1940, through September, 1941

was indicated as 26 years; the average height as 5′ 8½″, and the average weight as 152 pounds. While the average age was identical for the white and the Negro, the average height was 0.4″ taller for the white and the weight 2½ pounds greater. The distribution

TABLE 4. HEIGHT, WEIGHT, CHEST GIRTH AND UMBILICAL GIRTH OF REGISTRANTS
EXAMINED AT LOCAL BOARDS, BY RACE AND BY AVAILABILITY FOR MILITARY SERVICE[1]
NOVEMBER, 1940, THROUGH SEPTEMBER, 1941

Measurement	Average			Standard deviation[2]		
	White and Negro	White[3]	Negro	White and Negro	White[3]	Negro
Height, inches						
All men examined	68.43	68.47	68.08	2.800	2.792	2.845
General service	68.49	68.53	68.20	2.678	2.667	2.749
Rejected	68.32	68.37	67.92	2.976	2.973	2.967
Weight, pounds						
All men examined	151.99	152.15	150.77	22.65	22.97	19.99
General service	152.15	152.32	150.77	20.53	20.74	18.69
Rejected	151.74	151.87	150.77	25.59	26.06	21.70
Chest girth, inspiration, inches						
All men examined	37.09	37.22	36.09	2.524	2.530	2.238
General service	37.12	37.25	36.08	2.334	2.327	2.122
Rejected	37.05	37.17	36.12	2.794	2.821	2.395
Chest girth, expiration, inches						
All men examined	34.23	34.30	33.55	2.441	2.715	2.248
General service	34.19	34.27	33.49	2.300	2.307	2.122
Rejected	34.26	34.35	33.64	2.782	2.818	2.415
Chest expansion, inches						
All men examined	2.82	2.88	2.50	.789	.798	.711
General service	2.89	2.94	2.55	.736	.731	.670
Rejected	2.74	2.78	2.43	.883	.891	.758
Umbilical girth, inches						
All men examined	30.68	30.76	29.99	2.982	3.032	2.450
General service	30.54	30.62	29.86	2.680	2.715	2.257
Rejected	30.89	30.98	30.18	3.391	3.463	2.691
Number measured[4]						
All men examined	112,314	99,712	12,602			
General service	68,176	60,783	7,393			
Rejected	44,138	38,929	5,209			

[1] Based on measurements of registrants physically examined in 21 selected States.

[2] Approximately 68 per cent of the measurements can be expected to lie within a range of one standard deviation below the average and one standard deviation above the average.

[3] Includes all races other than Negro.

[4] Number whose height was measured.

of height and weight for whites is depicted in a three-dimensional chart, Figure No. 2.

The average rejection rates in relation to age are shown in Table No. 5.

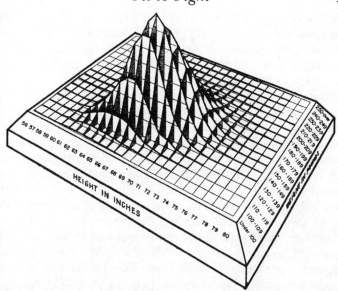

FIGURE 2. Three-dimensional chart showing distribution of heights and weights of white registrants physically examined at local boards from November, 1940, through September, 1941.

TABLE 5. LOCAL BOARD AND INDUCTION STATION REJECTION RATES PER 100 REGISTRANTS EXAMINED, BY YEAR OF BIRTH, NOVEMBER, 1940, THROUGH SEPTEMBER, 1941

Year of birth	Local board	Induction station[1]	Combined local board and induction station
Total	43.8	16.0	52.8
1919	32.8	13.1	41.6
1918	35.9	8.0	41.0
1917	37.3	8.8	42.8
1916	39.5	10.7	46.0
1915	42.5	12.8	49.9
1914	45.7	13.1	52.8
1913	48.3	21.3	59.3
1912	51.3	28.1	65.0
1911	54.3	28.0	67.1
1910	57.4	30.6	70.4
1909	60.1	28.1	71.3
1908	61.4	33.1	74.2
1907	64.5	34.7	76.8
1906	68.2	36.1	79.7
1905	69.7	34.9	80.3
1904	74.2	47.5	86.5

[1] Estimated from data on age distribution of inducted registrants supplied by the Machine Records Section, The Adjutant General's Office and data shown on Accumulative Progress Report of Classification and Induction through September 30, 1941.

When the figures from Medical Statistics Bulletin No. 1 were first presented, they met with great skepticism; however, the data from the next million men examined showed still higher rejection rates, 52.8 per cent. Subsequent analyses all support the high levels of incidence of defects and rejection rates.

While these figures are of the utmost importance from the military standpoint, since they limit military service within the age limits to 50 per cent of the total manpower in that range, they do not mean that the victims of these defects are always disabled or seriously ill. The standards for admission admittedly were high, and a large percentage of rejectees continued to carry on satisfactorily in civil life. In other words, many of these defects exercised slight or no limitation on normal activities in civil life, though they did disqualify the registrant for military service.

However, the figures do have national significance of exceptional and fundamental interest. They show an unduly high incidence or prevalence of defects and they indicate distinct and definite manpower limitations. In fact, the findings of Selective Service were of such importance that the President, in response, set up a definite plan for the rehabilitation of at least 200,000 of these rejectees to make them fit for military service.

The President's plan provided that this rehabilitation program should be under the auspices of Selective Service and its nationwide network of boards; that it should be carried out in the registrant's home community by Selective Service in conjunction with the local county medical and dental societies; and that it should be effected at a reasonable cost, for which adequate funds would be forthcoming.

Obviously the problem was extremely complex. It called for good judgment as well as adequate remedial measures, for cooperation on the part of all those interested in the healing art.

A meeting was called at National Headquarters by Selective Service, bringing together representatives of the schools and hospitals, the American medical and dental associations, the defense health and welfare services to the War Manpower Commission, the Council of National Defense, and certain Federal and social agencies. The problems of rehabilitation were thoroughly discussed and to some extent the interest and the role of each organization was defined.

Army experience teaches that only certain types of cases are susceptible of satisfactory rehabilitation, and consequently it was decided to limit rehabilitation to these types. In conference with the Surgeon General, it was further determined to limit rehabilitation to registrants who could be certified by the Army in advance as acceptable upon completion of the rehabilitation specified. This plan obviously eliminated all waste effort and expense and limited rehabilitation to those who could be accepted subsequently into the military forces.

More was involved in rehabilitation than the mere removal of the defects or deficiencies. Thus, it was possible to correct a hernia mechanically and yet this hernia might later be a cause for discharge from the Army. Compulsion at that stage would be out of the question, particularly compulsory surgery, since the resulting psychical response could be much more serious in Army life than the original disease which underwent correction. In addition, surgical risk must always be considered. It was thought wise, at that time at least, to rehabilitate as large a number as possible without resorting to surgery or entering any field where the results might be questionable. Naturally, those requesting surgery and willing to accept the responsibility were accorded every privilege.

Shortly after the rehabilitation program was suggested, the Japanese made their attack on Pearl Harbor. As a result, the pressure for fighting men became extreme and most of the registrants scheduled for rehabilitation were inducted *in statu quo* and without the correction of their defects. However, the plan was pilot-tested in Maryland and Virginia. The results were relatively meager. General Hershey decided, therefore, not to continue it and turned the whole problem over to the War Manpower Commission, which had been created in the interim.

The President's plan provided for rehabilitation of 200,000 men for service with the armed forces. It did not, however, solve the much greater problem of physical unfitness and the prevalence of deficiencies and defects among other men of military age, or among the civilian population as a whole.

In this connection, Selective Service offered its own plan, the plan of prehabilitation, which provided for a campaign of education concerning standard requirements in the Army; examination by the family doctor or dentist of men who fell short of those requirements; correction of remediable defects by the doctor or dentist concerned, and on the usual doctor-patient relationship;

and certification of prehabilitation by the doctor responsible for the correction of the defects.

This plan invited every registrant and every young man in the nation to fit himself in advance for examination, and if acceptable, for service with troops or industry. It emphasized the desirability of not permitting minor defects to defeat major objectives. It was particularly applicable in universities, colleges and schools all over the country, and in labor and industry. The fact that defects were rampant, as evidenced by the surveys of Selective Service, indicated a widespread need for improvement in physical fitness and health. This campaign accomplished much, particularly in making the nation conscious of health needs and in laying the foundation for programs of physical restoration training.

To sum up: Peacetime selection was a relative leisurely procurement program, with high standards for admission to the Army, which was created for defense in a national emergency. It involved two complete physical examinations, one by Selective Service and the other by the armed forces induction stations. The incidence of disqualifying defects was high and rejection rates approximated 50 per cent. Many problems called for solution. The experience constituted a splendid training for Selective Service boards and physicians for the more intensive program that lay ahead in wartime selection of men for the fighting forces.

Originally, Selective Service was concerned only with the procurement of men for a peacetime army of moderate proportions, a process of slow growth and expansion. With Pearl Harbor and the declaration of war came:

(1) the need for immediate and unprecedented expansion with a marked increase in the rate of inductions;

(2) the immediate lowering of the requirements for induction, in some instances temporary in nature;

(3) the use of 1-B men by the Army;

(4) a change in the character of examination for induction both in Selective Service and in the Army;

(5) the abolishment of enlistment by the Navy, and Selective Service procurement for the Navy;

(6) the correction of certain physical defects within the military establishment; and

(7) the extension in the age range of those liable for military

service—first 18 to 45, later 38, as contrasted with 20 to 28 in the pre-Pearl Harbor period.

The total number of 18 to 44 men registered at this writing is in excess of 29,000,000. The number eligible under existing regulations, between the ages of 18 and 38, is 22,000,000. The number of registrants examined for service is in excess of 13,000,000. The number classified as IV-F, or unfit for any form of military duty, is in excess of 4,000,000. These figures speak for themselves. By no stretch of the imagination can they be taken as indicative of satisfactory health and physical fitness among our registrants.

III

The advent of war resulted in a movement to increase the tempo of Selective Service and to enlarge the registered manpower pool to its maximum strength as rapidly as possible. The fourth registration, on April 27, 1942, required men between the ages of 45 and 65 to register, and on June 30 of the same year, persons between the ages of 18 and 20. In December, 1942, inductions were limited to men of 18 to 37 years inclusive.

In August, 1942, classifications 1-A (r) (remedial) and 1-B were eliminated, leaving IV-F as the only classification for registrants disqualified for military service.

From a medical point of view, the most important change concerned the type of medical examination given registrants by the local board examining physicians. Final responsibility rested in the Office of the Surgeon General for a complete physical examination, and the marked expansion of medical personnel in the Medical Corps of the Army and Navy plus increasing difficulty in obtaining adequate numbers of local board examining physicians led to the abolition of the Selective Service local board medical examination. In its place was substituted a preliminary physical examination, a screening test, whereby only those registrants with manifestly disqualifying defects were rejected. These defects were listed on D.S.S. Form 220.

This fundamental change in procedure elicited varying reactions: satisfaction in areas where medical service was difficult to obtain; dissatisfaction, and to some extent resentment, where medical service was still available. However, in the course of the next six months, the new system was found generally acceptable.

Notwithstanding the changed procedure, group team examinations still continued in larger centers. In Chicago and New York, the system culminated in mass examinations involving, in some instances, as many as 1,000 to 1,200 registrants per day.

As a result of the changed procedure and the increasing inductions, the relative rejection figures from local boards and induction stations were reversed. Under the final type of examination given, it was found that Selective Service was responsible for 41 per cent of the 50 per cent rejection rate. But under the screening examination, with the final examination given by the armed forces, Selective Service became responsible for rejections of only 5.6 per cent of the 46.9 rejection rate.

In its first three years of existence, Selective Service continued to collect blood for serological tests for syphilis, but discontinued this practice in the early months of 1944. Both the collection of blood and serological tests were taken over by the induction stations.

Beginning in January, 1943, Selective Service procured men for the Navy as well as for the Army. Enlistment, except under 18 and above 38 years of age, was abolished.

The standards for admission to the fighting forces were established by the War Department (more recently, after conference with the Navy) and adjusted from time to time to admit the maximum possible manpower pool. The level of the requirements depended upon the number of men needed in the military services, the urgency of need, the size of the manpower pool, and the relative need of men for military service and for production. Selective Service attempted at all times, through proper adjustment, to maintain the optimal balance in meeting manpower needs.

The impending necessity for the induction of fathers led Congress in 1943 to request the appointment of a committee of five physicians to determine whether the physical standards could still be lowered in relation to manpower needs. The committee found that further lowering of standards was inadvisable, except in certain minor respects, and would not materially increase the number of men available for induction into the military services.

The fact that the armed forces need to provide remedial medical and educational measures while in the midst of war points to the further fact that the medical and educational systems must meet the national requirements by medical and educational programs stressing physical fitness and better health. As a consequence of civilian failure, the armed forces were compelled, in their own interest, to initiate rehabilitation within the services.

With dental standards virtually abolished and dental defects waived, it became necessary to expand greatly the personnel of the Dental Corps of the Army and Navy and to provide facilities to meet the minimal dental requirements of the services. The results were completely satisfactory. Illiteracy had also failed of civilian solution, but illiterates in large numbers were inducted and educated within the services.

Rejections because of venereal disease reached such high levels that provision for suitable treatment facilities within the armed forces had to be made. Uncomplicated syphilis and gonorrhea cases were accepted as rapidly as facilities for treatment and cure could be provided. The same pattern was followed for treatment of hernias. Hernial defects (if not scrotal) were waived by the regulations and rehabilitated in the services, or the individual was placed on limited service.

The policy of waiver for defects and their correction within the military services exerted a marked effect on medical statistics. Dental defects, which stood first in peacetime selection, no longer appeared in the list of principal causes for rejection. Similarly, the rates for illiteracy, venereal diseases and hernia were greatly lowered. But other defects, especially nervous and mental diseases, then assumed relatively greater importance. Unfortunately, no one successfully set up an acceptable profile in these neuropsychiatric categories, nor were the armed services willing to accept such cases and attempt their correction within the ranks.

In the selection of men for a peacetime army, the rejection rate approximated 50 per cent. With all the changes incident to Pearl Harbor, the lowest rate ever attained was about 30 per cent. This occurred over a short period only, during the wholesale induction of men 18 to 19 years of age. For the teen-age registrants, the rate of rejections was 25.4 per cent; for whites, 23.3 per cent, and for Negroes, 45 per cent. The general rejection rate in mid-1944 approximated 45 per cent and was on an upward trend.

The most difficult problem of selection lay in the field of neuropsychiatry. Many plans were tried and a great number of possibilities suggested. The most important steps taken by Selective Service and the armed forces were as follows:

(1) Provision in D.S.S. Form 40 for the registrant's own statements relative to present or past mental difficulty.

(2) A course of indoctrination, which was given in the early days of Selective Service through an educational campaign of seminars, and Medical Circular No. 1.

(3) The local board's judgment based on knowledge or information acquired locally or through the local board examining physicians.

(4) The local board preliminary physical examination conducted by the local board physicians.

(5) Provision for information to the local board by affidavits from physicians or statements of governmental agencies.

(6) The Selective Service program covering the assembling of pertinent information, as set forth in Section 623.33 (e) of the Regulations.

(7) Examination at the armed forces induction station.

(8) Observation period of three days at the discretion of the armed forces examining board. This period may be too brief in some instances. Perhaps it could be extended to advantage—a viewpoint expressed by Dr. R. D. Gillespie on his visit here from England.

(9) After rejection by the armed forces, a special review of findings by a medical advisory board, if considered indicated and requested by the local board.

Despite all the various devices, rejection rates and discharge rates for nervous and mental diseases still continued unduly high. In February, 1943, a letter received by General Hershey from Secretary of War Stimson outlined the difficulties and called on Selective Service for a special program whereby information pertinent to selection or rejection or registrants be assembled locally and transmitted to the psychiatrists on the induction boards for their guidance in arriving at decisions.

As a result, a national program was developed. It involved the appointment of special advisers to each State Director, and the appointment of several thousand medical field agents, one or more to each local board, for the assembling of information, much of which was obtained from existing social and welfare agencies, the files of penal institutions, etc. Information was also obtained from school teachers or school records. By 1944, forty-six states had such a program in operation, and 8,000 medical field agents had been appointed. The program had the backing and support of the War Department, the Surgeons General of the Army and

TABLE 6. ESTIMATED PRINCIPAL CAUSES FOR REJECTION OF REGISTRANTS 18-37
YEARS OF AGE IN CLASS IV-F, AS OF APRIL 1, 1944

(PRELIMINARY)

Principal Cause for Rejection	Number	Per cent
Total	3,836,000	100.0
Manifestly disqualifying defects	403,100	10.5
Mental disease	601,300	15.7
Mental deficiency[1]	536,200	14.0
Physical defects	2,242,500	58.4
Syphilis	288,800	7.5
Musculoskeletal	287,500	7.5
Cardiovascular	246,800	6.4
Hernia	217,700	5.7
Neurological	200,900	5.2
Eyes	197,800	5.1
Ears	148,000	3.9
Tuberculosis	100,800	2.6
Lungs	65,600	1.7
Feet	48,800	1.3
Abdominal viscera	46,900	1.2
Kidney and urinary	39,000	1.0
Varicose veins	38,400	1.0
Genitalia	38,100	1.0
Endocrine	37,100	1.0
Teeth	35,400	0.9
Skin	23,400	0.6
Neoplasms	23,400	0.6
Nose	23,100	0.6
Gonorrhea and other venereal diseases	18,000	0.5
Hemorrhoids	15,500	0.4
Mouth and gums	10,800	0.3
Infectious and parasitic	4,000	0.1
Throat	3,800	0.1
Blood and blood-forming	3,600	0.1
Underweight, overweight and other	79,300	2.1
Non-medical	52,900	1.4

[1] Includes registrants rejected for educational deficiency before June 1, 1943 and for failure to meet minimum intelligence standards after that date, as well as those rejected for mental deficiency.

Navy, the United States Public Health Service and the Commissioner of the United States Office of Education. It was developed under the coordination of Lieutenant Colonel Louis H. Renfrow.

Before presenting the figures on psychotic and psychosomatic diseases, it may be helpful to consider the size and composition of the 4-F pool as it existed in mid-1944, thus providing a much needed perspective. The 4-F pool had grown steadily in the preceding year at a rate of approximately 85,000 per month, and it was continuing to grow despite the drastic lowering of standards. The size and composition of the 4-F pool as of April 1, 1944, is shown in Table No. 6.

The age distribution in this group is of special interest: 1,400,000 under 26 years of age, approximately 700,000 between the ages of 26 and 30 years, and 1,400,000 between 30 and 38 years of age. Above 38 years of age, experience has shown that there are few who can qualify and serve satisfactorily. Above 38 years, the rejection rate is more than 60 per cent and the discharge rate is unusually high.

Note particularly the figures presented on rejections for mental disease—601,300, or 15.7 per cent; for mental deficiency (including illiteracy), 536,200, or 14 per cent; for neurological disorders, 200,900, or 5.2 per cent. The total in these categories is 1,340,000, or about 35 per cent of the grand total of the rejected.

In addition, it should be stated that in 1943 the discharges from the fighting forces increased materially and numbered more than 500,000 in 1944. The rate for neuropsychiatry continued high, definitely above 40 per cent. The figure was 216,000 as of February 1, 1944.

The picture as a whole shows that, of some 13,000,000 to 14,000,000 examinations given, there were approximately 4,000,000 to 5,000,000 discards, rejectees, or men discharged from service. More than a third of the rejections, and more than 40 per cent of the discharges, were for neuropsychiatric reasons.

The question arises as to whether psychosomatic diseases should be included in this category. They are closely related in many instances, at least. They represent the visceral expression of disease, functional or organic in nature, rather than nervous and mental diseases *per se*.

The figures for psychosomatic disease during wartime selection

TABLE 7. DISTRIBUTION OF PRINCIPAL CAUSES FOR REJECTION AT LOCAL BOARDS AND INDUCTION STATIONS, FEBRUARY, 1943-DECEMBER, 1943 CONTINENTAL UNITED STATES

Principal Cause for Rejection	Local Board			Induction Station			Local Board and Induction Station		
	Total	White[1]	Negro	Total	White[1]	Negro	Total	White[1]	Negro
Total ....:	100.0	100.0	100.0	100.0	100.0	100.0	100.0	100.0	100.0
Eyes	2.4	2.6	2.3	6.1	6.7	4.2	5.5	6.0	3.7
Ears	2.0	2.5	0.5	5.6	6.8	0.9	4.9	6.1	0.7
Teeth	0.5	0.5	0.4	0.8	1.0	0.3	0.8	0.9	0.4
Mouth and gums	0.3	0.4	0.1	0.2	0.3	0.1	0.2	0.3	0.1
Nose	0.4	0.4	0.1	1.1	1.3	0.3	1.0	1.1	0.2
Throat	0.1	0.1	*	0.1	0.1	*	0.1	0.1	*
Lungs	2.3	2.6	1.5	2.3	2.5	1.6	2.3	2.4	1.5
Tuberculosis	3.4	4.0	1.8	3.3	3.6	2.3	3.3	3.7	2.0
Cardiovascular	5.3	6.1	3.2	8.5	8.5	8.7	7.9	8.1	7.3
Blood and blood-forming ..	0.1	0.2	*	0.1	0.1	*	0.1	0.1	*
Hernia	17.8	19.9	12.0	4.8	5.2	3.0	6.7	7.4	4.3
Kidney and urinary	0.6	0.7	0.1	1.6	1.8	0.8	1.4	1.7	0.7
Abdominal viscera	1.7	2.1	0.4	1.7	2.0	0.5	1.6	2.0	0.4
Genitalia	1.0	1.0	1.1	1.4	1.3	1.4	1.3	1.3	1.3
Syphilis	18.0	6.1	51.8	1.5	1.0	3.1	4.7	1.9	14.9
Gonorrhea and other venereal	0.3	0.1	1.0	0.4	0.1	1.3	0.3	0.1	1.2
Skin	0.6	0.6	0.5	0.8	0.9	0.6	0.8	0.8	0.5
Hemorrhoids	0.6	0.7	0.4	0.4	0.4	0.4	0.4	0.5	0.4
Varicose veins	1.3	1.4	0.9	1.1	1.2	0.8	1.1	1.2	0.8
Mental deficiency[2]	3.8	4.3	2.6	16.0	9.6	39.5	14.0	8.8	31.9
Mental disease	3.9	4.7	1.5	20.8	22.5	14.5	18.2	19.9	12.2
Neurological	9.7	11.9	3.2	4.2	4.4	3.3	5.1	5.6	3.2
Musculoskeletal	17.3	19.6	10.8	7.3	7.9	4.9	8.8	9.8	5.7
Feet	1.1	1.2	0.8	2.3	2.1	3.3	2.1	1.9	2.8
Endocrine	2.1	2.6	0.3	0.9	1.1	0.3	1.1	1.3	0.2
Neoplasms	0.6	0.6	0.5	0.8	1.0	0.3	0.8	0.9	0.3
Infectious and parasitic	*	0.1	*	0.1	0.1	0.1	0.1	0.1	0.1
Underweight and overweight	1.0	1.1	0.6	2.0	2.4	0.7	1.9	2.2	0.7
Other	1.4	1.5	1.3	0.8	0.8	0.6	0.8	0.9	0.6
Non-medical reasons	0.4	0.4	0.3	3.0	3.3	2.2	2.7	2.9	1.9

[1] Includes all races other than Negro.

[2] Includes registrants rejected for educational deficiency before June 1, 1943, and for failure to meet minimum intelligence standards after that date, as well as those rejected for mental deficiency.

* Less than 0.1 per cent.

TABLE 8. SELECTED PSYCHOSOMATIC DISEASE AMONG SELECTIVE SERVICE REGISTRANTS
IN PEACETIME[1] AND IN WARTIME[2]

(PRELIMINARY)

	Per 1,000 Registrants Examined		
	Incidence of Defect	Incidence of Defect in Rejected Men	Incidence as Principal Cause for Rejection
All Races			
Total	27.7 (17.7)[3]	23.8 (14.2)[3]	20.9 (9.2)[3]
Asthma	8.4 (4.8)[3]	7.5 (4.1)[3]	6.0 (3.2)[3]
Peptic ulcer	4.3 (3.3)[3]	4.3 (3.1)[3]	3.8 (2.7)[3]
History of peptic ulcer	3.4 (1.1)[3]	3.1 (0.7)[3]	2.3 (0.3)[3]
Gastro-intestinal syndrome ...	1.7 (0.7)[3]	1.6 (0.4)[3]	1.6 (0.3)[3]
Neurocirculatory asthenia	8.6 (3.4)[3]	6.4 (2.6)[3]	6.4 (1.5)[3]
Functional disorders of expressive movements	1.3 (4.4)[3]	0.9 (3.3)[3]	0.8 (1.2)[3]
White[1]			
Total	31.1 (18.8)[3]	26.4 (15.2)[3]	23.1 [4]
Asthma	8.5 (4.9)[3]	7.5 (4.2)[3]	6.0 [4]
Peptic ulcer	5.2 (3.6)[3]	5.2 (3.4)[3]	4.6 [4]
History of peptic ulcer	4.2 (1.1)[3]	3.8 (0.7)[3]	2.9 [4]
Gastro-intestinal syndrome ...	2.0 (0.8)[3]	1.9 (0.5)[3]	1.9 [4]
Neurocirculatory asthenia	10.0 (3.7)[3]	7.1 (2.8)[3]	7.0 [4]
Functional disorders of expressive movements	1.2 (4.7)[3]	0.9 (3.5)[3]	0.7 [4]
Negro			
Total	16.5 (7.7)[3]	15.5 (5.7)[3]	13.3 [4]
Asthma	7.8 (3.9)[3]	7.4 (3.4)[3]	5.9 [4]
Peptic ulcer	1.4 (0.6)[3]	1.4 (0.3)[3]	1.3 [4]
History of peptic ulcer	0.9 (0.4)[3]	0.8 (0.2)[3]	0.2 [4]
Gastro-intestinal syndrome ...	0.6 ..	0.6 ..	0.6 [4]
Neurocirculatory asthenia	4.5 (0.8)[3]	4.2 (0.6)[3]	4.2 [4]
Functional disorders of expressive movements	1.3 (2.0)[3]	1.1 (1.2)[3]	1.1 [4]

[1] Peacetime figures are from a sample of Forms 200 dated September 30, 1941, or earlier, for 15 States.

[2] Wartime figures are for November and December, 1943, and based on a random sample.

[3] Peacetime figures are shown in parenthesis.

[4] Race breakdown of rejection rates not available for peacetime data.

are shown in Table No. 8. For convenience of reference, we have included in this table (in parenthesis) some figures from a paper dealing with peacetime rejections, thus providing easy comparison.

Not only do defects abound, but the physical fitness of the youth of the nation is at a low ebb, so low that the President saw fit to create a National Committee on Physical Fitness. This committee has been working in close harmony with Selective Service.

The suggestion was then made, perhaps to aid in the solution of the problem, that a year of emphasis on physical fitness and better health be designated by the President or Congress, to be known as "the physical fitness and health year." Efforts must be devoted to the education of the public and the professions through radio, the screen and the press, and by leaders in medicine, dentistry, teachers' and parents' organizations, and the leaders of the nation. There should be developed a new system for the establishment of better health and physical fitness. It calls for new leadership. We hope that out of future experience there may develop a national health council and foundation to function in physical fitness matters as the National Research Council has done since the days of Lincoln. Such leadership should be non-political and without remuneration; it should be enlightened and, above all, unselfish.

In such an organization, medical leadership could be centered in the American Medical Association, the United States Public Health Service, the American Dental Association and the American Hospital Association. There should be a solid medical front devoid of all rivalry, and medical leadership representing all the nation's needs. It should afford wise guidance to the nation in all matters pertaining to better health and physical fitness. It should result in "better living through dynamic health."

Under the guidance of General Hershey, Selective Service fulfilled its original function satisfactorily—that of procurement of men for the armed forces. As a result, this country amassed the largest fighting force in its entire history. The troops themselves represented the cream of the crop of American manhood, physically, mentally and morally. They had the largest and best Medical and Dental Corps in the nation's history to administer to their care and welfare. But in procuring the necessary manpower, a great deal of hidden disease was uncovered, and appalling rates of rejections and of discharges became necessary. The discarded men were absorbed largely in industry, but no adequate national rehabilitation program to meet all national needs had been evolved as late as 1944.

In the utilization of manpower in war industries, Selective Service, along with the War Manpower Commission, also rendered a great national service, and industrial medicine was given a great impetus.

War is a hard taskmaster but a great teacher. The medical profession has given of its services voluntarily, and according to President Roosevelt, no other group has given of itself so liberally. It has learned to know the American people as it has never known them before. Medicine has learned much of the nation's strength, its steadfastness of purpose, its will to do, to win, to live and to be great and free.

But it has learned also of the innumerable physical and mental defects, deficiencies, disabilities, disorders and diseases that now beset us. Let us hope that the lessons learned will not only have helped this nation to win the war, but will also make us stronger and more productive in the postwar era.

If wisdom prevails, the war will not have been in vain. America of necessity has become aware of the need for more vigorous health, and medicine has learned much that is essential to better living, through more dynamic health. As a result of the war, medicine is in a better position now than ever before to guide the nation to a higher plane of individual and public health.

The work of the examining doctors and dentists associated with local boards, the members of the medical advisory boards, and the doctors at induction centers is staggering in sheer volume. Some 14,000,000 men have been physically examined, of whom more than 4,000,000 men were in Class IV-F by the middle of 1944, and there was a large movement in and out of the class each month requiring re-examination. The preliminary work to induction was performed by the badly depleted ranks of doctors and dentists, in addition to their care of the civilian population. It was an uncompensated service, freely and willingly given. It was an expression of patriotic character and the social obligation of mutual helpfulness. The doctor's function is to come to the aid of the sick and to maintain the health of the community in the individual and social interest.

Here, on a grand scale, the medical and dental profession continued to serve individuals and the community in the same spirit of service and sacrifice that perhaps is not always so clear in less troublous times. Doctors and dentists will carry on in the same spirit, and with wider knowledge and new knowledge, make America physically and mentally fit for the challenge of the new world which victory over the enemy assures.

When Japan struck at Pearl Harbor, the physicians of America had already been conditioned to the need for their service in war. The Army and Navy demanded physicians out of all proportion to the needs of the civilian population. Industrial production speeded to the utmost placed stress on the worker, so that there was more need for physical conditioning and physical care than at any other time. The entire civilian population, emotionally stirred and driven to its utmost capacity to meet the needs of war, wanted more medical help than at any other time.

The provision of doctors for all these purposes and for many others was a problem more difficult to meet than almost any other that confronted the nation, first, because the number of physicians is limited; second, because it takes so long to educate a young man for the practice of medicine; third, because teaching and care of the sick must go on constantly in peace as in war; and, lastly, because the Army could use only physicians who were young and physically fit for the vast majority of its tasks.

Since the problem was of such magnitude, a new agency was developed by a committee of physicians called to Washington at the request of the Coordinator of Health and Welfare, Mr. Paul V. McNutt. This committee of physicians recommended the establishment of a special agency known at first as the Procurement and Assignment Service for Physicians, Dentists and Veterinarians, and later expanded to include nurses, sanitary engineers and other medical personnel. On the regional board of five appointed by the President to conduct this service was Dr. Harold S. Diehl, already known as a medical and public health educator, widely known as dean of the University of Minnesota School of Medicine, member of many distinguished scientific organizations, and author of several important books.

On the Directing Board of Procurement and Assignment, his talent for systematization of regulations and for clear expression was quickly recognized. In the report which follows, Dr. Diehl tells how the physicians of America were allocated to meet the needs of the civilian population as well as those of the armed forces.

CHAPTER III

THE DOCTOR'S SERVICE — AT HOME, IN INDUSTRY AND AT WAR

By
HAROLD S. DIEHL, M.D.

*Member of the Directing Board, Procurement and Assignment
Service, and Dean of the School of Medicine, University of
Minnesota*

PRIOR TO THE war the United States had a greater number of physicians than any other country in the world. (Table 1.) Yet to those who foresaw the possibility that our country would be involved in World War II, it was apparent that this number would be insufficient to meet both the inevitable demands of the armed forces and the needs of the civilian population. Furthermore, although the total ratio of physicians to population for the country as a whole was good, certain rural areas, particularly in the South and Midwest, were even then inadequately supplied with medical services.

TABLE 1. POPULATION PER PHYSICIAN IN VARIOUS COUNTRIES*

United States	1 physician to		750	persons
Austria	1	"	"	880	"
Switzerland	1	"	"	1,250	"
Denmark	1	"	"	1,430	"
England and Wales	1	"	"	1,490	"
Germany	1	"	"	1,560	"
France	1	"	"	1,690	"
Norway	1	"	"	1,760	"
The Netherlands	1	"	"	1,820	"
Belgium	1	"	"	1,850	"
Sweden	1	"	"	2,800	"

* Figures for countries other than the United States from Final Report of the Commission on Medical Education, 1932, p. 99.

In June, 1940, the House of Delegates of the American Medical

Association created a Committee on Medical Preparedness to "establish and maintain contact and suitable relationships with all government agencies concerned with the prevention of disease and the care of the sick, in both civil and military aspects, so as to make available at the earliest possible moment every facility that the American Medical Association can offer for the health and safety of the American people and the maintenance of American democracy."*

At this same meeting of the American Medical Association, the Surgeons General of the Army, the Navy and the Public Health Service requested the Association to survey the medical personnel of the United States to determine the number of physicians available for service in various capacities and to assemble information which would be helpful in enabling the profession to render the greatest possible service in any national emergency that might develop. The Association authorized that this be done through its Committee on Medical Preparedness.

In September, 1940, with the approval of the President of the United States, the Council of National Defense established the Health and Medical Committee to advise the Council regarding the health and medical aspects of national defense, and to coordinate all health and medical activities affecting national defense. This committee consisted of the Surgeon General of the Army, the Surgeon General of the Navy, the Surgeon General of the United States Public Health Service, the Director of the Medical Science Division of the National Research Council, and as chairman and representative of the civilian physicians of the country, the President of the American Medical Association.

To aid in carrying out its duties, the Health and Medical Committee appointed six subcommittees, one of which was a Committee on Medical Education. This committee was asked what the medical schools could do to increase the output of doctors to meet the needs of the nation in case of war. The reply was that the training of physicians could be accelerated and the number of medical students slightly increased. It was pointed out, however, that the additions to the medical profession which would result from these measures could not possibly meet the increased demand

* Irvin, Abell, "The Medical Profession and Medical Preparedness," *Journal of the American Medical Association*, Vol. 117. p. 177, July 19, 1941.

for physicians in case of war. The committee therefore urged that consideration be given to the establishment of an agency which would be responsible in case of war for the effective distribution and utilization of the services of the country's physicians.

After preliminary consideration by the Health and Medical Committee, the suggestion was transmitted to the Committee on Medical Preparedness of the American Medical Association. This committee formulated the following resolution, which was approved by the House of Delegates of the American Medical Association at its meeting in May, 1941.

"Be it resolved:

"That the United States government be urged to plan and arrange immediately for the establishment of a central authority with representatives of the civilian medical profession to be known as the Procurement and Assignment Agency for physicians for the Army, Navy and Public Health Service and for the civilian and industrial needs of the nation."

On October 22, 1941, the Health and Medical Committee named a commission to draft a plan for the development of such an agency. This commission made the following recommendations:

1. That an office for the procurement and assignment of physicians, dentists and veterinarians be established.

2. That this office function as part of the Office of Defense, Health and Welfare Services, itself a part of the Office for Emergency Management.

3. That the function of this office shall be to procure personnel from existing qualified members of the professions concerned. The office shall receive from various governmental and other agencies requests for medical, dental and veterinary personnel. These requests shall indicate the number of men desired, the time during which they must be secured, the qualifications and limitations placed on such personnel. The office must then by appropriate mechanism arrange to secure lists of professional personnel available to meet these requirements, utilizing such existing rosters, public and private, as it may find acceptable. It shall also be authorized to approach such professional personnel as is considered available and to use suitable means to stimulate voluntary enrollment.

4. The Office of Procurement and Assignment shall consist of a board of five members, one of whom shall be chairman. This board shall be chosen from members of the medical, dental and veterinary professions and shall not include any salaried employees of the Federal government. This board shall function without salary but shall be entitled to actual and necessary transportation, subsistence and other expenses incidental to the performance of its duties.

5. The board shall appoint an executive secretary who shall serve also as executive officer and who shall be without vote in its deliberations and decisions. He shall serve as a full-time employee with salary (to be determined) and with such assistants as the board may deem necessary to carry out its functions.

6. The board shall be authorized to establish such advisory committees and subcommittees as may be necessary. These committees shall represent the various interests concerned, such as medical, dental and veterinary schools, hospitals, Negro physicians and women physicians. Members of such committees shall serve without salary but shall be entitled to actual and necessary transportation, subsistence and other expenses incidental to the performance of their duties.

7. The board shall also be authorized to request various agencies of the government using medical, dental or veterinary personnel to appoint liaison officers and representatives to advise the board in carrying out its functions.

8. In carrying out its functions, the board shall cooperate with such agencies as are now established under the Selective Service as well as other Federal agencies.*

On October 30, 1941, the following letter from the Director of Defense, Health and Welfare Services was approved by the President. This constitutes the authority under which the Procurement and Assignment Service has operated:

October 30, 1941.

My dear Mr. President:

The coordination of the various demands made on the medical, dental and veterinary personnel of the nation and the most efficient utilization of this personnel would seem to require the establishment

* Section on Medical Preparedness, *Journal of the American Medical Association*, Vol. 118, pp. 625–638, Feb. 21, 1942.

of a special agency capable of recording the qualified personnel available, of assigning or encouraging enlistment of such personnel in the services where most needed, and of giving every qualified physician, dentist and veterinarian an opportunity to enroll himself in some service demanded by the national need.

For these reasons I wish to propose that there be established as one of the principal subdivisions of the Office of Defense, Health and Welfare Services an office for the procurement and assignment of physicians, dentists and veterinarians. This office would be known as the Procurement and Assignment Agency.

The functions of the agency would be (1) to receive from various governmental and other agencies requests for medical, dental and veterinary personnel, (2) to secure and maintain lists of professional personnel available, showing detailed qualifications of such personnel, and (3) to utilize all suitable means to stimulate voluntary enrollment, having due regard for the over-all public health needs of the nation, including those of governmental agencies and civilian institutions.

The agency would consist of a board of five members, one of whom would serve as chairman. The board would serve without salary but would be entitled to actual and necessary transportation, subsistence and other expenses incidental to the performance of its duties.

A full-time executive officer (with salary to be determined) would be appointed, together with such assistants as would be required to carry out the functions of the Agency.

I recommend that the board be composed of Dr. Frank Lahey, chairman, Dr. James Paullin, Dr. Harvey B. Stone, Dr. Harold S. Diehl and Dr. C. Willard Camalier.

This communication is addressed to you in accordance with provisions contained in paragraph 4 of the Executive Order, dated Sept. 3, 1941, "Establishing the Office of Defense, Health and Welfare Services in the Executive Office of the President and Defining Its Functions and Duties," to the effect that the President shall approve the establishment of the principal subdivision of the Office of Defense, Health and Welfare Services and the appointment of the heads thereof.

In the event you approve the establishment of the Procurement and Assignment Agency, together with the board membership as recommended, I shall proceed immediately with the creation of the agency and will prepare budget estimates in the amount of approximately $50,000 for submission to the Budget Bureau to cover the costs of the Agency.

In addition I would propose to instruct the Agency to draft legislation which may be necessary to submit to the Congress providing for the involuntary recruitment of medical, dental and veterinary personnel, in the event the exigencies of the national emergency appear to require it.

Sincerely yours,
PAUL V. McNUTT, *Director*.

Approved.
FRANKLIN D. ROOSEVELT.

This letter was approved by the President on October 30, 1941, and the Procurement and Assignment Service was organized accordingly.

In general terms, the responsibility of the Service was to plan for the distribution of the services of the physicians, dentists and veterinarians of this country so as to meet as effectively as possible the needs of both the armed forces and the civilian population during the war.

Unfortunately, the ink was hardly dry on the President's executive order creating this service when we were plunged into war. This made it necessary for the Procurement and Assignment Service to formulate policies, develop its organization, and begin to function all at the same time. There was no blueprint to follow, no past experience to draw on.

Although its establishment antedated that of the War Manpower Commission, the Procurement and Assignment Service was transferred to that agency immediately upon its creation. This made the service the first functioning division of the War Manpower Commission. In 1943, the Director of the War Manpower Commission broadened the scope of the service to include sanitary engineers and nurses, and added one sanitary engineer and two nurses to the Directing Board.

Although official channels between the service and the War and Navy Departments went through the Director of the War Manpower Commission, the vast majority of relationships with the Army and the Navy were conducted directly and informally with the officers of the Surgeons General of those services. The Directing Board of the Procurement and Assignment Service held frequent meetings with the Surgeon General of the Army, the Surgeon General of the Navy, the Surgeon General of the United States Public Health Service, the Director of Selective Service and at times with representatives of other governmental agencies. The results of these conferences and informal relationships were so satisfactory that few communications through official channels were necessary. Without this splendid, understanding, and effective cooperation on the part of the military and other governmental services, the task of the Procurement and Assignment Service would have been an impossible one.

The administrative organization of the Procurement and Assignment Service consisted of a Directing Board, a Central Office in Washington, a sub-office in the headquarters of the American Medical Association in Chicago, Corps Area (Service Command) Committees and State Committees. At the "State level" separate committees were established for each of the professional groups with which the Procurement and Assignment Service was concerned.

In addition, the following advisory committees were established: the Allocation of Medical Personnel; Medical Education; Hospitals; Industrial Medicine; Public Health; Dentistry; Dental Education; Nursing; Veterinary Medicine; Sanitary Engineering; Women Physicians; and Negro Health.

The responsibilities of these several divisions of the Procurement and Assignment Service have been summarized as follows:

Directing Board

1. Establishment of policies and procedures for the Procurement and Assignment Service.

2. Maintenance of liaison with the appropriate governmental officials and agencies and with the various professional groups.

Central Office

1. Maintenance of contacts with Federal agencies relative to their needs for physicians, dentists, nurses, veterinarians and sanitary engineers, and consultations with these agencies regarding the possibility of revision of their requests in view of the limited supply of professional personnel in these fields.

2. Preparation of quotas of the minimum medical, dental, nursing, veterinary and sanitary engineering services which should be retained for the civilian population, including private practice, hospital service, public health service and professional education.

3. Preparation of quotas for allocating to the States the re-

quests for physicians, dentists, nurses, veterinarians and sanitary engineers needed for war service.

4. Maintenance of rosters of physicians, dentists, nurses, veterinarians and sanitary engineers to show: (a) total in the United States, (b) their qualifications, age, location and the like. From these rosters names of the professional personnel with certain qualifications will be obtained from time to time.

5. Secure information for the various governmental agencies in regard to physicians, dentists, nurses, veterinarians and sanitary engineers as to (a) availability for service other than in their present location, (b) their professional and other qualifications, (c) their willingness to serve in various capacities during the war emergency.

6. On the basis of this information, select the names of those who meet the specifications of the requisitioning agency.

7. Cooperate with the various governmental agencies in obtaining the applications of the individuals thus selected for service.

Chicago Office

1. Maintain, and keep up to date, information concerning all physicians, dentists and veterinarians with respect to character, type of practice, infringements of law, and so on, which must be considered by the Army, Navy or other services in deciding whether individuals are qualified for appointment. Confidential information would be obtained on request of the Army or Navy from the files of the American Medical Association.

2. Assistance of a consultative and advisory nature to the directing board and to the various committees of the Procurement and Assignment Service. This includes the utilization of statistical data collected over a period of many years by the medical, dental, nursing and veterinary medical associations.

Corps Area (Service Command) Committees

1. To supervise the work of the State committees in order that they may be reasonably uniform in the manner in which they carry out the policies of the directing board. This will require meetings of the corps area committees with State chairmen and visits by the corps area chairman to the States within his corps area.

2. To act as appeal board in cases in which the individual, his

community or his employing agency differs with the classification given by the State procurement and assignment committee.

State Committees

1. To obtain the over-all enrollment of the professions in the State. This will require the maintenance of rosters in the State offices of those who have enrolled with the Procurement and Assignment Service and those who have not. The former lists will be obtained from the central office.

2. Survey local needs for professional services in conformity with the policies laid down by the directing board. On the basis of these surveys, determine how many physicians, dentists, nurses, veterinarians or sanitary engineers are needed in the various communities of the States to care for the civilian needs, and how many can be released for service elsewhere.

3. Determine which particular individual physicians, dentists, nurses, veterinarians and sanitary engineers can be considered "available" for service elsewhere. In view of the changing circumstances, this will require constant reappraisal and obviously can be done only locally.

4. Pass on the availability, character and professional qualifications of individuals who are being considered for appointment for service elsewhere, e.g., for commissions in the Army or Navy.

5. Cooperate with the State offices of the Selective Service System in determining whether physicians, dentists, veterinarians and sanitary engineers who are subject to classification by Selective Service are essential in their local communities.

6. Maintenance of lists, to be transmitted from the central office, of those who have expressed their preference for service in industrial practice, civil practice in other communities, State and local health departments and institutions, and acting as liaison between these individuals and the industrial organizations, civilian communities, health departments and institutions desiring their services in a temporary capacity for the duration of the war.

7. The creation of such local, county, or district advisory committees as may be required to carry out the responsibilities of the State committees.

The members of these various boards and committees gave unstintingly of their time and services. Without compensation, at great personal sacrifice, and frequently in spite of uninformed or malicious criticism, these individuals rendered an invaluable and patriotic service to our country in its war effort.

Although the Procurement and Assignment Service has been concerned with dentists, nurses, veterinarians and sanitary engineers as well as with physicians, the discussion offered here will be limited primarily to its work with physicians. This was the foremost of its responsibilities and the program which was developed for physicians was later applied with but minor modifications to those other groups of health personnel.

In developing and carrying out its program, the service had close, though unofficial, relationships with the American Medical Association and the various State medical societies.

In 1941, the American Medical Association, at great expense and effort, prepared a roster of all the physicians in the United States, with detailed information concerning their training, experience and qualifications. This roster, which was turned over to the service immediately after its organization, provided the information upon which planning and operation have been based. In addition, the American Medical Association has made its staff and facilities available at all times to assist with the work of the service. State medical societies have not only cooperated wholeheartedly, but in many instances have carried much of the work and the expense of the Procurement and Assignment committees. Without this assistance and support, the service could not possibly have functioned effectively.

With the rapid expansion of our armed forces, the first responsibility of the service was clearly to cooperate with the Army and Navy in the recruitment of medical officers. Our men and women, whether in Africa, India, Guadalcanal, Australia, Alaska, Europe, or the continental United States, had to be provided with adequate medical care. Everyone agreed that the provision of medical services to those who were risking and in many cases sacrificing their lives in defense of the nation deserved first priority in the allocation of physicians.

Second, probably, came the need of the medical schools for teachers to train more physicians under the accelerated program of medical education. These institutions, which were mobilized

100 per cent for the war effort, served as the only source for additions to, or replacements of, physicians for both the armed forces and the civilian population.

Next, in order of priority, came the provision of medical care for workers in war industries. These workers had to be kept on the job, producing the materials of war without which armies and navies are helpless in modern warfare.

This left the needs of the general population for medical services at the bottom of our priority list. It does not follow, however, that the civilian population was expected to get along with what was left after the armed forces, the medical schools and the war industries had taken all the physicians they wanted. The effective prosecution of a modern war requires the mobilization of all the resources of the nation in support of the war effort. Under such circumstances, it was clearly necessary that a sufficient number of physicians be retained to provide essential medical services for the civilian population. Recognizing this, the Army and the Navy agreed not to grant commissions to physicians declared essential by the Procurement and Assignment Service for civilian medical care. Local Selective Service boards were directed by National Headquarters to secure the recommendation of the service whenever they considered the classification of physicians, dentists or veterinarians. The result was that physicians whom the service considered essential for civilian medical care were not drafted into, nor accepted by, the military services.

At the beginning of the military preparedness program in 1940, the medical departments of the Army and the Navy together contained only 2,386 medical officers.

On the outbreak of war in December, 1941, 13,000 medical officers were on active duty in the Army and the Navy. By the end of 1942, approximately one year later, this number had increased to almost 42,000. The recruitment of so many physicians in a short period of time was a colossal undertaking. There was no authority to compel physicians, except for a few single men under the jurisdiction of Selective Service, to go into the service. Recruitment was entirely on a voluntary basis. The Procurement and Assignment Service had no authority to say to a physician that he must go into the service or that he must stay at home.

Early in 1942 it seemed that some physicians were slow in responding to the call for their services. But by the end of the year, more than 50 per cent of the practising physicians under 45 years of age had entered the armed services. No other professional group in this country has ever been called upon for such public service nor responded to a call so magnificently.

During the First World War, the recruitment of physicians for the Army and the Navy was carried on with little or no consideration for the needs of the civilian population. Many areas and communities were left without medical service, while in other areas excessive numbers of physicians remained in civilian life. To prevent a similar situation this time, the service established quotas as to the number of physicians each State was expected to supply in 1942. These quotas represented the proportionate share of the 42,000 medical officers requested by the armed forces, which it seemed equitable for each State to provide, taking into account the population of the State, the number of physicians in civilian practice, their ages, distribution, etc. These quotas for States with relatively few physicians in relation to population represented 10 to 15 per cent of the practising physicians, while the quotas of States relatively well supplied with physicians, such as New York and Illinois, called for 25 to 30 per cent of the physicians engaged in civilian practice. The country as a whole and all but five individual States met or exceeded the quotas assigned to them for 1942.

With the advent of 1943, an analysis of the physicians of the country disclosed that the statement about our having 180,000 physicians was misleading and that withdrawals from this group were already approaching the limit of the available supply. The figures show approximately 180,000 physicians registered in the United States. Of these, however, approximately 15,000 occupied full-time positions in public health departments, medical schools, insurance companies, or other governmental or private agencies not engaged in the practice of medicine; 28,000 were over 65 years of age, and for planning purposes were counted as only one-third effective by the service. It was estimated also that approximately 5 per cent, or a total of 7,000 of the physicians under 65, were completely or partially ineffective, that some 3,000 were resident physicians in hospitals, and that approximately 42,000 were in the armed forces at the beginning of the year. This left only about 94,500 effective physicians in civilian practice. (Figure 3.) On a basis of an over-all ratio of one physician for 1,500 population, approximately 83,000 of this number were required to provide essential medical services for the civilian population. This left only 11,500 physicians in civilian practice who could still be considered "available" for military service.

During 1943, approximately 5,000 of these entered the military services, leaving an estimated 6,500 still available. This is a theo-

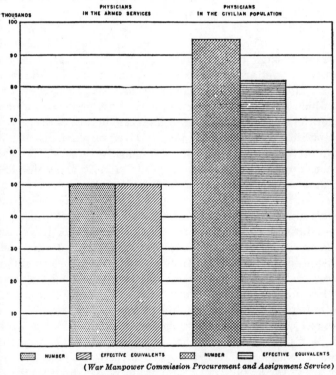

FIGURE 1. Physicians (number and effective equivalents) in military service and caring for the civilian population, 1944

retical number based on the national average. To determine the number of physicians actually available, it is necessary that the physicians in each local community be classified as either essential for civilian medical care or available for military service. During the latter part of 1943 and the early months of 1944, this was done county by county and State by State. These totals listed approximately 7,000 physicians under 45 years of age as available for military service. This does not mean that all of them could be expected to enter military service: some were physically or otherwise unacceptable to the services; some were deferred by Selective Service for various reasons; and some had adequate personal reasons for remaining at home.

In addition to the physicians recruited from civilian life, between 4,000 and 5,000 hospital interns and residents became available to the Army and Navy each year. These, together with the recruitments from civilian practice, raised the total of physicians in Army and Navy service to 52,000 early in 1944. This is an exceedingly large proportion of the active physicians in the country. Yet our armed forces reached such a size that the ratio of medical officers to total strength was only about 60 per cent of that which in the past has been considered necessary by responsible authorities to provide adequate medical care in time of war.

From time to time reports were received of physicians in the Army or Navy who were not professionally employed or who were making but little use of their special training and skills. The Procurement and Assignment Service was alert to improper or under-utilization of physicians by the armed forces. With the over-all supply inadequate to meet both military and civilian demands during the war, it became essential that the services of the available supply be utilized effectively and economically. Both the Surgeons General of the Army and the Navy appreciated that fact and reduced tables of organization for medical officers, revising the duties assigned to them so that, as far as possible, medical officers were utilized only for professional medical work. Thousands of medical administrative officers were trained by the Army, and Pharmacists' Mates by the Navy, to carry duties formerly assigned to medical officers. The more extensive use of nurses and even of WAVES and WACS also made physicians' services go farther. In addition, the medical corpsmen of both services were better trained than ever before to perform many services under the direction of medical officers.

In order to safeguard civilian medical care, the chairmen of State Procurement and Assignment Committees were directed to designate as "essential" those physicians considered necessary for the maintenance of essential civilian medical services. As a guide to State chairmen in making these classifications, "criteria of essentiality" for the several categories of civilian medical service were prepared by the Directing Board with the aid of its advisory committees.

The importance of maintaining and, if possible, of increasing the supply of physicians was recognized at the beginning of our program of national mobilization and military training. Medical schools responded promptly to this need by the discontinuance of vacations, by increasing enrollments as much as their facilities would permit without serious prejudice to the quality of instruction, and by reducing their requirements for admission from three or four years to two years of premedical college work.

Medical schools were also called upon to release members of their faculties for service, in many instances highly specialized service, with the armed forces. Other members of their staffs were requested to devote their time in whole or in large part to war research. The medical schools met these demands promptly and willingly, in spite of the fact that they were faced with the heaviest teaching responsibilities in their history.

The concern of the Procurement and Assignment Service with recruitment from medical faculties was to assure the retention of adequate teaching staffs for the conduct of a sound program of medical education during the war. To accomplish this, each medical school was requested to appraise its teaching faculty periodically, marking as "available" those who constituted the minimum staff necessary to carry teaching responsibilities satisfactorily.

Analysis of the medical school lists of "essential teachers" showed that, up to July 1, 1942, 21 per cent of the physicians on medical school faculties were in Army or Navy service, as compared with 12 per cent of all physicians in the United States. In addition, the medical schools listed as "available" 25 per cent of the physicians of military age remaining on their staffs.

Some schools appeared to have released too many members of their faculties and to have retained insufficient staffs for the instruction of their students. This could only mean a sacrifice in the quality of the training of the medical students in those institutions. Other schools were more conservative and were requested to release additional physicians toward meeting the quotas of medical officers neeeded for service with the armed forces.

Some people have suggested that medical teaching in wartime might be done by practitioners who are over military age or are physically disqualified for military service. Such suggestions indicate a failure to realize that medical teaching has become an important specialty and that in many schools younger men not only carry most of the teaching load but also are the most effective teachers. Before the war, considerably more than half the physicians teaching in medical schools were under 45 years of age, and these men on the average were devoting more time to teaching than were their older colleagues. Furthermore, most practitioners have been too busy during the war to assume much more, if any, teaching responsibilities. It was essential, therefore, that some of the effective younger teachers who were devoting all or a large part of their time to teaching be retained on the faculties of the medical schools. There they could render their most valuable war service.

Lists of "essential teachers" as submitted by the medical schools were reviewed by the Medical Education Committee of the Procurement and Assignment Service. The opinions of this committee in regard to the lists were then transmitted to the chairmen of the respective State committees of the service, who were responsible for decision as to the "availability" or "essentiality" of the individual physicians in their States. Appeals from the decisions of State committees could be made by the dean of the school, or by the physician concerned, to the corps area committees, or even to the Directing Board of the service. The objective of this program was to retain adequate teaching staffs for the medical schools, but to do so without withholding from military service more than a minimum number of men physically qualified for such service.

An adequate and uninterrupted supply of qualified medical students is necessary if there is to be a continuing output of physicians from the medical schools. Realizing this, the Director of Selective Service early in 1941 advised local boards that medical and premedical students in good standing and making normal progress toward graduation should be considered eligible for deferment of military service. In 1942, the Army and Navy became concerned about the continuing supply of young medical officers and authorized the granting of commissions on inactive status to students who were in, or had been accepted for, the next entering class in approved medical schools.

On July 1, 1943, these students were placed on active duty under the Army Specialized Training Program, or the Navy College Program. Tuition, subsistence and the regular pay of enlisted men were provided for these students.

In a few schools group housing and messing were provided, but the majority of the students were given subsistence allowances and permitted to make their own living arrangements. All were under military jurisdiction, but military duties were at a minimum and interfered little, if at all, with their medical training. Army, Navy and civilian students were all in the same classes. The curriculum was unchanged from peacetime, except for the addition by some schools of courses in war medicine and tropical medicine.

The College Training Program of both the Army and Navy provided also for premedical education, the Army's premedical program consisting of five terms of 12 weeks each and the Navy program of five terms of 16 weeks each. Selection for, and advancement in, these programs were based on competitive examinations and careful "screening" procedures. From those who successfully completed these programs, the Army and Navy expected to fill the places in medical schools for which they contracted.

In December, 1942, it was agreed by the Surgeons General of the Army and Navy and the Directing Board of the Procurement and Assignment Service that classes admitted to medical school during the war should be made up of the following groups: Army students, 55 per cent; Navy students, 25 per cent; and civilian students, 20 per cent—the last-named group to be made up of women and of men ineligible for military service. Selective Service policy still provided for the deferment of premedical students who were accepted for admission to medical school and would complete their premedical studies within 24 months, but few such students were deferred.

The Directing Board of the Procurement and Assignment Service formally expressed its concern over the failure of this plan to provide an adequate number of replacements for physicians to serve the civilian population. In spite of this, the plan was adopted because of the priority given to the needs of the armed forces for medical officers.

Early in 1944, when these programs were just beginning to function smoothly, the Army decided to terminate its college training program except for students in medical schools, premedical students already in the program and selected to continue with premedical training, and a few advanced students in engineering. No additional students were admitted to the program after April 1, 1941. It was estimated that the number of premedical students remaining in the program would be sufficient to fill about half the places in medical schools for which the Army had contracted. The Navy would continue to fill the places for which it had contracted, 25 to 31 per cent of the total. At about the same time that the Army curtailed its Specialized Training Program, the Director of Selective Service issued instructions discontinuing the deferment of premedical students except for those who could be enrolled in medical schools before July 1, 1944.

The curtailment of the Army Specialized Training Program increased by 27 per cent the number of places in medical classes to be filled by civilian students, while the discontinuance of Selective Service deferments for premedical students cut off the supply of such students.

The Directing Board of the Procurement and Assignment Service was deeply concerned over this situation lest it should be impossible to keep the supply of doctors constant and adequate. Already the ratio of physicians to population in 1944 had reached the minimum considered safe by the service and the United States Public Health Service. Still more serious was the progressive reduction of this ratio, due to the death of approximately 3,500 civilian physicians annually, with fewer than 1,200 replacements available from medical graduates ineligible for military service.

Presentations of the dangers inherent in this situation were given to the Director of Selective Service, to the War and the Navy Departments, and to the Division of War Mobilization. The decision of these groups, however, was that the immediate need of the armed forces for physically acceptable men superseded the prospective need of the country for these young men as doctors in 1949 or thereafter.

Most of the physicians on hospital staffs practised in the community and were designated as "available" or "essential" on the basis of the importance of their services to the community as a whole rather than to an individual hospital. In large charity and teaching hospitals, on the other hand, certain residents and physicians in charge of special services, such as the x-ray and laboratory departments, were deemed essential both for the clinical instruction of medical students and for the adequate care of the hospital patients. With this group, the problem was to release as many as possible for service with the armed forces and still retain the minimum number essential for the proper functioning of the institution. To accomplish this, hospitals were requested to prepare lists of the residents and other physicians on their staffs, indicating which ones they considered the minimum essential staff of the hospital. These lists were reviewed by the Hospital Advisory Committee and the respective State committees of the service.

In normal times a considerable part of the medical work in hospitals, and particularly in large charity hospitals, is done by the intern and resident staffs. Prior to the war, most internships were one year but many were 18 months to two years in length. For further training, particularly in the specialties, many interns continued as hospital residents for one to five additional years. with two- or three-year residencies most common.

In 1940, 7,200 interns and 6,150 residents were on duty in the hospitals of this country. With the outbreak of war, many of these young physicians went into military service, and in conformity with Army and Navy policy, all hospitals were requested to reduce the length of internships to 12 months.

By January, 1943, almost all the students being graduated from medical schools were under the jurisdiction of the Army or the Navy. Each of these graduates was permitted only 12 months of hospital internship before being ordered to active military duty. For civilian hospitals this meant the loss of all the experienced resident physicians except a few women and physically disqualified men.

To improve this situation and safeguard the welfare of hospital patients, the Directing Board of the service formulated, and the Surgeons General of the Army and the Navy approved, a plan which reduced the length of internships to nine months, but provided that one-third of the interns under the jurisdiction of the Army and the Navy could be deferred for a second nine months to serve as assistant residents, and that one-half of these could be deferred for a third nine months to serve as residents in civilian hospitals. This has been known as the "9-9-9 program."

This program assured a limited supply of interns and residents for civilian hospitals. The next problem was to provide for an equitable distribution of this number to the hospitals in need of

their services. To accomplish this, the service established quota
of interns and residents for the civilian hospitals of the Unite
States. In general these quotas represented 60 to 70 per cent of th
number of interns and residents on duty in the hospitals on Marc
15, 1940. Certain adjustments were made for hospitals with larg
teaching programs and for hospitals with large increases in patien
loads.

The chief objection to this plan was that it did not provid
adequate internship or residency training. Judged by peacetim
standards, the objection is well founded. On the other hand, wit
the armed forces urgently in need of young medical officers, th
plan represented the most liberal deferment of commissione
officers to serve as assistant residents and residents in civilian ho
pitals that could be approved by the Army and Navy. Had 12
month internships been continued, hospitals would have bee
forced to operate without any commissioned officers as resident
The "9-9-9 program" thus provided the most efficient use of recen
medical graduates, assured young physicians the best hospit
training possible under wartime conditions, and permitted th
widest possible coverage of house officers to all hospitals.

The initiation of this plan called for a reduction from mor
than 8,100 approved internships of one to three years' length, an
nearly 6,000 approved residencies of similar length, to 6,000 ir
ternships and 4,200 residencies of nine months' duration. The su
cessful operation of the plan reflects the cooperation of all co
cerned and is evidence of the willingness of American medicin
to make the adjustments and sacrifices required of a nation at wa

Industrial medical services assume increasing importance i
time of war. Accidents and illnesses among industrial workers an
their families curtail war production and must be kept to a min
mum. This requires an expansion of industrial hygiene an
medical services for which unfortunately most industries depen
primarily upon young physicians in the age group and with th
qualifications most desired by the armed forces.

In order to safeguard essential health services in industry, whil
cooperating with the armed forces in the recruitment of medic
officers, the Procurement and Assignment Service Committee o
Industrial Health formulated, and the Directing Board approve
the following criteria as to the conditions under which physician
should be considered "essential" for industrial health services.

A physician employed in industrial medicine is deemed to be not available for military service when the following conditions exist:

A. Full-time industrial physician.

　　1. The physician is employed by an industry which is manufacturing war materials exclusively or under priority ratings, and

　　2. The physician gives his full time to the industry or 40 or more hours weekly; has been so employed for at least two years or has been especially trained for that purpose, and is carrying on an acceptable health maintenance program, and

　　3. The physician is performing the functions of a medical director or department head or a specialist or is the only physician employed.

B. Assistant physicians who perform routine functions under direction, and are employed on a full-time basis, are deemed essential until they can be replaced within a reasonable time (three to six months).

C. Part-time industrial physician.

　　1. The physician serves part time or more industries engaged exclusively in the manufacture of war materials or under priority ratings, providing his total part-time service is the equivalent of 40 or more hours weekly.

D. The physician serves a State industrial hygiene bureau on a full-time basis.

Note: The physician who serves on call only is not deemed to be essential.

In the application of these criteria, the service insisted that important industrial medical services be continued but that physically fit physicians of military age serving in industry be replaced as rapidly as possible by those who were not physically fit or were otherwise ineligible for military service.

Public health services must be maintained for the protection of the health of both the armed forces and the civilian population. Yet the staffs of these services normally include many physicians with training and experience urgently needed by both the Army and the Navy. Epidemiologists, parasitologists, bacteriologists, statisticians and public health administrators were needed for the prevention and control of disease among soldiers and sailors serving in all parts of the world.

In order that public health services might be maintained and yet as many as possible of these specialists released to the armed forces, all States, city and county health departments were requested to prepare lists of personnel, indicating which ones of military age could be released for service and which ones were considered "essential" for the effective functioning of the health department. These lists were reviewed by the Public Health Committee of the service, with recommendations to State chairmen. On the basis of these recommendations, individual physicians in public health work were listed either as "available" for military service or as "essential" for the continuation of essential civilian health services. (Figure 4.)

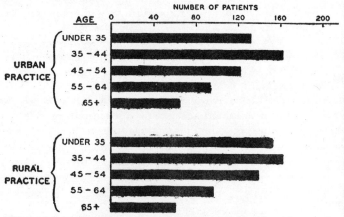

FIGURE 2. Average number of patients seen in 1 week by white male general practitioners in urban and rural practice.*

* Antonio, Ciocco, and Isadore Altman: "The Patient Load of Physicians in Private Practice," *Public Health Reports*, Vol. 58, pp. 1329-1351, September 3, 1943.

Prior to the war, the civilian population of this country was better supplied with physicians than the people of any other country in the world. National mobilization and the subsequent increase in the size of the armed forces changed all this. By the end of 1943, approximately two-thirds of the physicians under 45 years of age who were physically fit for military service were serving in the armed forces. This is the age group which is most active in medical practice and carries the largest load of medical care. With these no longer available, it was inevitable that the public should feel a shortage of medical service. (Figure 5.)

At the beginning of the war, there was approximately one effective private practitioner of medicine to every 1,022 persons in the United States. By the end of 1942, this ratio had increased to one to 1,361, and by the end of 1943, to approximately one to

1,500. (Figure 4.) It is reported that England has one physician to approximately 230 persons in the armed forces, and one to 2,700 civilians. In this country the corresponding figures in 1944 were approximately one to 200 with the armed forces, and one to 1,500 in the civilian population. From this one can only conclude that the United States was still relatively well off in terms of medical care both for the civilian population and for the armed forces.

WORK LOAD OF PHYSICIANS (Patients Seen Each Week)

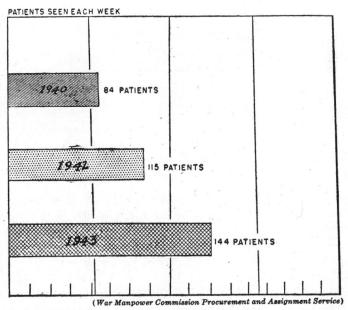

FIGURE 3. There will be corresponding increase in 1944-45 work load, which means increase in deaths and partial and complete incapacitations, because the load is being carried by physicians 10 years older on the average than those carrying 1940 load.

In order to maintain essential medical services for the civilian population, it was the policy of the Procurement and Assignment Service to declare "essential" for civilian practice a sufficient number of physicians to meet the needs of the population in the various sections of the country. The Army, Navy and United States Public Health Service honored these ratings and refused commissions to physicians listed as "essential"

In most communities this policy resulted in a sufficient number

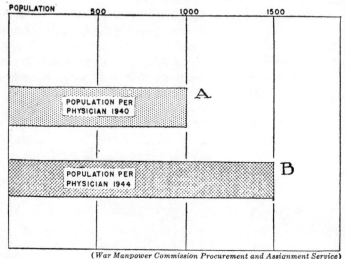

(*War Manpower Commission Procurement and Assignment Service*)

FIGURE 4. Number of civilians per physician, 1940 and 1944

A. P & A S. was removing physicians when each one cared for 1,000 people.
B. P & A S. must now remove physicians when each one cares for 1,500 people.

of physicians being retained to provide essential medical services. On the other hand, from a few areas, particularly in the South, too many physicians went into the service. Some of these held commissions in the Reserve Corps of the Army or Navy and were called to active duty at the outbreak of the war; others volunteered before the Procurement and Assignment Service became operative; others were released by the State Procurement and Assignment Service committees because it seemed that a sufficient number of physicians remained to care for the civilian population. In some instances these calculations were upset by the illness or death of remaining physicians, or by the unanticipated influx of large populations connected with war industries or war activities. One county in North Dakota had three physicians before the war. The youngest of these was declared "available" for military service. Subsequently one of the two remaining physicians died and the other had a "coronary attack," which seriously limited his ability to practise medicine. The result was that this county was critically short of medical services. (Table 2.)

Other problems resulted from the fact that approximately six

TABLE 2. ACTIVE PHYSICIANS IN THE UNITED STATES 1940 AND 1944

	Total Physicians 1940[1]	Ratios[2]	Total Physicians 1944[3]	Ratios[4]
United States	140,755	935	98,960	1,286
Alabama	1,682	1,684	1,273	2,135
Arizona	526	949	263	2,165
Arkansas	1,400	1,392	1,109	1,565
California	9,241	747	6,441	1,224
Colorado	1,304	861	818	1,305
Connecticut	2,191	780	1,709	1,023
Delaware	292	913	169	1,619
District of Columbia	1,615	411	1,073	761
Florida	1,875	1,012	921	2,185
Georgia	2,251	1,388	1,561	1,907
Idaho	369	1,422	232	2,040
Illinois	10,013	789	7,635	991
Indiana	3,298	1,039	2,345	1,443
Iowa	2,448	1,037	1,738	1,310
Kansas	1,600	1,126	1,184	1,418
Kentucky	2,150	1,324	1,416	1,600
Louisiana	1,938	1,220	1,449	1,599
Maine	746	1,136	626	1,250
Maryland	2,274	801	1,552	1,279
Massachusetts	6,206	696	5,284[5]	775
Michigan	5,170	1,017	3,806	1,413
Minnesota	3,093	903	1,797	1,405
Mississippi	1,224	1,784	45	2,113
Missouri	3,780	1,001	2,672	1,319
Montana	465	1,203	353	1,332
Nebraska	1,327	992	966	1,217
Nevada	146	755	109	1,199
New Hampshire	504	975	388	1,168
New Jersey	4,943	842	3,208	1,272
New Mexico	374	1,422	260	1,885
New York	22,589	597	14,469	860
North Carolina	2,374	1,504	1,696	1,973
North Dakota	446	1,439	344	1,560
Ohio	7,451	927	5,007	1,340
Oklahoma	1,789	1,306	1,482	1,341
Oregon	1,176	927	838	1,396
Pennsylvania	11,117	691	8,025	1,156
Rhode Island	781	913	658	1,056
South Carolina	1,214	1,665	876[5]	2,043
South Dakota	388	1,657	283	1,925
Tennessee	2,319	1,257	1,705	1,653

[1] Total physicians in private practice and with full-time appointments less 2/3 of those 65 yrs. and over, less physicians in regular Army, regular Navy, public health service and interns and residents.

[2] Using population figures, U. S. Census Bureau, April, 1940.

[3] As of January 1, 1944, excluding Class IV physicians.

[4] Using population estimate figures, U. S. Census Bureau, November 1, 1943.

[5] Data in process of being revised.

Note: These figures and ratios are based on total active physicians, while the figures in Figure 4 are based on active physicians in the civilian practice of medicine.

TABLE 2. ACTIVE PHYSICIANS IN THE UNITED STATES 1940 AND 1944—*(Continued)*

	Total Physicians 1940[1]	Ratios[2]	Total Physicians 1944[3]	Ratios[4]
Texas	5,151	1,245	3,420	1,836
Utah	492	1,119	387	1,508
Vermont	425	845	257	1,230
Virginia	2,287	1,171	1,312	2,111
Washington	1,708	1,017	1,190	1,601
West Virginia	1,551	1,226	1,123	1,543
Wisconsin	2,819	1,113	2,352	1,252
Wyoming	233	1,078	144	1,637

million Americans moved their homes as a result of the war. Many towns experienced mushroom growth in connection with war industries or military installations. In some of these cases, there was a critical shortage of medical care. Many articles have been written about these areas, frequently with gross exaggeration as to number and seriousness. In many instances the workers in these war industries were recruited from residents of the area; or if the influx of population had not been excessive, the physicians in the community were able to provide necessary medical care. On the other hand, there are other areas in which the shortage of medical services was really critical. I visited one community which in a little more than a year had increased from 15,000 to 65,000 population. It was still growing and was expected to reach 100,000. Another area of approximately 40,000 population before the war had 110,000 in the spring of 1943 and was expected to reach 145,000.

In 1942 a number of agencies in Washington became concerned about the shortage of medical services in these areas, and numerous conferences were held to define lines of responsibility and to outline procedures to deal with the situation. On the basis of these conferences, the Directing Board of the service formulated certain policies in regard to the investigation of the need and provision of medical care in critical shortage areas. These policies, which were approved by the United States Public Health Service, by the Trustees and the War Participation Committee of the American Medical Association and by the War Manpower Commission, placed the primary responsibility for the investigation of these areas and for the formulation of plans to meet their needs upon the Procurement and Assignment Service and the local medical profession, with the cooperation and assistance of the United States Public Health Service.

To meet these responsibilities, the Directing Board requested detailed reports from State chairmen concerning changes in population, the medical personnel and the medical and health facilities available and needed in communities or areas in which there were war industries or war activities, or in which there was a known or expected shortage of medical services. In investigating the needs of these areas, the State Procurement and Assignment committees were advised to seek the "cooperation of the State medical societies, the State dental societies, the State health officers, of industry, of organized labor, and of other agencies, such as the State Defense Council, which should be able to make significant contributions to the solution of this problem." In addition, the United States Public Health Service was charged with the responsibility of cooperating in the conduct of these investigations. When they revealed a need for additional physicians or other medical or health facilities or personnel, it was provided that:

Whenever possible, civilian needs as determined by these committees should be met through local arrangements, resources and agencies. In case assistance is needed for the organization, administration or financing of necessary medical services in these areas, the responsibility for formulating the plan best suited to each particular situation should devolve upon an agency which should include representatives of the State health department, the State medical society and the State dental society with the cooperation and support—financial and technical— of the appropriate Federal agencies; the administration of such plans to be delegated to the appropriate official State agency. It is recognized that the United States Public Health Service is the Federal agency which will be responsible for the provision of funds or personnel which may be required to provide the necessary health services in these areas.

In the formulation and execution of this program, there was complete harmony and effective cooperation between the Directing Board of the service and the United States Public Health Service as represented by its Surgeon General, Thomas Parran, and Assistant Surgeon General Warren Draper.

Surveys have indicated that in some areas the need was not for more physicians but rather for hospitals, nurses or public health services. In a considerable number of areas, local medical societies, in cooperation with public health departments and housing and welfare groups, were able to meet the need for physicians either by having the doctors in nearby communities give specific amounts of time to the shortage area or by inducing other physicians to move into the area.

From January, 1942, to March 31, 1944, State chairmen of the Procurement and Assignment Service reported 510 areas as being critically short of medical personnel. Of these areas, the needs for medical personnel were met in 281 communities, 55 per cent of the critical areas. Relocations of physicians were effected in 195 of these communities, and the needs of 146 communities were met by other means, such as inducing retired physicians to resume active practice, changes in types of medical practice, and "freezing" of medical personnel in civilian communities.

Altogether 2,900 physicians took positions in war industries or moved into "shortage areas" between January, 1942, and 1944, and reports indicate that approximately two-thirds of those moves were the result of efforts of State or local Procurement and Assignment chairmen or committees.

The main obstacles to permanent solutions for some communities were to be found in such factors as these:

(1) To a large extent, relocations had to be effected within the various States themselves owing to restrictions in medical license laws which prohibited outside physicians from practising.

(2) It was very difficult to find qualified older physicians who were not already firmly established and who were willing to move to other areas where their services were needed.

(3) Some physicians, though professionally qualified, were not acceptable to local communities.

(4) The distribution of medical personnel for civilian purposes had to be voluntary. As a result, it was sometimes impossible to persuade physicians to move to certain communities considered unattractive. Equally difficult to counteract was the movement of physicians from some rural areas where their services were needed to urban areas with better financial opportunities.

Although the ratio of one doctor to 1,500 population was utilized for planning purposes by the service as the over-all number of physicians required to provide essential medical services to the civilian population, in shortage areas a ratio of 1 to 3,000 was accepted as the coverage beyond which the situation should be considered critical. Some "boom town" communities not only had ratios below this but also were in need of other health personnel and facilities, such as nurses, dentists, hospital beds, etc.

The responsibility for formulating plans to meet these needs was placed jointly upon the Procurement and Assignment Service, the United States Public Health Service, and State and local medical societies. Most of the residents of these areas were earning good incomes and should have been able to support physicians on a private practice basis. Under a recent law, the United States Public Health Service was enabled to pay a subsistence allowance of $250 a month for three months plus transportation expenses to physicians being relocated, provided the local community paid one-fourth of the total cost. In some areas, pre-payment plans for medical services under the supervision of the State medical society met the need. In rare instances, it was necessary to assign an officer of the United States Public Health Service to practise temporarily in the area. Such assignment, however, was made only as a last resort and upon the joint recommendation of the Pro-curement and Assignment Service and the United States Public Health Service. Less than half a dozen Public Health Service officers were so assigned.

An editorial writer on one of our leading newspapers proposed from time to time that medical officers of the United States Public Health Service be assigned to care for the civilian population in all areas in which shortages of physicians existed. Such a proposal implied that the Public Health Service had or could secure a sufficient number of medical officers for such assignments. Actually this service had difficulty in recruiting enough medical officers to meet its regular responsibilities; and it is fantastic to assume that physicians would seek appointments in the Public Health Service for the purpose of practising medicine in rural areas of North Dakota or Mississippi.

It would have required a National Service Act with the authority to draft physicians for civilian medical care even to inaugurate such a plan. On the other hand, if Congress had enacted a National Service law, the program of the Procurement and Assignment Service could have functioned more effectively.

Except for a few physicians who were subject to induction by Selective Service, the Procurement and Assignment Service was forced to use only "moral pressure" to induce physicians either to enter the armed forces or to move to areas where their services were needed for civilian medical care. While the voluntary program under which the service functioned had many advantages, a National Service Act would have made it possible to recruit a few more medical officers for the armed forces and to provide physicians for many areas in which critical shortages of medical services existed.

Even with authority, it would have been difficult to require a physician who was well established in a community to leave his home, his office and his practice to move to some other community. On the other hand, there were several hundred young physicians, physically ineligible for military service, who left hospital internships or residencies each year to enter civilian practice. Many of these established themselves in large cities where there were splendid opportunities but no critical need for their services. Some authority requiring such physicians to locate in rural areas or to accept positions in war industries would have made it possible to improve many unsatisfactory situations.

The authority to practise medicine is granted by individual States through Boards of Medical Licensure. The result is a lack of uniformity in licensure, in laws and regulations, and definite limitations on the migration of physicians. In normal times this causes little difficulty, but it was a handicap to the relocation of physicians in certain "shortage areas" during the war. To meet this situation, the Directing Board of the service and the Executive Council of the Federation of State Medical Boards jointly made the following recommendations to State Boards of Licensure:

Statement of Principles Reccommended to State Boards of Registration and Education in Medicine for the Temporary Licensure of Physicians during the War Emergency.

I. The need for relocation or assignment of physicians or dentists shall be determined by the Directing Board of the Procurement and Assignment Service with the aid of the State Committees of the Procurement and Assignment Service and other agencies and on agreement with the State Boards of Registration and·Education in Medicine and Dentistry.

II. These needs shall be met as far as possible by the relocation of physicians and dentists holding licenses within the State.

III. Whenever possible, needs shall be met by taking full advantage of existing provisions for reciprocity between the States and inter-State endorsement.

IV. Whenever existing laws make impossible the granting of temporary certificates, State Boards should recommend to the Governor and to the State Legislatures the earliest possible enactment of a bill designed to make possible the utilization of physicians and dentists under temporary certification.

V. When existing measures for relocation of physicians or dentists prove inadequate, State Boards of Registration and Education may request the Directing Board of the Procurement and Assignment Service to certify to them the names and qualifications of physicians and dentists who have volunteered or who may be otherwise available for relocation, at which time also such physicians or dentists may be notified that their names have been sent to the State Boards making such requests.

VI. The physician or dentist who accepts relocation shall agree to assignment to the specific area in which services are required and to acceptance of a certificate which limits the duration of such service to the period of the emergency and for such additional time as the State Boards may prescribe.

VII. In view of the emergency character of this action, the Committee representatives, the Directing Board of the Procurement and Assignment Service, and the Federation of State Medical Boards of the United States recommend that fees for such certification be waived or reduced to a minimum.

These recommendations led to liberalization of the laws and regulations governing licensure in certain States and resulted in the relocation of some physicians in "shortage areas" within those States.

To sum up: The Procurement and Assignment Service represented an experiment in cooperation between the Federal government and the medical profession. The results were generally most satisfactory, considering the difficulties and problems involved. Certainly, no other professional group was called upon to do or to sacrifice so much in support of the war. The medical profession met those demands and responsibilities magnificently.

The doctor of today is either a general practitioner or a highly specialized authority in some medical branch. Most of the need of the Army has been for what is known as the battalion medical officer—the doctor who is with a small detachment and who serves all their medical needs. Nevertheless, the Army Medical Department early recognized the importance of assigning every physician to the work for which he was best fitted, and for distributing physicians throughout the world on a great many battle fronts so that they could do for the wounded men and the health of our soldiers the most that could possibly be done.

From the very first, after our entrance into the war, Dr. George F. Lull was in charge of personnel, a position in which his genial character, his understanding and his sympathy did much to endear him to the men over whom he had control. When Major General Norman T. Kirk was appointed Surgeon General of the Army, George F. Lull was also appointed a major general, and was given the position of Deputy Surgeon General in which he carried on his previous duties and took on a good many more. General Lull's military career has been distinguished from the first. He was commissioned an officer in the Medical Corps of the United States Army in 1912; he has been decorated with the Purple Heart; he has served all over the world.

In his article in this volume, Major General Lull explains the manner in which the medical manpower of the nation was mobilized and brought to bear on service in this war.

CHAPTER IV

FIFTY THOUSAND DOCTORS AND HALF A MILLION PERSONNEL

By
MAJOR GENERAL GEORGE F. LULL
Deputy Surgeon General

THE MEDICAL SERVICE of our Army has worked under serious handicaps for many years. It was inadequate, both in matériel and personnel, until long after the Spanish-American War. In a report to President McKinley following that war, the Dodge Commission noted the deplorable lack of medical personnel existing in 1898, and as a result an Act of Congress approved on February 2, 1901, increased the Medical Department's size. But the move was totally inadequate.

President Theodore Roosevelt wrote a letter to both Houses of Congress on January 5, 1905, urging further legislation to increase personnel, but nothing was done until 1908, when at last a law was passed which increased the strength of the Medical Corps to seven medical officers for every thousand men in the Army. This ratio was maintained by Section 10 of the National Defense Act of 1916, and lowered again to 6.5 by the amendment of June 4, 1920, although a quota of 0.5 Medical Administrative Corps officers for each thousand men was provided at the same time.

The ratio was discarded in favor of a definite number by Act of June 30, 1922, and thereafter the proportion varied until the Act of April 3, 1939, which authorized 1,424 officers over a period of years—equivalent to 6.33 physicians for each thousand enlisted men.

An enormous expansion took place, however, when the small peacetime department was required by the national emergency to furnish medical service for nearly eight million men. The figures in Table 1 indicate this expansion more graphically than words. To grasp what took place between 1939 and January 1, 1944, consider how amazing would be the growth of a business which jumped from little more than 11,000 employees to more than 600,000 in slightly more than four years.

TABLE 1. MEDICAL DEPARTMENT EXPANSION—PEACETIME AND JANUARY 1, 1944

Corps	Peacetime Strength	Approximate Strength Jan. 1, 1944
Medical	1,230	40,200
Dental	267	15,000
Veterinary	126	2,073
Sanitary	None	2,300
Medical Administrative	72*	15,000
Army Nurse	949	38,000
Enlisted Men Medical Department	8,643	512,000

* Now the Pharmacy Corps regular Army.

All the corps of the Medical Department participated in the expansion. The Sanitary Corps, for instance, exists only in the Reserve during peacetime, and when the expansion began, it contained all types of skilled and unskilled men who had been given commissions in that corps because there was no other place to put them in the Medical Department. Some more properly belonged in the Medical Administrative Corps. New regulations were prepared to limit this corps to sanitary engineers, supply procurement personnel, bacteriologists, entomologists, chemists, statisticians, food and nutrition experts, and similar specialists.

After the war began, many bills were introduced in Congress to add certain other corps to the Department. Physical therapy aides and dietitians were given commissions similar to those for nurses. Other groups singled out legislatively included optometrists, chiropodists, chiropractors, x-ray technicians and morticians. The bill creating the Pharmacy Corps affected only the Regular Army and provided for seventy-two officers in that corps.

Before the war, the Military Personnel Division of the Office of the Surgeon General was a relatively small organization. It was divided into two sections, one for Regular Army personnel, the other for Reserve Officers. This Reserve section felt the load first when the Army began its expansion. On January 1, 1941, there were only 2,149 Medical Reserve officers and 515 National Guard medical officers on extended active duty, during the early training period. Great efforts were made to secure personnel to help to train the Medical Department troops. During this period, officers with Reserve Commissions were requested to accept active duty. Such procedure had to be followed because officers below the grade of captain could resign if ordered to active duty, provided they had dependents and no income other than their Army pay (Pub. Res. 96, 76th Congress).

There was extreme difficulty in getting a sufficient number of trained officers to staff the newly opened Medical Department Training Centers, first at Camp Lee, Virginia, and later at Camp Grant, Illinois, Camp Barkeley, Texas, and Camp Robinson, Arkansas. Calls came for officers for overseas garrisons and only volunteers could be sent.

The entire file of Reserve officers was searched to select professional personnel for a few general hospitals. When a suitable man was located, he was asked by letter whether he would be willing to accept active duty. Lieutenant Colonel John M. Welch, M.C., was instrumental in staffing the first nine hospitals, and they were ideally staffed. Each man was considered on the basis of his personal characteristics and his professional ability. Never before nor since have any Army general hospitals been so well provided with professional staffs as were these units of our Medical Department.

Almost every doctor who accepted active duty wanted to be assigned to a hospital; he took it as a reflection on his professional ability if he got any other kind of assignment. Officers assigned to tactical units were much disgruntled over the dearth of purely professional work. They did not want administrative duties; they wanted diagnosis, surgery and treatment of the sick. On February 4, 1941, a policy of rotating the services of medical officers was announced (Let. AG 353 Med. [10-31-40] MMG). Officers who had spent six months with tactical units could apply for duty with hospital installations. The result was a mass of letters from doctors with tactical units, and only two from officers on hospital assignments. Consequently few people were reassigned.

New recommendations were submitted to provide a more generalized and workable method by increasing the period of service to one year, but the advent of war killed this proposal before it ever became effective. Officers assigned to tactical units did not realize how important their work would be with those units, because there was no fighting to be done at that time. Many who have since seen service in theaters of operations now appreciate this fact. They have also been made to realize that not only is physical stamina needed for tactical duty, but also a broad knowledge of the practice of medicine.

Before the outbreak of war, the Preparedness Committee of the American Medical Association formulated plans for an orderly supply of physicians for the armed forces. This plan was approved, with minor modifications, by the War Department on December 19, 1941. Later the President, by Executive Order, placed operation of the plan under the Federal Security Administrator as the Procurement and Assignment Service. This service circularized all physicians, requesting information about their desire for service, and State quotas were established. The service had no authority to force a physician to accept military or naval service.

Although considerable work was done by the Central Executive Committee and by State and county officers, volunteers were often not plentiful enough for the needs of the service. After several conferences with the War Department General Staff and the Procurement and Assignment Service, Army recruiting parties were sent to recruit doctors and dentists. These boards were organized early in 1942 and continued to function until late in the same year, when they were discontinued at the request of the War Manpower Commission, under which the service was functioning.

The recruiting boards operated in a unique manner. They would establish themselves in a locality, and after an applicant had been interviewed, he would be given a physical examination locally, be cleared by the State Procurement and Assignment Service men attached to the board and, if his physical examination was satisfactory, be commissioned on the spot. As far as we know, it was the first time in the history of the Army that commissions were ever issued in that manner.

If we actually followed a ratio of seven doctors per thousand strength, it would mean 61,600 men for an army of 7,700,000. This number is considered ideal for the highest type of medical service. Early in the war, however, authorities realized that the

Army would never be able to secure this number without seriously affecting the care of the civil population. Consequently, requirements were reduced and every effort was made to conserve medical manpower. There was, moreover, constant criticism that not all medical officers were as busy as they should be. Actually, many of them were in positions similar to those of paid employees of a city fire department. They had to be on the job and trained, ready to act when the emergency arose.

In April, 1942, there were three thousand fewer physicians on active duty than there were in the First World War five months after our entry. Requirements were reduced to a point beyond which the Surgeon General thought it dangerous to go. Recruiting lagged behind requirements. In November, 1942, the Executive Board of the Procurement and Assignment Service voted to furnish the Army with 575 doctors each month, exclusive of interns and residents. This was to last for a period of one year. The Surgeon General of the Army accepted the proposal, and as a result 10,337 names of doctors were submitted as available. Of this number, 52.9 per cent refused to file applications, and the average monthly rate of procurement for the year was 268 instead of 575.

The Women's Medical Association repeatedly made overtures to the Surgeon General about commissioning women in the military service, but a ruling of the Comptroller General held that moneys appropriated for Army pay could not be used to pay women. These women physicians were offered positions as contract surgeons, but few would accept them. They felt that the Office of the Surgeon General was discriminating against them. Finally, legislation was introduced and passed by Congress authorizing the commissioning of women. This legislation became effective April 16, 1943. The response was not so great as expected; on January 1, 1944, there were only 41 women physicians on active duty.

From the start, an effort was made to assign medical officers to positions for which they were most suited. This was difficult in some instances because there were many positions not comparable to civilian specialties. For example, the physicians assigned to combat units during the training period performed little medical practice except for sick call, emergencies, etc. In the Army there was no need for such specialists as obstetricians, gynecologists or pediatricians. Let it be said of this group, however, that they volunteered to do anything they could for the war effort. Many of them became able medical administrators or filled positions concerning which they had some knowledge, but which were not associated with their specialties in civil life. A constant shortage of doctors compelled the use of medical men to fill vacancies regardless of their specialties.

All Reserve officers were called to duty in the grades they held when the war began. Many well-qualified men who had neglected to keep up their peacetime work in the Reserve Corps found themselves on duty in low rank. Any number of qualified specialists came on duty as first lieutenants. Others, not so well qualified professionally, had taken correspondence courses and summer training and had been promoted to higher grades. This condition was further aggravated when physicians from civil life who were not members of the Reserve Corps were called to Army service. Certain rules were laid down, based on age, education and training, and the kind of work performed in civil life. Applications were considered carefully by a committee in the Office of the Surgeon General and appropriate commissions were given the applicants. This was generally satisfactory as far as the applicants were concerned, but it naturally caused concern to many of the Reserve officers already on active duty.

The problem of proper professional classification of medical officers was recognized long before the war began. The Classification Questionnaire for Medical Officers (A. G. Form 178-2) was the first form used to obtain information about the professional ability of individual officers. These records were being assembled in 1939. A simple system of classification or grading was instituted. Symbols were given the specialists, such as S for Surgery, M for Medicine, S (Ortho) for Orthopedic Surgery. The figures 1, 2, 3 and 4 were used to show degrees of ability within a specialty. Later, the numerals were changed to letters A, B, C and D.

The four grades or degrees of ability included, first, officers with civilian or military backgrounds who had outstanding ability in their specialties. Officers who were professors or heads of departments and associate professors in large teaching centers were in this group. These specialists were officers who could operate without professional supervision.

Next came officers with superior training and demonstrated ability. Classification in this group indicated that the doctor had had a training period of one year as an intern and a three-year residency or fellowship devoted to his specialty in a recognized teaching center. Officers with mature experience and demonstrated ability were classified in this group even though they did not have the formal training indicated. Those who had been certified by the American Specialty Boards were classified in this group or higher, although absence of certification did not prohibit inclusion. These officers functioned within their specialties without professional supervision.

A third group included officers who had recently completed periods of training including one year as an intern and from two to three years' residency in their specialties. It comprised also officers with shorter periods of training, but with backgrounds of mature experience.

The fourth and last group were officers who had recently completed periods of training including one year as an intern and one year of residency; officers who had demonstrated some ability in their specialties; and officers with shorter periods of training but with minor proportions of practice devoted to specialties—for example, a general practitioner who had given particular attention to a specialty for a period of at least three years.

All physicians of any given specialty had their cards filed together. In addition to the professional ability of the officer, the card indicated his ability to speak a foreign language and another card appropriately filed in the cross-index covered the particular language. This proved to be of great value when demands were made for officers who spoke unusual languages. Later, when an individual officer completed a special course of training, either military or professional, that information was entered on his classification card and another card prepared for filing in the cross-index covering the special training course.

Through cooperation with the American Medical Association and the American College of Physicians, surveys of all physicians practising in the United States were made. Outstanding physicians in every State were chosen as central groups to evaluate physicians within their States and report upon them. This survey was accomplished with the expenditure of considerable amounts of time and money by civilian physicians and organizations. In addition to the professional evaluation, the possible value of the doctor to the military service was considered. As these records were confidential, they were filed at American Medical Association Headquarters and a liaison officer was assigned to act between that Headquarters and the Office of the Surgeon General.

When the Procurement and Assignment Service began to function, the notices of a doctor's availability were sent to Chicago. There they were reviewed by the Army liaison officer to determine whether the doctor's record was clear; if he was fully qualified, a notice was sent promptly to the Surgeon General.

But this information was of little use if it lay in the file. It had to be placed in the hands of the office which assigned the officer after he reported for duty. Plans were drawn whereby the classification record of the physician applying for a commission was routed through the Chicago office, where it was stamped and sent on to the officer's station.

Classification of the doctor did not depend on any one statement; it was formulated from records of his membership in professional societies, personal knowledge of the doctor by consultants who came to the office and gave freely of their time, and from other sources.

The proper assignment of a doctor in the armed forces depended on many factors. The wishes of the doctor himself came rather low on the list of these factors, and there was inevitably a certain amount of dissatisfaction. There were many jobs to be done in the Army which had no civilian counterpart, and the men chosen to do them had to learn new specialties. Too much praise cannot be given to those specialists who gave up lucrative practices to do their bit.

In developing officers for key administrative positions, the well-qualified professional men, in the vast majority of cases, made the most able executives. In other words, a mediocre doctor would remain mediocre no matter where you placed him. There were certain exceptions on both sides, but they only proved the rule.

Nearly 22,000 physicians were classified as having some special skills, and the analysis of the entire corps, as of January 1, 1944, is shown in Table 2, page 104.

Promotion in the Regular Army Medical Corps in peacetime is

based on total years of commissioned service. In the early fall of 1941, some promotions of Regular Army officers were made by selection from the top of the lineal list. By this time it had been determined that it would probably be necessary to continue most of the Reserve officers on duty longer than one year, as originally contemplated. Many of these had been called to duty as first lieutenants and captains and were men who justly deserved promotion.

On April 30, 1941, a directive was issued promoting National Guard Medical Department officers according to length of National Guard service, regardless of assignment. The result was that nearly all combat divisions had an excess of officers in the upper grades. One division had five colonels, Dental Corps, whereas the Table of Organization called for but one lieutenant colonel. Another had three or four colonels, Medical Corps. These officers had to be reassigned to corps areas and given precedence over many Reserve officers who were just as well qualified but in lower grades.

The Surgeon General was deeply concerned over the plight of the Reserve officers and made a number of overtures to the War Department about them. One of these requests was for authority to promote 200 captains and 1,600 first lieutenants to fill positions authorized in the Troop Unit Basis, on the assumption that the provisions of mobilization regulations regarding promotion in time of emergency could be put in force before the declaration of war. Recommendations were called for from the field and carefully reviewed in the Office of the Surgeon General; 351 captains and 1,277 first lieutenants were promoted.

In February, 1942, the long-awaited War Department policy of promotion by selection to fill authorized position vacancies was announced by War Department Circular No. 1, dated January 1, 1942 (later modified by Circulars 3, 161, 214, 417, series 1942, and finally superseded by AR 605–12, dated February 3, 1944). Circular No. 1 was not actually distributed until about the 10th of February, 1942. The new system of promotion began the long process of decentralization of personnel control.

Under this policy, the commanding generals of armies, defense commands, corps areas, overseas theaters, bases, chiefs of services and similar major elements were authorized to submit recommendations for the temporary promotion of officers serving under their immediate jurisdiction. The Surgeon General was immediately deprived of control over the promotion of all officers of the Medical Department who were not serving in one of his overhead installations, which at that time included general hospitals, the Office of the Surgeon General, the Medical Field Service School and the Medical Replacement Training Centers.

The Army was reorganized in May, 1942, into three major commands, and the general hospitals and Replacement Training Centers were placed directly under control of the service commands. This meant that control of medical personnel was decentralized to the Commanding Generals of the Army Air Forces, Army Ground Forces and Service Commands. The Surgeon General coordinated assignments among these various components, but had to secure concurrences on all moves of personnel.

There were two groups of physicians in the United States which caused the Office of the Surgeon General much concern. These were the foreign school graduates and graduates of the so-called unapproved or substandard schools. Many of these men were qualified for certain duties, and the physicians who had already given up their private practices to enter the service objected to having these two groups exempt from service, because most of them were deferred by their draft boards as being essential in their communities. It was decided that some of these men would be taken.

In the case of the foreign school graduate, the following requirements had to be met:

1. It was necessary that the applicant be a citizen of the United States; proof to be included if citizenship had been acquired through naturalization.

2. He was required to furnish a transcript of premedical education equivalent to the requirements for admission to an approved American medical school (with certified translation).

3. He was required to include a photostat of a medical diploma that had been awarded after four years' academic instruction in medicine (with certified translation).

4. He was required to include a photostat of license to practise medicine in a State, Territory or the District of Columbia (State licensure could not be waived for appointment); also a

license or registration authorizing practice of medicine in the country in which medical education had been obtained.

5. He was required to furnish a certificate of approved internship of not less than one year's duration.

The Surgeon General then determined whether or not the graduate of the school in question was eligible for appointment.

The graduate of an unapproved school was obliged to furnish the following, in addition to the regular data furnished by all other applicants:

1. A letter from the dean of his medical school, verifying the fact that the applicant had satisfactorily completed a four-year course of regular medicine and had been granted an M.D. degree.

2. A letter from the superintendent of a hospital, verifying at least one year of rotating internship on the part of the applicant.

3. A photostatic copy or certification by an Army officer on active duty that he had seen the applicant's license to practise medicine in one of the States of the Union or in the District of Columbia.

4. Letters from three physicians who were graduates of approved medical schools and were practising in the county of the applicant's residence, stating that they knew the applicant to be engaged in the ethical practice of medicine. The writer of each of these letters was to state his school and year of graduation, in addition to information concerning the applicant's professional qualifications.

It was also necessary that the applicant be a member of his local County Medical Society or present a letter from the Secretary of the District or County Medical Society, as follows:

Place...

Date ....

Dr. .... of .... is known to this Society as a graduate of .... Medical School, located in ...., ... He is engaged in the practice of medicine in ...., ..., having been licensed by this State since ....

He is, so far as is known, an *ethical* practitioner of medicine. He would be eligible to apply for membership in the .... Medical Society if he had been in practice for .... years. Having attained such membership, he would be accredited to the .... County (District) Medical Society.

Signed .... District

Secretary, ... County

Medical Society.

N. B. The applicant should bring his diploma and certificate of licensure to the District or County Secretary when requesting such certification.

The Surgeon General determined whether or not the graduate of the school in question was eligible for appointment.

Graduates of certain unapproved schools were not accepted under any circumstances.

On November 22, 1939, the Secretary of War authorized the organization of thirty-two general hospitals, seventeen evacuation hospitals and thirteen surgical hospitals. These units were to be sponsored by medical schools and large civilian hospitals, and were to be known as "affiliated units." In so far as possible, institutions were invited to sponsor units of the same number and type as those sponsored by them in World War I. The response was most enthusiastic. In fact, many institutions approached the Surgeon General with requests to form some type of unit. As a result of these requests, the Surgeon General asked for authority to form certain additional units, which authorization was granted in July, 1940.

Officers were given special Reserve commissions (affiliated unit) and were carefully chosen for the positions they were to occupy in the units. The main objection to these units, it was later discovered, was that the staffs were top-heavy with skilled personnel and, in many instances, the second or even third man on a medical or surgical service was well qualified to be chief of a service just as important. This factor was made use of later by Chief Surgeons of Theaters of Operations, who adjusted staffs of various types of hospitals in such a way as to insure a proper balancing of specialized personnel.

Credit for the enormous amount of work in connection with

the formation of these units should, in the main, be given to Colonel Francis M. Fitts, M.C. He devoted a large part of his time for several months to the helpful guidance of medical directors and deans in making these hospitals splendid units.

As a result of combat experience, and owing to the receipt of requisitions for particular types of units, various changes were made in certain units to make a more efficient medical service.

Individual officers assigned to these units were urged to ask for active duty early, as individuals, prior to the call to active duty of their units. Many of the officers took advantage of the opportunity, and the results were mutually advantageous to the service and to the individual.

Beginning shortly after Pearl Harbor, a few units were called to active duty for training, followed by the rest at later dates. Moves to Ports of Embarkation were slow in many instances, owing to the movements of the enemy and the problems of logistics involved. It was not until early in 1943 that the final units were activated for service.

Many stories can be told after the war of the valuable work done by these units in all parts of the world.

Table 3 shows the sponsoring units and the officers who assumed responsibility for organizing the units. (Page 105.)

The medical profession of the United States can take great pride in the fact that through a purely volunteer system its members offered their services in such large numbers. Many men who had to remain at home in essential positions were bitterly disappointed that they could not participate as members of the armed forces.

It would not be just to close this chapter without mentioning the doctors in the older age groups who volunteered in such large numbers. Many of them who were sixty years of age traveled long distances to Washington to plead that they be given a chance to enter the Army. They, as well as their fellows in the service, can be proud of their profession's war record.

TABLE 2. SPECIALTY CLASSIFICATION—MEDICAL OFFICERS

Specialty	A & B	C	D	Total
General Surgery	723	2,289	2,363	5,375
Orthopedic Surgery	304	387	666	1,357
Physical Therapy	6	21	29	56
Urology	180	315	182	677
Plastic Surgery	33	52	51	136
Thoracic Surgery	25	51	100	176
Proctology	8	47	30	85
Neurosurgery	42	82	123	247
Anesthesia	50	180	518	748
Ophthalmology and Otolaryngology	141	295	156	592
Otolaryngology	291	162	127	580
Ophthalmology	285	173	98	556
Pathology	107	90	161	358
Bacteriology	10	15	10	35
Chemical Laboratory	14	27	115	156
Internal Medicine	568	1,449	1,207	3,224
Pediatrics	330	386	247	963
Gastro-Enterology	24	82	56	162
Cardiology	63	174	169	406
Dermatology and Syphilis	106	154	114	374
Neuropsychiatry	237	386	326	949
Neurology	4	6	12	22
Psychiatry	55	53	177	285
Radiology	380	193	527	1,100
Obstetrics and Gynecology	219	446	366	1,031
Tuberculosis	15	151	114	280
Public Health	110	137	86	333
Tropical Medicine	27	69	599	695
Allergy	13	58	64	135
Venereal Disease	42	50	94	186
Laboratory, Unclassified	23	35	404	462
Grand Total				21,741

TABLE 3. AFFILIATED MEDICAL DEPARTMENT UNITS
GENERAL HOSPITALS

Number of Unit	Sponsoring Unit	Unit Director
1st General	Bellevue Hospital, New York City	Lt. Col. J. H. Mulholland
2nd General	Presbyterian Hospital, New York City	Lt. Col. Wm. B. Parsons
3rd General	Mt. Sinai Hospital, New York City	Lt. Col. Herman Lande
4th General	University Hospital, Cleveland, Ohio	Lt. Col. J. M. Hayman
5th General	Harvard University, Cambridge, Massachusetts	Lt. Col. T. H. Lanman
6th General	Massachusetts General Hospital, Boston	Col. T. R. Goethals
7th General	Boston City Hospital, Boston, Massachusetts	Col. R. C. Cochrane
9th General	New York Hospital, New York City	Lt. Col. R. F. Bowers
12th General	Northwestern University, Chicago, Illinois	Lt. Col. M. H. Barker
13th General	Presbyterian Hospital, Chicago, Illinois	Lt. Col. E. M. Miller
17th General	Harper Hospital, Detroit, Michigan	Col. H. R. Carstens
18th General	Johns Hopkins Hospital, Baltimore, Maryland	Lt. Col. G. G. Finney
19th General	Rochester General Hospital, Rochester, New York	Col. E. Wentworth
20th General	Hospital of University of Pennsylvania, Philadelphia	Lt. Col. I. S. Ravdin
21st General	Washington University, St. Louis, Missouri	Lt. Col. Lee E. Cady
23rd General	Buffalo General Hospital, Buffalo, New York	Lt. Col. C. B. Brown
24th General	Tulane University, New Orleans, Louisiana	Lt. Col. I. M. Gage
25th General	University of Cincinnati, Cincinnati, Ohio	Lt. Col. J. McGuire
26th General	University of Minnesota, Minneapolis	Lt. Col. L. H. Fowler
27th General	University of Pittsburgh, Pittsburgh, Pennsylvania	Lt. Col. H. E. Feather
29th General	University of Colorado, Denver	Lt. Col. E. G. Billings
30th General	University of California, San Francisco	Lt. Col. G. K. Rhodes
31st General	Denver General Hospital, Denver, Colorado	Lt. Col. E. Durbin
32nd General	Indiana University Hospital, Indianapolis	Lt. Col. C. J. Clark
33rd General	Albany Hospital, Albany, New York	Lt. Col. E. H. Campbell
36th General	Wyane University, Detroit, Michigan	Lt. Col. W. C. C. Cole
37th General	Kings County Hospital, Brooklyn, New York	Lt. Col. G. G. Dixon
38th General	Jefferson Medical College, Philadelphia	Lt. Col. B. L. Keys
39th General	Yale University Medical School, New Haven, Connecticut	Lt. Col. J. C. Fox
42nd General	University of Maryland, Baltimore	Lt. Col. M. C. Pincoffs

TABLE 3. AFFILIATED MEDICAL DEPARTMENT UNITS—*(Continued)*
GENERAL HOSPITALS—*(Continued)*

Number of Unit	Sponsoring Unit	Unit Director
43rd General	Emory University, Atlanta, Georgia	Lt. Col. I. A. Ferguson
44th General	University of Wisconsin, Madison	Lt. Col. F. L. Weston
45th General	Medical College of Virginia, Richmond	Lt. Col. J. P. Williams
46th General	University of Oregon, Portland	Col. J. G. Strohm
47th General	College of Medical Evangelists, Los Angeles, California	Lt. Col. C. Courville
50th General	Seattle College, Seattle, Washington	Lt. Col. H. T. Bruckner
52nd General	Syracuse University, Syracuse, New York	Lt. Col. R. S. Farr
58th General	Western Pennsylvania Hospital, Pittsburgh	Lt. Col. F. R. Bailey
64th General	Louisiana State University, New Orleans	Lt. Col. M. Gage
65th General	Duke University, Durham, North Carolina	Lt. Col. E. L. Persons
67th General	Maine General Hospital, Portland	Lt. Col. R. B. Moore
70th General	St. Louis University, St. Louis, Missouri	Lt. Col. C. H. Lohr
71st General	Mayo Clinic, Rochester, Minnesota	Lt. Col. C. W. Mayo
79th General	Long Island College of Medicine, Brooklyn, New York	Lt. Col. W. O. Moore
105th General	Harvard University, Boston, Massachusetts	Major A. Thorndike
108th General	Loyola University, Chicago, Illinois	Col. G. T. Jordan
118th General	Johns Hopkins Hospital, Baltimore, Maryland	Lt. Col. J. Bordley, III
127th General	University of Texas, Galveston	Lt. Col. W. M. Moore
142nd General	University of Maryland, Baltimore	Major H. V. Langeluttig
297th General	Cook County Hospital, Chicago, Illinois	Lt. Col. C. Guy
298th General	University of Michigan, Ann Arbor	Lt. Col. W. G. Maddock
300th General	Vanderbilt University, Nashville, Tennessee	Major J. A. Kirtley

EVACUATION HOSPITALS

2nd Evacuation	St. Luke's Hospital, New York City	Lt. Col. W. F. MacFee
7th Evacuation	New York Post Graduate Hospital, New York City	Lt. Col. R. B. Lobbab
8th Evacuation	University of Virginia, Richmond	Lt. Col. S. D. Blackford
9th Evacuation	Roosevelt Hospital, New York City	Lt. Col. F. B. Berry
12th Evacuation	Lenox Hill Hospital, New York City	Lt. Col. O. C. Pickhardt
14th Evacuation	City Hospital, New York City	Lt. Col. P. K. Sauer
16th Evacuation	Michael Reese Hospital, Chicago, Illinois	Lt. Col. P. Lewin
21st Evacuation	Oklahoma State University, Oklahoma City	Lt. Col. H. D. Collins
25th Evacuation	West Suburban Hospital, Oak Park, Illinois	Lt. Col. W. J. Potts
27th Evacuation	University of Illinois, Chicago	Lt. Col. C. B. Puestow
30th Evacuation	University of Texas, Galveston	Major D. M. Paton

TABLE 3. AFFILIATED MEDICAL DEPARTMENT UNITS—*(Continued)*
EVACUATION HOSPITALS—*(Continued)*

Number of Unit	Sponsoring Unit	Unit Director
38th Evacuation	Charlotte Memorial Hospital, Charlottesville, North Carolina	Lt. Col. P. W. Sanger
48th Evacuation	Rhode Island Hospital, Providence	Lt. Col. W. A. Mahoney
51st Evacuation	Sacramento County Hospital, Sacramento, California	Lt. Col. O. S. Cook
52nd Evacuation	Pennsylvania Hospital, Philadelphia	Lt. Col. H. P. Brown
56th Evacuation	Baylor University, Dallas, Texas	Lt. Col. H. M. Winans
59th Evacuation	San Francisco Hospital, San Francisco, California	Lt. Col. C. Mathewson
73rd Evacuation	Los Angeles County Hospital, Los Angeles, California	Lt. Col. E. E. McEvers
77th Evacuation	University of Kansas Hospital, Kansas City	Lt. Col. E. H. Hashinger
92nd Evacuation	St. Mary's Hospital, Colorado Springs, Colorado	Major P. M. Ireland

On June 1, 1943, Major General Norman T. Kirk became Surgeon General of the Army, succeeding Major General James C. Magee, who was Surgeon General when we entered the war and who retired with an excellent record for leadership and a high standard for military medical service. By that date the Army had grown in size and importance beyond anything ever previously anticipated.

Brigadier General Kirk, when he took over the office of Surgeon General with the rank of major general, relinquished the position of commanding officer of the new Percy Jones General Hospital at Battle Creek, Michigan. In 1919, General Kirk was in the surgical service at Walter Reed Hospital and later had duty at the Johns Hopkins University Hospital, the Massachusetts General Hospital and the Station Hospital at Fort Sam Houston, Texas, where he became chief of the surgical service. He served subsequently as chief of the surgical service at Sternberg General Hospital in Manila, the Station Hospital at Fort Mills in the Philippine Islands, again at Sternberg and the Walter Reed General Hospital in Washington.

General Kirk is distinguished as an orthopedic surgeon and, in fact, had operated during the course of his career on both Secretary of War Stimson and Major General Brehon Somervell. After he became Surgeon General of the Army Medical Department, General Kirk visited every one of the fighting fronts, flying in practically every instance. His picture of the service rendered by the doctors to our armed forces throughout the world is an inspiring record of achievement.

CHAPTER V

THE ARMY DOCTOR IN ACTION

By
MAJOR GENERAL NORMAN T. KIRK
The Surgeon General, United States Army

I

WITH THE SIGNING of the Armistice between France and Germany
on June 22, 1940, the conquest of Continental Europe by the Axis
seemed near completion. Russia alone remained to be taken. The
Battle for Britain began. The people of the United States, whose
sympathies had been openly declared, marveled at the dogged
determination and the valiant fight of the R.A.F., whose pitiful
material inadequacies were more than made up by their fliers'
strong, gallant hearts, which have since earned the lasting homage
and undying tribute of all lovers of freedom throughout the world.

During this ominous period, our own United States Army was
alarmingly small, numbering only about 250,000 men. The Medical Corps at this time had 1,578 officers, of whom 1,164 were of
the Regular Army. By the end of August, 1941, our forces, though
still totally inadequate, had grown to approximately a million
and a half men, including some ten thousand in the Medical
Corps. This growth had occurred as the result of the Selective
Training and Service Act, but, because of the Act's one-year service
clause, it did not assure a stable increase in the size of the Army.

In the latter part of August, 1941, with the approval by Congress of the Selective Service Extension Act of 1941, the rapid,
progressive and stable expansion of the Army was assured. Only
three months later, on December 7, our country was precipitately
thrown into a war for which she was incompletely prepared. At
that time, the Army numbered 1,613,000 men, with 11,390 Medical Corps officers.

The rapid rate at which the strength of our Army reached into millions during the ensuing months is now history. Recalling those fateful days of 1940 and 1941 emphasizes the seemingly impossible feat that has been accomplished in such a relatively short period of time through the sheer will, concerted effort, and singleness of purpose of the American people.

At the outset of the emergency, the Medical Department clearly understood its role in the gigantic undertaking facing the country. Its essential function was the conservation and maintenance of the Army's fighting strength at the peak level required to assure combat superiority, by providing the most healthful conditions and the best and most modern methods of preventing and treating disease and injury. The number of soldiers kept firing guns and the number of sick and wounded returned to the fighting ranks are measures of its efficiency. The fact that the health of the Army has been the highest and the mortality of the wounded the lowest in the history of the nation is impressive evidence of the manner in which the Department met these responsibilities.

This gratifying record was achieved through a carefully planned program which involved a number of factors, among the most important of which were rapid mobilization, intensive training, intelligent organization of personnel, provision of adequate medical supplies and equipment, advancing hospital facilities far forward in order to render the earliest and best medical care possible, an efficiently organized system for safe and speedy evacuation of the sick and wounded, application and utilization of the most effective therapeutic measures known to medical science, and a carefully planned and highly effective program of immunization and preventive medicine.

As would be expected of a profession in which duty is always placed before personal ambition or gain, the doctors of this country responded wholeheartedly to the call to arms. Remunerative practices were forfeited, professional ambitions cast aside, coveted teaching positions relinquished; the prime question in the mind of every American physician became: Am I needed? The answer to this question was sought by inquiries to local agencies, as well as to the Office of the Surgeon General. The younger men of the profession, knowing the answer to the question in their own cases, simply applied for commissions. Medical schools requested and received authorization to organize affiliated hospital units, the staffs of which were composed of many younger, highly trained and skilled men who had been holding teaching positions. All services of these university units were headed by men with mature surgical or medical judgment. Important names in American medicine and surgery appeared in ever-increasing numbers in the swelling card index of the personnel section at the Office of the Surgeon General.

Thus the professional medical personnel of the Army Medical Department expanded rapidly to its enormous 1944 figure of more than 40,000 medical officers. This figure, when those in other branches of the service are added, makes a total comprising approximately 40 per cent of the usable medical personnel in the country.

It was necessary to indoctrinate each of these men into military custom and practice so that the underlying reasons for certain necessary differences between military and civil life would be clearly understood by everyone. The training of medical officers was accomplished by several methods and in various types of military installations. Thousands were trained in the Medical Field School at Carlisle Barracks, Pennsylvania, the traditional training ground for tactical and field service. Others got their military training, though less extensive, at camps and officer pools in various new general hospitals to which they were assigned upon entering the service. These hospitals also served as liaison agencies in facilitating the staffing of new hospitals and special medical service organizations. There was also special training of selected officers in such professional subjects as preventive and tropical medicine, orthopedic surgery, anesthesia, chest surgery, neurosurgery and plastic surgery. This was made possible by the cheerful and cooperative efforts of a number of medical schools throughout the country.

Other medical officers were given detailed and intensive courses in chemical warfare and the peculiar problems encountered in the management of gas casualties, at the Chemical Warfare School of Edgewood Arsenal. Still others were trained as Flight Surgeons at the School of Aviation Medicine, prior to their assignment with the expanding Army Air Forces.

The rapid, thorough and efficient manner in which this extensive training problem was initiated and accomplished was due in great measure to foresight and detailed planning by the Army Medical Department's leaders, and to the wholehearted cooperation of other Army organizations, the National Research Council, the medical universities of the country, and other civilian groups and individuals who were intimately concerned with the Medical Department of the Army.

One of the pressing problems quickly appreciated and squarely confronted from the outset was the proper classification and assignment of physicians according to their professional qualifications. This tremendous undertaking was efficiently administered by a staff which proved its capabilities. In an organization that mushroomed in growth from less than fifteen hundred members to more than thirty times this number within a period of less than two years, and which spread to practically all corners of the world, occasional honest administrative errors are bound to occur. That these have been kept at a minimum is shown by a survey which disclosed that 90 per cent of specialist personnel in the Army Medical Department had been properly assigned. Moreover, the correction of occasional malassignment was vigorously pursued. This was accomplished by repeated review and study of appropriate forms on which were entered all the data required for proper classification and assignment according to professional ability and training.

Another questionnaire was distributed on which was recorded by each medical officer a detailed account of his duties in his present assignment. As these forms were returned to the Service Command Headquarters and the Office of the Surgeon General, each was carefully reviewed, and these data, together with the information already available on the professional qualification forms mentioned above, were appraised in order to detect malassignments. Prompt action was taken in these instances to rectify errors, and they were remarkably few considering the enormous size of the Medical Corps. The distribution and adjustment of personnel in order to effect the most economical and efficient utilization of professional talent is a task which required the continuous efforts and unrelenting attention of the Office of the Surgeon General. But it is one considered particularly important.

In accordance with their professional and military training some of these 40,000 doctors were assigned as attached medical, as battalion surgeons with infantry or artillery battalions, as flight surgeons, as squadron surgeons, or as paratroop battalion surgeons. Others commanded, or were assigned to and operated, the medical battalions which evacuate battle casualties and sick from the front line to evacuation hospitals. These were manned by officers experienced in traumatic surgery, in the treatment of shock, and in other specialties which one recognizes in the hospitals at home. Still other medical officers were assigned according to their training to the many large station and general hospitals at home and overseas. Others commanded hospital ships and hospital trains, and still others were assigned to overseas evacuation of battle casualties by air.

To assist these men in carrying out their missions, more than 2,000 officers who, in civil life, were specialists in hospital administration, bacteriology, chemistry, sanitary engineering and other technical specialties and ancillary branches of medicine were commissioned in the Sanitary Corps. More than 13,000 laymen were commissioned in the Medical Administrative Corps. About 11,000 of these were trained at Officer Candidate Schools run by the Medical Department. These officers were assigned as adjutants, mess officers, and to certain other administrative capacities in order to relieve medical officers of their duties and allow them to devote more time and effort to professional work. Two thousand Medical Administrative Corps officers finished a second course of training to prepare them to serve as assistant battalion surgeons and assistant sanitary inspectors in order to free a similar number of medical officers for more pressing professional duties.

About 15,000 dental officers were commissioned in the Dental Corps to serve with medical officers on the various fronts and to carry on their function in making the soldier physically fit for military service, and to provide our Army with adequate dental care.

The Veterinary Corps, also a part of the Medical Department, had 2,081 commissioned officers whose job was the inspection of meat and dairy products so that the Army would be properly fed, and the medical care of horses, dogs and other animals used in the Army.

Forty thousand nurses were recruited, trained and assigned to various stations where they were needed to assist in the care of battle casualties, the accidentally wounded and the sick.

More than 500,000 enlisted men were assigned to the Medical Department for training with field units, and for duty either in hospitals at home or overseas. More than 70,000 of these men were trained in technical schools as x-ray laboratory, dental, medical and surgical technicians. Thousands of clerks and typists, mess sergeants and cooks, as well as chauffeurs and motor repair mechanics, were prepared for their assignments by Medical Department training centers.

These figures emphasize the scope and magnitude of the problems confronting the Medical Department in its responsibility for maintaining the health of the Army and providing adequate medical care. An efficient organization was required to develop this rapidly expanding personnel and coordinate various functions into a smoothly working team to provide a chain of medical care which extended to every fighting front in a global war. This organization was, to a large extent, the product of detailed study and planning that had begun long before the onset of war, and later proved its value.

The medical services within the United States, and the Defense Commands and Theaters of Operation, were coordinated by the Office of the Surgeon General through the Service Command and Theater Surgeons, each of whom was responsible for the medical activities of the respective regions. These men, with their staffs, determined policies in accordance with local circumstances and were charged with the maintenance of the highest possible standards of medical and surgical care in the medical installations and other units under their jurisdiction. The men occupying these positions, as well as those heading the various services and divisions of their staffs, were selected because of their outstanding qualifications for these particular assignments.

Attached to the staff of each of these surgeons, to assist and advise him in all professional matters, were professional consultants in medicine, surgery, neuropsychiatry and other specialties in certain circumstances. It was their function to evaluate, promote and improve the quality of medical care by every possible means and to interpret the professional policies of the Surgeon General and aid in their implementation. The proper performance of these functions necessarily involved an appraisal of all factors concerned with the professional care of patients, including particularly the organization and program of professional services in medical installations; the quality, distribution and assignments of professional personnel; the diagnostic facilities;

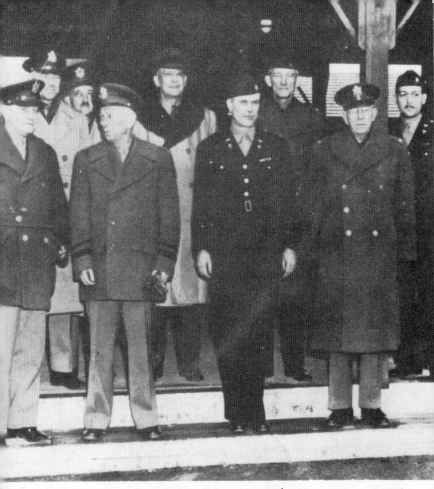

THIS PICTURE WAS TAKEN DURING THE SURGEON GENERAL'S VISIT TO ETO, IN 1943. Left to right, front row: *Major General Paul R. Hawley, Chief Surgeon, ETO; Major General Norman T. Kirk, Surgeon General; Lieutenant Colonel Ralph S. Muckinfuss, Commanding First Medical General Laboratory; Colonel Robert E. Thomas, Surgeon, Southern* Base Section. *Left to right, second row: Lieutenant Colonel R. S. Dukes; Colonel Rex L. Dively; Colonel Thompson, neuropsychiatry consultant; Dr. E. A. Strecker, Consultant to the Secretary of War; Colonel Edward C. Cutler; Lieutenant Colonel D. Murray Angevine.*

(MUSEUM AND MEDICAL ARTS SERVICE)

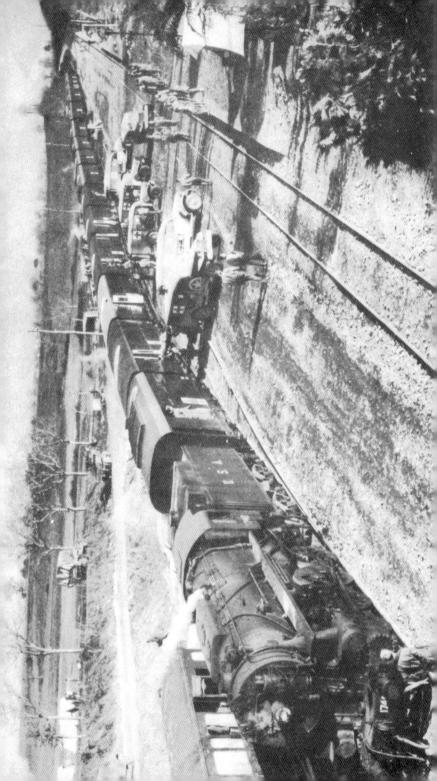

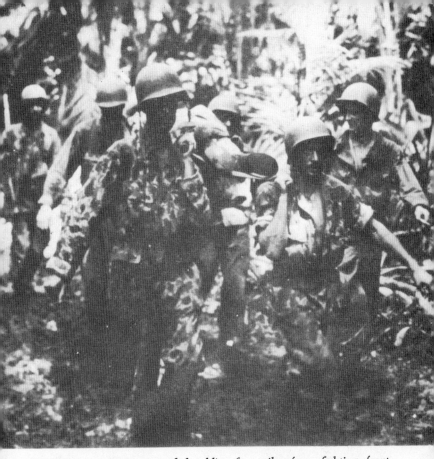

Litter-bearers carry a wounded soldier five miles from fighting front on New Georgia into advanced first-aid station. From there on, wounded men were transported by jeeps and boats. (SIGNAL CORPS PHOTO)

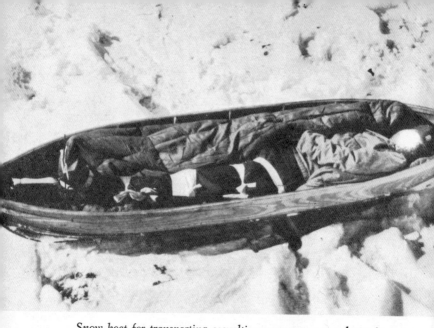

Snow boat for transporting casualties over snow-covered terrain.
(SIGNAL CORPS PHOTO)

Pontoon rafts sometimes transport patients over water. This picture was taken somewhere in the Southwest Pacific.
(SIGNAL CORPS PHOTO)

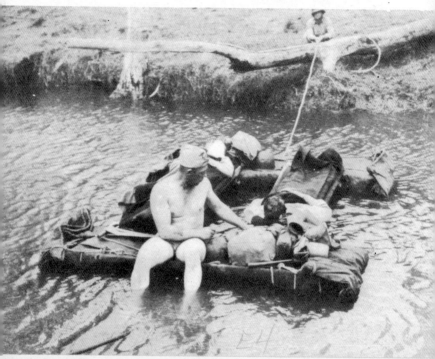

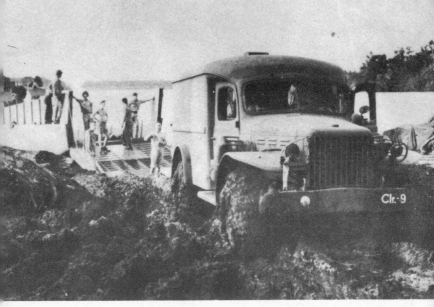

Ambulance which has just received patients starts down muddy road to a division hospital. (SIGNAL CORPS PHOTO)

American field hospital near the Mediterranean Sea in Sicily. On landing field nearby, hundreds of casualties were evacuated daily to Africa in C-47 and C-46 transport planes. (SIGNAL CORPS PHOTO)

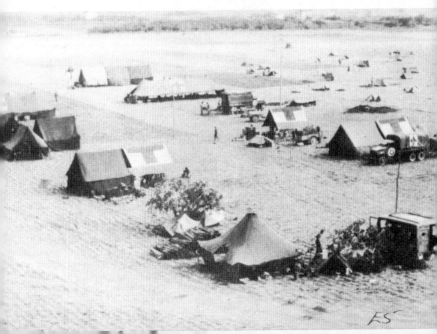

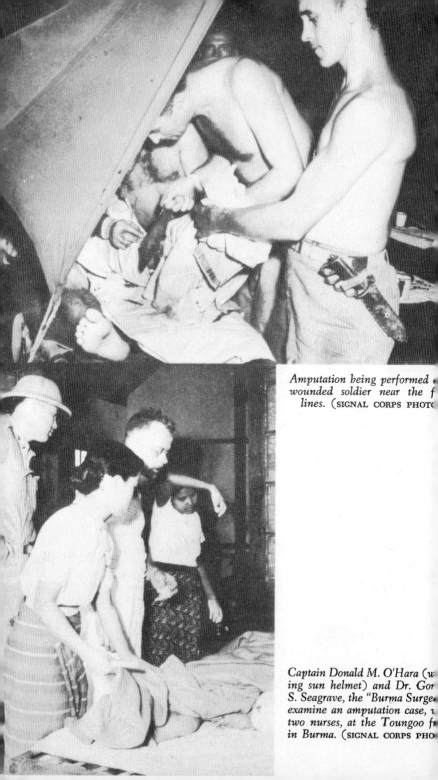

Amputation being performed [...] *wounded soldier near the f*[...] *lines.* (SIGNAL CORPS PHOT[...]

Captain Donald M. O'Hara (*w*[...] *ing sun helmet*) *and Dr. Gor*[...] *S. Seagrave, the "Burma Surge*[...] *examine an amputation case,* [...] *two nurses, at the Toungoo f*[...] *in Burma.* (SIGNAL CORPS PHO[...]

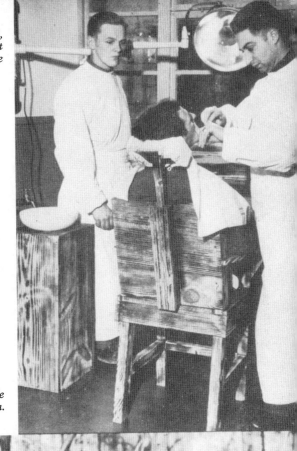

al clinic in a station hospital,
where in the Southwest
ic. The chair has been made
from old lumber.
(SIGNAL CORPS PHOTO)

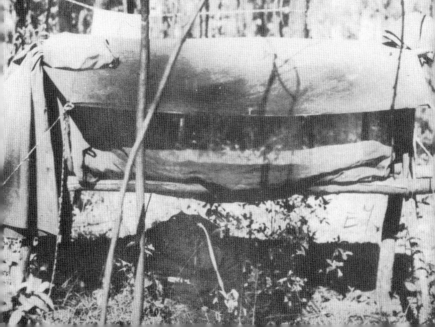

e-type bed used by a portable
tal detachment in Australia.
(SIGNAL CORPS PHOTO)

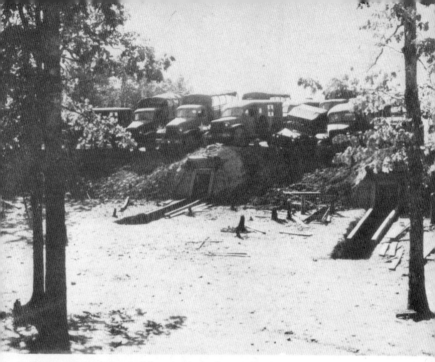

A three-ward underground hospital complete with x-ray equipment and facilities for surgery, dug out of sand, stone and solid rock. Exterior view shows tunnel entrances, with entire motor pool on top of structure. (SIGNAL CORPS PHOTO)

Laboratory of a hospital, somewhere in the Southwest Pacific. (SIGNAL CORPS PHOTO)

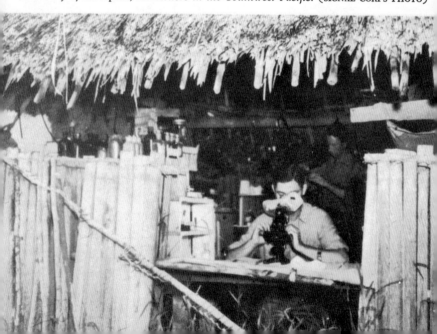

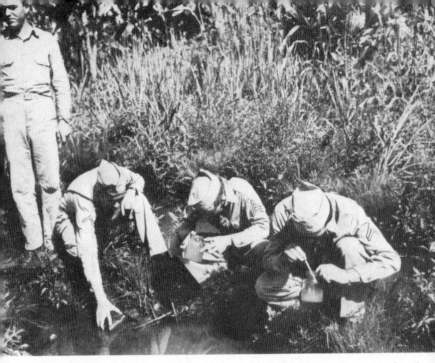

Dipping specimen jars into a roadside puddle, these Medical Corps "mosquito boys" search for larvae of the malaria-carrying mosquito. (SIGNAL CORPS PHOTO)

1st Lieutenant William G. Matteson, Jr., Dental Corps, at work on a patient in the field in Australia. (SIGNAL CORPS PHOTO)

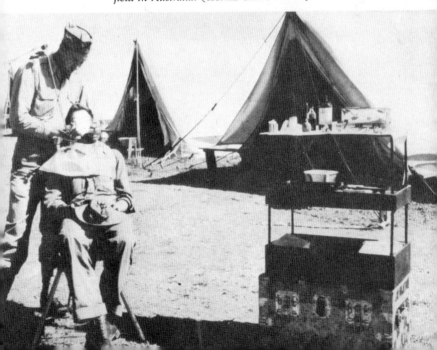

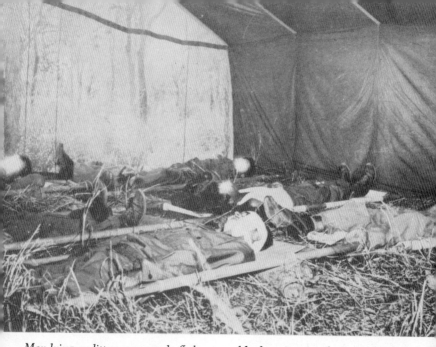

Men lying on litters supported off the ground by logs, in a ward tent made of airplane cloth, Australia. (SIGNAL CORPS PHOTO)

Shock ward after a heavy storm in Italy. (MUSEUM AND MEDICAL ARTS SERVICE)

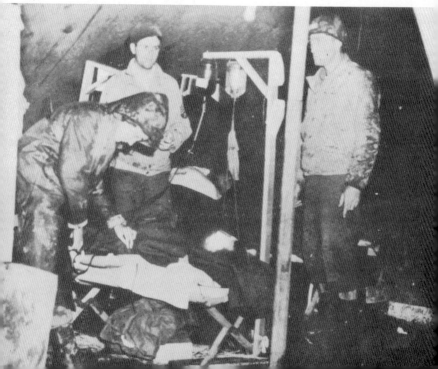

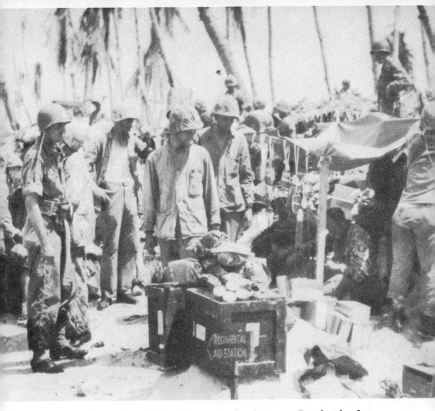

First-aid station established soon after landing on a Pacific island.
(OFFICIAL MARINE CORPS PHOTO)

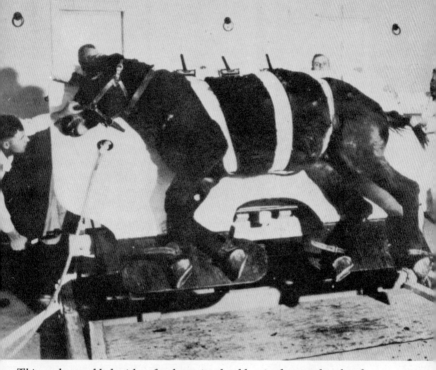

This mule, troubled with a fistula on its shoulder, is about to be placed on operating table at Veterinary Station Hospital, Fort Bliss, Texas. (SIGNAL CORPS PHOTO)

the availability and suitability of equipment and supplies for professional needs; and the nursing care, dietary provisions, recreational and reconditioning facilities, and other ancillary services essential to the welfare and morale of patients.

These professional consultants exercised their functions by assisting and advising the Service Command and Theater Surgeons on all matters pertaining to professional practice, by giving advice on professional subjects in general and on newer developments in diagnoses and treatment and technical procedures by stimulating interest in professional problems and aiding in their investigation, and by encouraging educational programs such as conferences, ward rounds and journal clubs. The execution of these functions involved periodic visits to all medical installations and other units concerned with the medical care of military personnel within their command.

It is apparent from these considerations that these consultants had to be highly qualified and especially competent persons with special training, extensive background and experience, and an established reputation in their field of endeavor. The excellent manner in which they executed their functions, the industry and zeal which they manifested, and the high standards of medical care in Army hospitals which they helped to establish, were indeed gratifying.

The functional units of the Medical Department's organization at home were the station and general hospitals. The former were present at every camp and station and were equipped and staffed to provide hospitalization and definitive medical and surgical care for minor illnesses and injuries, including emergency treatment in case of accidents, both ground and air, among the personnel at the base, station, camp or area where the hospital was located. Normally, a station hospital received patients from dispensaries at, or in the vicinity of, the station where it was located. Cases representing particularly complex problems, or ones requiring highly specialized care, were not treated in these installations but were transferred to the nearest general hospital.

As of 1944, there were about sixty general hospitals conveniently distributed in all parts of this country, providing more than 100,-000 beds. To supplement these beds, if others were needed, there were about 200,000 beds in station hospitals. These beds were used to hospitalize the sick and injured during the training period but, as troops completed their training and went overseas and posts and camps closed, these beds became available for other use. The general hospitals were specially staffed and equipped with men representing the best professional talent in the Army. They afforded facilities for the observation, treatment and disposition of complicated or obscure cases, and provided beds for patients evacuated from overseas and for those from station hospitals, as might be required. Some acted as debarkation hospitals at the various ports where the sick and wounded arrived by hospital ships, transports and air transports. Patients here were sorted and distributed to the general hospital or specialized center nearest their homes, where they received definitive treatment. Those not transportable were treated at the debarkation hospital until their condition permitted transportation. Certain of these hospitals were designated as specialized centers for the treatment of patients with certain conditions in which a high degree of specialization was necessary. The type and number of these specialties were as follows:

Chest surgery	6
Plastic surgery	6
Blind	2
Deaf	3
Amputations	5
Neurosurgical	18
Vascular surgery	2
Tuberculosis	2
Arthritis	1
Psychiatric	5
X-ray and radium therapy	4

These services established in general hospitals as noted above were carefully staffed with personnel who were professionally capable of offering the sick and wounded the most authoritative attention in these fields of medicine and surgery. The wisdom of this policy, which insisted on the transfer of complex cases to installations capable of rendering the most expert care, was demonstrated repeatedly. An illustration of this policy is the treatment of amputations in the Army.

The following circular letter (S.G.O. No. 91, April 26, 1943) directed the type of amputation and the care that would be given the amputee during his hospitalization:

Subject: Amputations.

1. The guillotine or open circular method of amputation is the procedure of choice in traumatic surgery under war conditions and is especially indicated in gunshot wounds and in controlling infection. Primary suture of all wounds of the extremities under war conditions is never to be done; it is permitted after débridement in certain abdominal, chest and maxillo-facial injuries only.

2. Primary amputation should be performed at the lowest possible level which permits removal of all devitalized and contaminated tissue regardless of stump length. Revision of the stump in accordance with prosthetic considerations may be subsequently performed. The flap type *open* operation may be done only in cases in which early evacuation is not contemplated and subsequent closure at the same station is deemed possible.

3. Skin traction to the stump should always be applied immediately following the amputation and continued until healing occurs.

4. All major amputees will be transferred as early as practicable after the primary amputation to general hospitals designated as amputation centers for revision of stumps or fitting of prosthesis. All cases, except disarticulations of the hip, the shoulder or those with equivalent stumps, will be fitted with a proper temporary prosthesis before discharge from the Army.

5. Before discharge, an upper extremity amputee will be fitted with an acceptable prosthesis and taught its use as well as to write, dress and otherwise care for himself with his remaining hand.

6. Lower extremity amputees will be properly fitted with a standard temporary prosthesis, taught its use, and will be able to walk on level ground without the aid of crutch or cane; also, and before discharge, a refit will be effected after the original shrinkage has occurred. Each amputee will be issued three light wool stump socks (obtainable through Veterans' Facilities). Six months later the patient will report to Veterans' Facilities for fitting of permanent type prosthesis.

Another circular letter (S.G.O. No. 115, June 25, 1943) designated these five general hospitals as amputation centers:

Bushnell General Hospital.................Brigham, Utah
Lawson General Hospital.................Atlanta, Georgia
McCloskey General Hospital.................Temple, Texas
Percy Jones General Hospital.......Battle Creek, Michigan
Walter Reed General Hospital...........Washington, D.C.

It also directed the type of prosthesis that would be used for each type of amputation of the upper and lower extremity. The prostheses adopted by the Army for this work were approved by the Orthopedic Committee of the National Research Council. The prosthesis used for the lower extremity was one built of fiber which was easily adjustable to fit the rapidly changing stump following the amputation or secondary revision of the stump. It was easily aligned, could be put into quantity production, was readily available as required, and had the same mechanical features as the accepted American prosthesis. The leather socket was likewise easily readjusted as shrinkage of the stump occurred so that the prosthesis fitted while the amputee was being trained in its use.

In the upper extremity, the split mechanical hook was found to be the best working tool. Various types were made available so that the amputee might select the one that best suited his needs. Interchangeable with this hook was a dress or mechanical hand, which was likewise supplied as desired by the amputee.

Excellent orthopedic shops were constructed and equipped at each of these centers. The Army began training brace makers and leg fitters in its orthopedic shops in 1941. Soldiers who had had training as machinists or mechanics, and all trained and experienced brace and limb mechanics who had joined the Army from civil life, were transferred to the Medical Department and assigned to these centers. The best-qualified specialists in civil life, serving as medical officers in the Army, were assigned to the orthopedic services at these amputation centers. These officers were responsible not only for the surgery of the amputee, but for the proper prosthetic fitting of the stump and the instruction of the amputee.

Training films were made and issued to these centers to assist in the instruction of the amputee.

The circular type of guillotine amputation is the amputation of choice in war, as well as when amputation is indicated for trauma in civil life. This is true whether the amputation is indicated for the control of hemorrhage, to remove a hopelessly destroyed extremity, or where traumatic amputation has occurred and only débridement of the remaining stump is necessary. It is likewise the amputation of choice as a life-saving measure to control infection, such as gas gangrene, an infected joint or an uncontrolled osteomyelitis. This amputation is done at the lowest possible level, conserving all tissue that is viable after the trauma. It is a two-stage amputation; the resulting stump, when healed, will require revision or reamputation, depending upon its length, before it is fitted with its prosthesis.

This is ordinarily a minor procedure. Skin traction, following this type of primary amputation, is just as essential as the original surgery removing the extremity. With the use of sulfa drugs and penicillin, the period of time before the guillotine stump can be repaired has been markedly reduced. This procedure can be carried out as soon as the edema has disappeared and pathogenic organisms are no longer present in the unhealed area. If infection is present in the stump, it can be controlled by the use of those drugs and the interval between operations thereby materially shortened.

If closed amputations are done following trauma under war conditions, the stump is likely to develop severe infection and osteomyelitis during evacuation from the front, with increased danger to the patient's life. Loss of length in the stump is also occasioned by performance of closed amputation under war conditions, since the limb must be shortened to avoid the site of trauma and in order to close the wound.

The number of amputees under treatment in each of the five amputation centers ranged, during the first six months of 1944, from 100 to 350. These cases were ready for fitting within six weeks after the stump had been repaired, or following closed amputation, which could be done under aseptic conditions for indications other than that of trauma. Thus, it may be observed from this consideration of amputations how the organization of specialized centers and the coordination of their functions with those of other units permitted the highest level of professional care possible.

In theaters of operation, the station hospitals cared for the static troops in the communication zone in much the same manner as this kind of installation is employed in this country. On occasion, however, that policy was altered according to the particular situation.

General hospitals represented the other type of relatively fixed installation in theaters of operation. Ahead of these were the mobile evacuation and field hospitals. Other installations—such as the clearing company with attached auxiliary surgical groups, or the portable surgical hospital—carried surgery as far forward as was compatible with effective function. Even further ahead of these were the collecting companies, and finally the battalion aid stations themselves, which were located virtually on the battlefield.

The positioning of these overseas installations from the most forward battalion aid station to the most rearward general hospital was carried out with a clear concept of the functions of each of these units. As the casualty passed rearward, the degree of definitive care also progressed. The more forward mobile installations were concerned with the preservation of life by prompt treatment of shock and prevention of severe infections, while the general hospitals dealt with definitive treatment and return of function. Casualties which, because of the nature of their wounds, required longer than 90 to 120 days' hospitalization were evacuated, as soon as their condition permitted to Zone of Interior Debarkation Hospitals, where each case was checked and sent to an appropriate specialized center for definitive care.

The gaps between these overseas installations were bridged by every type of transportation imaginable owing to the variety of terrains on which our forces were engaged in combat. Every effort was made to reduce as much as possible the time required for evacuation between installations. The extensive use of the airplane in expediting evacuation whenever feasible was evidenced by the fact that, by the end of 1943, approximately 173,000 sick, injured or wounded soldiers had been transported by this means. During the Tunisian and Sicilian campaigns, more than 27,000 soldiers with all types of wounds were evacuated by air, covering a total of 8,000,000 miles with only one death. Entire hospitals were moved by this means.

II

The factor of supply is one on which the efficient functioning of every branch of an Army and Navy depends. In a war of global proportions, in which the lines of communication extend over 56,000 miles, the tremendous problem of logistics is apparent.

There is much more to the subject of supply, however, than the expeditious distribution of required matériel to the consumer, which in itself has always been one of the greatest problems in any war.

The development of new items of equipment and the solving of details of wholesale manufacture and production add to the complexity of this factor, which influences so positively the services rendered by an organization such as the Medical Department. Among the many important and often life-saving items developed, or for which wholesale production methods were worked out, were plasma, penicillin, tetanus toxoid and an effective delousing powder, to mention only a few.

The immensity of the medical supply program may be better appreciated by a brief consideration of the enormous volumes of certain everyday medical and surgical supplies that were required by the Medical Department. The quarterly issue of plaster of Paris for the preparation of plaster bandages by hospital installations was 800,000 pounds. This did not include the tremendous number of prepared bandages of this type procured for certain overseas installations not in a position to prepare their own. The quarterly issue of gauze bandages was 600,000, and that of adhesive plaster amounted to 14,000,000 yards, or a sufficient amount every nine months to encircle the world. Eighty thousand pounds, or 40 tons, of sulfonamides were issued quarterly to the various medical units of the Army. This did not include the amounts of these drugs incorporated in prepared ointments and other compounded preparations.

The following figures on the boxed equipment of one general hospital emphasize further the magnitude of the problem. The aggregate weight of this equipment was 642,000 pounds. The shipping space required for the equipment of one such installation was 18.7 freight cars, or 1,122 ship tons. It should be remembered that these were only examples of the hundreds of installations operated by the Medical Department and a few of the thousands of items procured by the Supply Division for the maintenance of such installations.

The development, manufacture, procurement and distribution of supplies required by the Medical Department involved the efforts of thousands of civilians working in factories, laboratories, Red Cross blood donor centers, drug houses, surgical instrument shops, and all other places where medical supplies are produced. Tribute is due these patriotic men and women whose work contributed so generously to the welfare of the American soldier.

The Medical Department received invaluable assistance in many of its manifold problems from organizations not in the Army. During the early and exigent phase of mobilization, it became apparent that the Medical Department's activities would be increased commensurately in magnitude and responsibility. Many problems which it recognized and faced and others which it would inevitably encounter and must prepare for created an urgent demand for mobilizing the best scientific minds and medical talent of the country.

Accordingly, at the request of the Surgeon General of the Army, the Division of Medical Sciences of the National Research Council under the able direction of its chairman began early in 1940 the establishment of special committees consisting of distinguished civilian specialists to act in a consultative and advisory capacity to the Surgeon General. They began to function promptly and efficiently and, as the country passed through the period of emergency into the period of complete mobilization, the need for additional committees increased and was quickly met. Despite the added burden imposed upon the members of these committees by the depletion of their staffs through the entrance of assistants and associates into the armed services, they continued to give cheerfully and unstintingly much of their time and effort in the performance of these duties.

Included among their numerous achievements and invaluable contributions are the prewar critical evaluation and classification of civilian doctors in terms of their usefulness to the armed forces; the preparation of reports, bulletins and monographs for use by the armed forces, covering the prevention, diagnosis and treatment of various diseases and injuries; and the provision of a prompt, authoritative and unbiased opinion regarding controversial questions in diagnosis and treatment.

Perhaps the most important contribution of these committees was the organization, supervision and coordination of laboratory investigations and research work on fundamental aspects of Medical Department problems, which the armed forces in general were not prepared to perform. These suggested research programs were implemented through the organization, by the President, of the Committee on Medical Research. This organization was considered one of the most effectual agencies established by this government to help the Medical Department of the Army in the development of its weapons for effectively fighting disease. The Committee on Medical Research, operating under the forceful and efficient guidance of its chairman and strongly supported by the Director of the Office of Scientific Research and Development, had authority delegated by the President to approve, put into action and finance specific research projects. It afforded a means not otherwise available to the Army of developing new and more effective methods for the control and treatment of the diseases and injuries of war.

A considerable number of research projects were started and carried out. Dealing with almost every phase of surgery, internal medicine, aviation medicine and preventive medicine, many of these projects were carried to a successful and productive conclusion. The laboratory research of this powerful agency gave to the armed forces and to the civil population three great groups of discoveries: blood plasma and blood substitutes, penicillin, and new insecticides and insect repellents. The development of blood plasma saved more lives than we shall ever know and undoubtedly was one of the great factors contributing to our record low mortality rate in battle casualties. This development, by opening a new field of investigation, disclosed a number of by-products, such as fibrin foam and fibrin film, which showed promise of great practical significance. Penicillin grew in a few short months from a little-known laboratory curiosity into an eagerly sought life-saving drug for use in many formerly hopeless afflictions, and promised to revolutionize the Army's entire program for the treatment of gonorrhea and syphilis. In the control of serious wound infection, and as an adjunct to surgery, it established its value in hospitals at home as well as on the fighting fronts.

In the field of preventive medicine, the new insecticides and insect repellents, developed by the Bureau of Entomology of the Department of Agriculture, were so effective against the insect vectors of disease that we now have high hope of eventually controlling many of these disabling maladies of tropical regions. These agents included the so-called freon pyrethrum bomb, which was being used in every one of our tropical theaters for the killing of adult anophelines, and our Army insect repellent, which was used wherever troops were annoyed by biting insects. The value of this material alone to the war effort cannot be estimated in dollars and cents.

New methods for combating the louse, which had been previously feared as a vector of epidemic typhus fever, were developed. First, there was developed the efficient methyl bromide procedure for delousing clothing. This was rapidly followed by the discovery and production of the standard Army louse powder known as MYL, which formerly was furnished to all soldiers sent to areas where this disease existed or might be a problem. The development of new uses for the well-known chemical, which is now referred to as DDT, has provided an even better agent. The tedious work of investigating new adaptations of this chemical, of testing its toxicity under the conditions of its new uses, and of increasing its production has been a momentous job. By adding DDT to the standard MYL louse powder, its effectiveness was greatly increased. The value of the new powder was conclusively proved by the United States of America Typhus Commission, which stopped what was potentially one of the great typhus epidemics of history by using the powder in powder blowers to delouse, "on the hoof," the more than a million susceptible civilians in Naples. This is only one of the important uses of DDT.

In the field of aviation medicine, the Committee on Medical Research and the National Research Council continually provided us with clinical and physiological information of inestimable value to the Air Forces. Consistent improvement of the safety and efficiency of flying personnel was made possible either by the actual development of equipment or by furnishing physiological data necessary for design. Included in this category was equipment required for supplying aviators the additional oxygen necessary at high altitudes, the oximeter so widely used in the altitude training program, and the improved safety harness that provided the pilot with greater protection.

Closely related to the problem of adequate oxygen supply was the constant danger of carbon monoxide poisoning in aircraft, and here valuable assistance was given in the development of means for estimating the concentration of this gas in the blood and in aircraft inclosures. The National Research Council also made an important survey of this potential danger in existing types of aircraft. Information concerning the physiological causes of 'blackout" in aerial maneuvers resulted from studies carried out under the civilian agencies, and this information led to the development of anti-blackout suits which enabled flying personnel to withstand the effects of accelerational forces on the circulation of blood to the brain.

The vital role that the American Red Cross played in the collection of blood for the plasma procurement program was especially important. The fact that this involved over 100,000 bleedings weekly emphasizes the magnitude of the program. This valuable contribution of the American Red Cross to military medicine can be measured only in terms of lives saved.

The organization of this huge personnel and the tremendous supply of medical equipment were essential in providing the network of medical facilities which spread to all corners of the globe. They were necessary in fulfilling the Medical Department's mission. The accomplishment of this mission had to depend upon the functional performance of men and women of the Department. The excellent manner in which they performed their function, the difficulties they encountered and overcame, and the many dangers they unflinchingly faced will some day form one of the most stirring chapters of this war. The many lives they saved and the untold suffering they relieved through their untiring energy, their unceasing devotion to their cause, and their valiant determination and many acts of heroism in the face of the most hazardous circumstances and adverse conditions—all this can never be adequately described.

During the Tunisian campaign, I was in North Africa and met ambulance drivers who had carried the wounded to evacuation hospitals under difficult blackout conditions for so many hours that their fatigue caused them to stagger like drunken men as they stepped from their vehicles to unload. There were litter-bearers working at the front who had carried the wounded as many as fourteen miles, and there were those in the evacuation hospitals who had got blisters on their hands from the unceasing execution of this most arduous task. Doctors were working for eighteen and twenty-four hours without rest. Nurses slept in tents, did their own washing, and wore soldiers' coveralls as uniforms and GI shoes as they waded around in the ankle-deep mud during the winter months of this campaign. There were no self-claimed martyrs or heroes and no complaints among these valiant men and women of the Medical Department, whose only concern was the expeditious and adequate care of the wounded and sick.

I should like to quote from the report of a portable surgical hospital which I received some time ago from the Southwest Pacific. This is the story of one of those small groups of men who pick and hack their way through the jungle as they maintain close contact with the fighting troops. This particular group was being transported by boat to the point at which they were to set up initially before proceeding inland:

"At 7 P.M., large numbers of Jap Zeros and 3 dive bombers attacked the four boats. The . . . leading had reached a point ½ mile from shore, about 300 yards northeast of . . ., on the . . shore, about 2½ miles away from the Jap positions in the . . . area. There were about 180 persons including 40 natives aboard the boat. The enemy planes strafed, bombed, burned and sank all four boats. The entire equipment, all personal equipment and all records of the . . . portable surgical hospital were destroyed and lost in this action. The surviving hospital personnel escaped by swimming to shore through bombs and continued strafing. The chief surgical technician, though wounded with shrapnel in the back, was outstanding in rendering surgical treatment on shore. Lieutenant . . . saved Captain . . .'s life while swimming ashore, and there were many unrecorded acts of heroism by other members of the unit. The . . . had been heavily loaded with over 30 tons of ammunition, which continued to burn and explode for 12 hours. There was no naval or air protection for the boats.

"The . . . portable surgical hospital lost 4 men killed or missing in action and 4 seriously wounded in the action of . . . . An additional man was less seriously wounded by shrapnel. Both clerks were killed. All records were lost. Only one body was recovered. Total casualties were therefore:

4 men K.I.A. or M.I.A.
5 men W.I.A.
—
9 out of a total of 29; 31% casualties.

Eight of these have been permanently lost to the unit by death or evacuation to Australia, seriously wounded.

"The . . . portable surgical hospital survivors cared for their own casualties and all other casualties from the [first ship]. Other casualties were cared for downshore by . . . hospital at . . ., several miles away. The only available medical equipment was two medical chests which fortunately were saved from a barge which was brought to shore. Additional help came from . . . at . . ., who supplied litters and did remarkable work. All casualties were collected along the shore, given treatment in the jungle, and littered to a small village several hundred yards towards . . . . With no blankets, and minimal medical equipment, they were treated through the night under native huts."

Two days after this harrowing ordeal, the battle began and the survivors of this group had reorganized themselves and proceeded to render medical and surgical care to the sick and wounded!

In another report from a similar type of installation, the following experience is described:

"On our next move, only the portable supplies were taken, supplemented by a few extra tent flies. All other properties were ordered turned over to the regimental supply depot, which had just moved up with other regimental troops. These supplies were supposedly to be forwarded to us, but were never returned to us. Loading and the movement up the coast was started after dark and again in a heavy rain, with many of the boats off their course and finally landing us about a mile below the proper area, thus necessitating our carrying the equipment through the jungle for the jump-off a couple of days later. We fed well at . . . and the last day here we had both fresh steak and hamburger, the fourth time we had had fresh meat in over four months and the last time until we reached . . . about the first of September. When the night arrived for the big jump, we again divided into two sections and loaded on separate Higgins boats. We were to land in the second wave with the Battalion Aid Station ahead of us, but in the darkness and heavy rain there was much confusion and we jammed upon the beach at almost the same time. A heavy sea was running and the boats were swept sideways, out of control, and it was with great difficulty that the men and property were landed safely. Being unable to locate any designated area, the men fell exhausted in the brush near the beach to get what rest they could until daylight. Headquarters was located soon after it became light, an area designated for the hospital, and the operating room erected a fly stretched for a ward and litters used for beds. Only one section of the personnel and about half of the equipment landed that night, the other boatload arriving about 30 hours later, having had difficulty in getting started, and then getting lost.

"Wounded began to come in and we worked steadily until late that night, being greatly hampered by only having part of the equipment and personnel. Half of the surgical instruments were available, but it was necessary to sterilize them by boiling them in a frying pan. Many other makeshift methods were used.

"Somehow, during the day, we had found time to dig slit trenches and we finally lay down beside these in an attempt to sleep, feeling rather glad that orders had been issued that under no circumstances would there be any movement after dark and so no more patients could be brought into the hospital. There was very little rest, however, for the rifle fire and grenade explosions were terrific. Our perimeter was very small and bullets were coming from all directions, so that the remainder of the night was spent in the slit trenches fighting mosquitoes.

"As soon as light appeared and it was safe to move, casualties came pouring in and the small area was soon overcrowded and although we worked steadily, when the task force surgeon came rushing up and began moving all patients to the beach for evacuation, there were quite a few who had not been properly treated. Fortunately, the rest of one portable surgical hospital and the collecting company had arrived on the boats which were to be used for evacuation (about 11 A.M.), which relieved the congestion somewhat, although patients continued to come in during the day.

"The following morning, 18 were buried and the location of more bodies was known (unofficial), but no patient treated at the portable died, due almost entirely to the fact that they were operated upon very soon after their injuries."

An officer in command of a regiment in the Southwest Pacific reported the following incident in a letter to me:

"An instance which I observed may be of interest to you as it also serves to illustrate the splendid work of your corpsmen. Blood plasma was being administered to a badly wounded man in an improvised aid station hastily set up in a small native shack in the jungle. The container was suspended from a nail in an upright. Suddenly another wave of dive bombers came in. Under supervision of the surgeon, two soldiers grasped the litter while a medical aid man secured the plasma container. Quickly, but gently, the wounded man was carried to a foxhole close by which was large enough for the litter. Nearly everyone flattened out as they heard the swish of a big bomb, the aid man stood erect holding up the container to insure the continued flow of the life-restoring fluid.

"The bomb (a 500-pounder) hit some fifty yards distant, but due to the dense jungle the aid man escaped injury, although a fragment went through an empty water can less than ten feet away. Our battalion aid men are always there when the going is tough and they hold a warm spot in the regard of all the fighting dough-boys. Your young surgeons, also, are playing the game in fine style . . . muddy, bewhiskered and sleeping as best they can on the ground along with the others in the advanced combat areas. I believe, also, that your department is doing a good job in getting its supplies and equipment where they are most needed."

The manner in which one medical officer carried on in the face of great difficulties won for him the D.S.C., the Silver Star and a promotion, all within one week. The following letter to one of his friends was written while he was convalescing in one of our general hospitals here at home from a severe wound sustained during the same eventful week:

"My examination reveals that the radial nerve is completely severed with considerable scar tissue intervening. They hope to operate soon, removing the scar and attempting to suture the nerve and to remove the shell fragments from my knee and foot.

"I certainly want to thank you for giving me the most interesting year of my life and the best command in the entire Medical Corps.

"During the last six months the . . . Field Hospital worked in Italy on the Anzio beachhead and I am proud to report we received two commendations, two citations and the 5th Army plaque. We did over 4,000 major operations and I am sure saved many lives. The 5th Army has had the finest medical care of any Army to date.

"Our unit supported an Army corps in Italy and at Anzio. One.

platoon of our field hospital supported each division, working in the advance combat zone alongside the divisional clearing station. The patients received were the non-transportable; hence, we did purely surgical work, taking care of those critically wounded who could not safely be transported back to an evacuation hospital. Our surgical organization for each platoon consisted of four general surgical teams and two shock teams. The surgeon heading up each team was certified by the American Board of Surgery.

"Each platoon was well equipped with x-ray, autoclaves, anesthesia machines, refrigerators and power light units, with suction apparatus, orthopedic tables, oxygen therapy and all the necessary equipment.

"It was found that whole blood was absolutely essential to supplement plasma. In our six months of operation in the three platoons of the field hospital, we gave over 3,500 whole blood transfusions. The bleeding was done, "on the hoof," either from Medical Department men in the detachment, a list of fifth available to donate being maintained, or from walking wounded. Our daily needs varied. Sometimes up to one hundred pints were required. A blood transfusion unit was attached to us before we landed on the Anzio beachhead."

Three members of our Army Nurse Corps have received the Silver Star for gallantry in action, which has been described a follows:

TO: ROE, Elaine Arletta, 2nd Lt., Army Nurse Corps

ROURKE, Rita Virginia, 2nd Lt., Army Nurse Corps

FOR: Gallantry in action on . . . February, 1944, near . . . Italy During a concentrated shelling of the . . . Field Hospital by heavy caliber enemy artillery, the entire hospital area was sprayed with shell fragments which killed two nurses and wounded other military personnel. Electric wires were cut and lights extinguished. Working with flashlights, Lt. Roe and Lt. Rourke immediately began the orderly evacuation of forty-two patients while quieting others who had become alarmed and were attempting to leave their beds. Throughout the shelling, which included many air bursts, they exhibited remarkable coolness and courage and carried on with complete disregard for their own safety. The quick thinking, competence under unnerving conditions and the loyal consideration of Lts. Roe and Rourke for the welfare of their patients, prevented confusion which might have been critical, and were an inspiration to the enlisted men working under their supervision. Their actions reflected the finest traditions of the U. S. Army and Army Nurse Corps.

TO: ROBERTS, Mary L., 1st Lt., Army Nurse Corps

FOR: Gallantry in action on . . . February, 1944, in an Evacuation Hospital, near . . . Italy. On that date the Evacuation Hospital was heavily shelled by enemy artillery while Lt. Roberts was on duty as Operating Room Chief Nurse. The operating room tent in which she was working was hit. The tent and its equipment were damaged and two enlisted men were wounded by shell fragments from air bursts which continued for approximately thirty minutes. Lt. Roberts exhibited exceptional coolness and outstanding leadership, reassured the nurses under her charge and encouraged and urged them to greater efforts. Despite the impairment of facilities and the prolonged shelling, the vital work at three operating tables was continued under the inspiration of her conduct and example. The actions of Lt. Roberts in a critical situation assured the uninterrupted continuation of activities and contributed in a large measure to the success of the operations. Her bravery and unfaltering devotion to duty and complete disregard for her own welfare are in the best traditions of the military service and reflect the highest credit on herself and the Army Nurse Corps.

These are only a few of the many experiences which exemplify the undaunted spirit and the magnificent manner in which the officers and men of the Medical Department carried on their work under the most trying and hazardous circumstances.

The commendations of the Medical Department for its outstanding performance are a source of pride to every man in the organization. In a letter to me dated September 25, 1943, Lieutenant General Mark Clark, Commanding General of the Fifth Army, wrote the following words about his medical service:

"I desire to express the highest commendation for the wonderfully fine work performed by the medical units of this Army. Their devotion to duty under the hazardous and trying circumstances of the landing in Salerno Bay and their skill and efficient administration reflect the best traditions of the service. Many wounded officers and men, who will eventually be restored to full health, would have died but for the effective work of the Medical Corps. I am especially well pleased with the performance of the Surgeon Fifth Army. He has done a magnificent job.

"From the first landing to the date of this letter, 3,335 casualtie have been admitted to Fifth Army hospitals. The first hospita opened within 3 to 5 miles of the front lines. The next hospita began to function the following day still closer and under the most difficult conditions. Neither hospital had any nurses when opened. Thus far, there have been only 42 deaths in the hospitals Thirty-two of these cases were those of U. S. personnel who died but would never have reached a hospital alive had the hospital been located at a normal distance from the front.

"Two thousand and sixty-one cases have been evacuated to North Africa by air and sea.

"The beach medical service was superior. One Medical Bat talion distinguished itself on the beaches under heavy fire earl in the operation. I shall recommend that the unit be cited fo its gallant work under terrible conditions.

"The medical supply system began to function according to plan with the assault wave, and despite the most difficult condi tions it rapidly developed to the highest state of efficiency.

"Among the difficulties with which the medical services hav had to cope were the loss of the entire equipment of our thir evacuation hospital and the bombing of a hospital ship which was bringing the nurses. Fortunately, only one nurse was injured and all are again on their way to Italy to rejoin their units.

"The whole performance of the Fifth Army medical service has been most heartening to me and has been of incalculabl aid in the operation. I have been so favorably impressed with their performance that I cannot forbear to write you this persona letter to tell you of my gratitude and admiration."

The Commanding General of the Northwest Service Command which comprises that cold country in which the Alaska Highwa is situated, as well as part of Alaska itself, expressed his view concerning the work done by the Medical Department in hi Service Command as follows:

"One of the satisfying memories of my service with the North west Service Command is the work of the Medical Departmen

"While the natural health condition of the large number c men engaged in this operation has been remarkably good, th work of your representatives has been outstanding. Withou regard for self and with an excellence which; under the condition has been amazing, your medical personnel has gained the admiration and appreciation of all. No difficulties were too great and no effort too much for them to be and to perform whenever their services might be required.

"The operation on a soldier for concussion with carpenter's tools in the middle of the Rocky Mountains with the leading elements of the road-building group, the airplane landing on a sand bar at night during stormy weather to perform a successful appendectomy were but two of many similar occurrences. The records of the manner in which they functioned show the excellence of their execution.

"It is my pleasure to share with you the grand feelings that such actions engender."

But in the final analysis, accomplishment must be the measure of the Medical Department's success. The health record of our Army and the low mortality rate from disease and injury are unequaled in the history of warfare. Despite the fact that our troops have been scattered over the four corners of the world, fighting in regions where disease is rife, no yellow fever, typhoid, leprosy, typhus, plague or other diseases which can cripple and decimate the fighting strength of an army ever developed. This was due to the efficiency of our preventive medicine program, which has applied intensive immunization and every other combative measure known to medical science in the control of these serious diseases.

The development of greatly improved insecticides and insect repellents which will keep away mosquitoes, flies, fleas, chiggers and similar disease-carrying pests was an important contribution to this program. Typhus is a disease which, in the past, has been an inevitable accompaniment of wars, famines and disasters of all sorts. Typhus vaccination and effective delousing facilities virtually eliminated the disease, and typhoid fever, too, was practically eliminated. Another example of our strikingly effective immunization program is the fact that no authenticated case of tetanus was reported in an American soldier who had received proper immunization. The control of venereal disease was especially significant. As of 1944, the venereal disease rate in our Army was 30 per thousand per annum—incomparably superior to any previous rate in any army at any time.

The treatment of disease when it occurred also provided an extraordinary record of achievement. Examples of this outstanding performance would fill pages, and only a few can be given here. Meningitis and pneumonia were among the most feared diseases in the last war, and rightly so, for they were accompanied by a very high mortality rate. Thus, 38 per cent of patients with meningitis in the last war died, whereas in this war only 4 per cent of such patients died. Similarly, in pneumonia, the case fatality rate was 28 per cent in contrast to a rate of 0.7 per cent in this war. Tuberculosis caused an admission rate of 12 per 1,000 per annum in the last war and, in this war, less than 1.2 per 1,000 per annum. Thus, the annual death rate per 1,000 for all disease in the Army, excluding surgical conditions, was lowered from 15.6 in the last war to only 0.6 in this war. Translated into other terms, this means that a division of 10,000 men would experience 156 deaths per annum from disease (excluding injuries) in the last war, whereas in this war the division would lose only six men by death from disease, a reduction greater than 95 per cent! This is the extraordinary record of our Army doctors. No better proof is needed to demonstrate the high level of professional competence in internal medicine in the Army.

Our surgeons, too, established a record in the care of the wounded which is unparalleled in the history of warfare and little short of miraculous. As of 1944, the over-all mortality rate among the wounded in the Army was approximately 3 per cent, which means that we saved 97 of every 100 soldiers wounded in battle, contrasted with a figure of more than 8 per cent in the last war. The high standard of surgical care provided the wounded may be emphasized even further by consideration of the mortality in some of the more serious types of regional wounds. Thus, in abdominal injuries, which even under the most ideal conditions have always been associated with a high mortality, the death rate in our Army in 1944 was about 25 per cent, in contrast to the figure of more than 50 per cent in the last war. Similarly, in penetrating chest wounds, the mortality was less than 15 per cent, whereas in the last war it was almost 50 per cent. In head wounds, too, the fatality rate was reduced to approximately 4 per cent from 14 per cent in the last war.

These figures demonstrate impressively the high level of surgical proficiency in our Army. Not only have our surgeons saved more lives among the wounded than ever before, but they performed near miracles in reconstructive and rehabilitative surgery. No higher degree of specialized surgical care can be obtained anywhere else in the world.

Outstanding as a medical investigator, great medical scientist and epidemiologist is Brigadier General James S. Simmons, who has been, since the beginning of this war, chief of the preventive medicine division of the United States Army, Office of the Surgeon General. So conspicuous has been the record in the prevention of disease that General Simmons has been virtually covered with honors in recognition of his accomplishments.

Dr. James S. Simmons, specially trained as a bacteriologist, was graduated by the University of North Carolina School of Medicine and later received the doctor of medicine degree from the University of Pennsylvania. Following an internship in the University of Pennsylvania Hospital, he entered the Army, devoting himself early in his work to laboratory service and the teaching of bacteriology. His achievements in this field brought him the honorary degree of doctor of philosophy from George Washington University Medical School in 1934, the degree of doctor of public health from the Harvard School of Public Health in 1939, and the honorary degree of doctor of science from Duke University and the University of Pennsylvania in 1943. He has published distinguished books in the fields of bacteriology, laboratory technic, tropical medicine and global epidemiology.

Dr. Simmons is a doctor who prevents disease rather than one who is chiefly concerned with its cure. He received a special citation for meritorious service in connection with the work of the American Typhus Commission, which he himself founded and which he organized as a joint undertaking between the Army Navy and Public Health Service. He was awarded the Sedgwick Memorial Medal of the American Public Health Association, and also the Sternberg Medal named in honor of Surgeon General Sternberg. He has been decorated with the Order of Carlos J Finlay by the president of Cuba. He is a member of the Advisory Board of the National Foundation for Infantile Paralysis and is also a member of practically every scientific organization in his field.

Brigadier General Simmons tells how the Army prevents war's epidemics, improves nutrition and inoculates against all sorts of infections. His account of preventive medicine in this war is a noteworthy record of medical progress.

CHAPTER VI

PREVENTIVE MEDICINE IN THE ARMY

By
BRIGADIER GENERAL JAMES STEVENS SIMMONS,
M.D., PH.D., D.P.H., SC.D. (HON.)
Chief of the Preventive Medicine Service, United States Army

I

GOOD HEALTH IS essential to any military force, and convinced that "an ounce of prevention is worth a pound of cure," the Medical Department of the United States Army has conducted an aggressive program of preventive medicine.

It is the primary mission of the Medical Department to protect the health of the American soldier in order to keep him fit to fight. A large force is required to perform this important task. As of 1944, the Department included the following branches: Medical Corps, Dental Corps, Veterinary Corps, Nurse Corps, Sanitary Corps, Medical Administrative Corps, Pharmacy Corps, the Physical Therapy aides, and Dietitians. These branches were composed of more than one hundred thousand officers and several hundred thousand enlisted men—a total force larger than the entire regular Army prior to the war.

This great medical organization has followed the soldier and guarded his health in all the far-flung places where our troops have been stationed throughout the world. The services which it performed were numerous and complex. It was actively concerned with the health and welfare of the soldier from the time of his arrival at the induction station until he returned to his home and civil life. It established and maintained the physical standards which were used in order to select only strong, healthy military personnel, and it examined every soldier admitted to the service. It saw to it that he was provided with satisfactory hygienic shelter, that he was furnished an adequate, scientifically balanced diet, and that he took the necessary healthful physical exercises. It was concerned with his personal habits and hygiene, with the sanitation of his entire environment, with his vaccinations against certain infectious diseases, and with innumerable other measures required to protect his health. If, in spite of these precautions, the soldier became sick or was injured, it provided him with expert surgical and medical attention in one of the Army's well-equipped modern hospitals, and when he left the service, he was given a careful final physical examination. Thus the Medical Department of the Army was responsible for the care of the soldier throughout the entire period of his military life.

One of the most spectacular wartime activities of the medical officer was the surgical and medical care of the wounded and their evacuation from the combat zone. An officer on duty in an active theater of operation led a life which was filled with drama intense enough to satisfy the most romantic and adventurous crusader.

The devotion to duty of our medical officers and soldiers has always reflected credit on the profession. Their heroic achievements in snatching the injured from the brink of death and returning the wounded to active duty constitutes a thrilling epic of war. Moreover, it affords a pleasing contrast to the necessary but unpleasant task of destruction which is a basic part of all wars. (See Figure 1.)

There is, however, another aspect of military medicine which, while less spectacular, is equally or more important. It is with this, the preventive aspect, that we are concerned here. In order to keep the maximum number of men in condition to perform their military duties at all times, the men must be protected from the numerous health hazards which surround them continuously—hazards which, if not controlled, may so seriously deplete manpower as to render military operations ineffective or impossible. An Army weakened by disease, like a sick individual, cannot be expected to cope with a strong, healthy enemy, and history affords innumerable tragic examples of the role played by disease in determining the outcome of battles and campaigns, and thus affecting the survival of nations.

We may admire the scientific technological advances that have produced the marvelous weapons of today, but one factor which has not changed since the day of the cavemen is the need for manpower to operate these modern instruments of destruction. The Second World War has been no exception to the generalization that the protection of the health of troops is an essential part of any well-planned military operation. For this reason, the Medical Department of our Army placed increasing emphasis on its strong, aggressive program of military preventive medicine.

The evolution of this program of prevention in our Army has been gradual but continuous. All our wars have been fought by rapidly mobilized civilian armies, and in each instance the Medi-

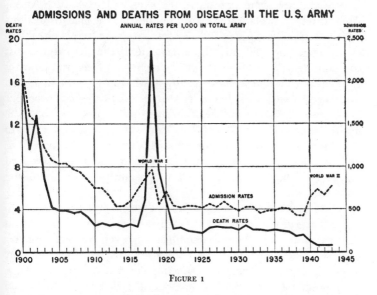

ADMISSIONS AND DEATHS FROM DISEASE IN THE U.S. ARMY

ANNUAL RATES PER 1,000 IN TOTAL ARMY

FIGURE 1

cal Department has been composed largely of civilian doctors. Therefore, the increasing effectiveness of the Army's preventive medicine program has closely paralleled the development of modern scientific medicine in the country.

The rapid improvement in civilian public health facilities since 1900 has contributed richly to the health and vigor of the nation and has been a factor in the establishment and maintenance of our position as one of the great civilized powers of the world. During the same period, the Army made remarkable advances in the science of military preventive medicine. When we entered the war in 1941, we were armed with many effective methods and facilities for the prevention of disease. This factor alone played an essential part in making possible the rapid organization and training of our great military and naval forces, and in the mobilization of the army of industrial workers who supported them.

The progress which has been made in the Army's health program can be appreciated by recalling conditions which existed during earlier wars. During the American Revolution, the War of 1812, the Mexican War and the Civil War, when the microorganisms which cause infections were still unknown, our troops were frequently weakened by disease and often the mortality from this cause alone was appalling. Even as late as the Spanish-American War, when the bacteria responsible for many infections had been discovered, certain diseases, particularly typhoid fever, caused crippling epidemics, thus reflecting the inadequate state of contemporary knowledge about their epidemiology and control. During World War I, when many advances had been made in military preventive medicine, the Army established an excellent health record, except for the serious influenza pandemic of 1918, against which there was no known protection. It is important to recall that in that war our troops fought only in temperate regions and therefore were not exposed to many of the serious tropical diseases which constituted such an important problem beginning with 1941.

When it appeared that the United States might be drawn into another world war, the Surgeon General began necessary revision and expansion of plans to establish a preventive medicine organization adequate to protect American troops wherever they might be sent. The small peacetime regular Army, living in permanent posts, had enjoyed a long period of excellent health, and its hospital admission and death rates were the lowest on record. Past experiences had shown, however, that one could not expect this good record to be maintained under the difficult conditions imposed by war, unless unusual preparations were made to meet the new situation. At that time, it was impossible to predict what diseases might attack our troops, as no one knew into what areas it might be necessary to send them. Therefore, the wartime plagues of all countries and of every climate and season were considered potential hazards, and careful plans were made to combat them. Subsequent events justified this foresight; American forces were soon spread throughout the world. (See Figure 2.)

In 1939, the Surgeon General began the organization in his office of the Preventive Medicine Service and arranged to utilize the total civilian health resources of the nation to assist in perfecting the Army's health program. By 1944 the service consisted of the following divisions: Medical Intelligence; Epidemiology; Venereal Disease Control; Tropical Disease Control; Laboratories; Sanitation and Hygiene; Sanitary Engineering; Nutrition; Occupational Health; and Civil Public Health. It also included the Board for the Control of Influenza and other Epidemic Diseases in the United States Army. This board, composed of more than 100 expert

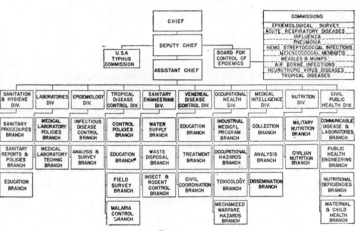

FIGURE 2

civilian consultants to the Surgeon General, was divided into ten special commissions, each of which was concerned with a specific problem of disease control. The Preventive Medicine Service also had associated with it the U.S.A. Typhus Commission, which is a joint Army, Navy and Public Health Service organization administered through the Secretary of War.

The Preventive Medicine Service has had as its objective the maintenance of good health in the Army through the elimination of sanitary, occupational and other health hazards, and the prevention and control of infectious diseases. It advanced toward this objective by careful planning, based on estimates of future possibilities, by the constant accumulation of all available scientific knowledge, by vigorous application of the most promising control plans available, and by initiating research on problems of immediate significance to the armed forces. It utilized every available facility, enlisted the services of many highly qualified persons, and maintained close liaison with numerous governmental and civilian health agencies. These included the National Research Council, the Committee on Medical Research, the United States Public Health Service, the Bureau of Medicine and Surgery of the Navy, the Pan-American Sanitary Bureau, the United States Department of Agriculture, the Coordinator of Inter-American Affairs, the American Red Cross, the International Health Division of the Rockefeller Foundation, and most of the scientific institutions and societies in the fields of biology, medical and public health.

II

The nature and extent of the Army's Preventive Medicine program can be visualized by considering (1) some of the more important general measures used to safeguard the soldier's health; (2) measures employed to protect him against the specific diseases to which he was exposed at home and abroad; and (3) the extensive research activities which have been carried on in the search for more effective methods for control of diseases which might attack him.

The general health measures carried out in the Army by 1944 included the physical selection of healthy recruits; the provision of healthful clothing, housing, nutrition and physical training; intensive instruction and training in hygiene; and careful sanitation of the soldier's environment.

Since the effectiveness of an army depends upon the physical stamina of its personnel, care was exercised to avoid bringing into the military service any individual with physical defects which might prove to be a handicap either to him or to the military organization. The Surgeon General maintained careful supervision over the physical standards and examinations given to all persons before admission into the Army. While this function was not performed under the immediate supervision of the Preventive Medicine Service, it was an important part of the Army's health program. It not only served to eliminate crippled and physically weak individuals, but it prevented the induction of persons suffering from acute and chronic infections which might spread and cause serious outbreaks of disease among troops.

A striking example of the value of such physical selection is the experience with tuberculosis. Since the First World War, improved methods have been developed for the early detection of tuberculosis. When drafting began for World War II, all selectees were examined for this disease by a rapid film x-ray method which made it possible to detect and eliminate a large proportion of infected individuals. This improved selection resulted in a decreased prevalence of tuberculosis in the Army. The hospital admission rates for tuberculosis for World War I were 13 per 1,000 every year, as compared with only 1.2 during the first two years of World War II.

On the other hand, during both wars the Army accepted individuals infected with gonorrhea or syphilis. This policy was adopted because persons infected with these diseases can be rendered non-infective by immediate treatment, thus eliminating the danger of spreading the infection among troops. The Army had highly effective drugs, namely, the sulfonamides and penicillin, with which gonorrhea can be cured in a short time while the soldier remains on a full-duty status. This program was an additional advantage in that it relieved civilian health agencies of a great treatment problem and at the same time provided the Army with thousands of additional soldiers.

The minimum physical standards adopted for the Army were changed from time to time, depending on military needs and the availability of manpower in the country. For example, in order to build up a strong, highly trained nucleus, the standards used during the early period of mobilization were higher than those for the First World War or those later in use. These differences in standards made it difficult to estimate changes in the health status of the civil population by comparing the proportion of individuals rejected physically during the two wars.

The physical selection of personnel was of great importance not only to the Army but to the health of the whole country. Its primary purpose was, of course, the screening out of unfits in order to give the Army a healthy population. However, by exposing the physical defects of the large group of rejected individuals, it provided a unique opportunity to correct many health deficiencies in the civilian population.

The Quartermaster Corps was responsible for the procurement and supply of all clothing furnished the troops. The Medical Department cooperated and was concerned in so far as the soldier's clothes might affect his health. Because of the global nature of military operations, it was necessary to develop many special types of clothing to insure the comfort and health of our troops under a wide variety of conditions of climate and warfare. These included the various special types of uniforms, shoes and personal equipment used by aviators, paratroopers and ski-troopers; impregnated garments to protect troops against enemy gas attacks; cool insect-proof jungle clothes for the tropics; and warm equipment to prevent frostbite and death in the frozen north. Intensive research on this subject and the development of improved garments for our soldiers were continued throughout the war.

The soldier not only must be clothed but he must be properly housed. Here again the Medical Department was responsible for seeing that the shelter provided by others was adequate from the viewpoint of his health. It advised those responsible for construction about the location and types of barracks and tents to be used in various climates, particularly about heating, ventilation and sanitation. It also recommended policies to prevent overcrowding and to mimimize the spread of contact infections. It was the policy of the War Department to provide for the soldier in barracks at least 50 square feet of floor space per man, except in emergencies, when it could be reduced temporarily to 40 square feet per man. The authorized normal capacity of a pyramidal tent with a floor space of 256 square feet is six men, or for temporary emergency purposes, eight men. The normal capacity for standard hutments with 800 square feet of floor space is eighteen men in the Zone of the Interior and twenty men overseas.

The Army's food was procured and distributed by the Quartermaster Corps. The Medical Department cooperated actively in the program, and assisted in insuring the adequacy and safety of the soldier's rations. The Nutrition Division of the Surgeon General's Office cooperated with and advised the Quartermaster on the medical aspects of all nutritional problems. The Veterinary Corps also performed an important function by maintaining an extensive organization for the sanitary inspection required to insure the safety of all meat and dairy products. One important aspect of this work was the Army policy requiring that all fresh milk furnished American troops had to be pasteurized.

The Army developed a number of different rations to meet

various military conditions. These were as follows: (1) *"The Garrison Ration,"* which was essentially the peacetime ration, with a fixed monetary value based upon the cost of a specified list of food items; (2) *"The Filipino Ration,"* which was prescribed for Philippine Scouts and was predicated on food preferences of Filipinos; (3) *"The Travel Ration,"* for troops while traveling otherwise than by marching and separated from cooking facilities; and (4) the various types of *"Field Rations."*

There were several types of field rations. *"Field Ration A"* was a complete ration of fresh and canned foods corresponding as nearly as practicable to the components of the garrison ration, including anything that the market afforded and which could be distributed to messes. *"Field Ration B"* corresponded as nearly as possible to the components of Field Ration A, except that nonperishable processed or canned products replaced perishable items. *"The Overseas Hospital Ration"* represented essentially the addition of a special supplement to existing Expeditionary Force Menus (Field Ration B). *"Then Ten-in-One Ration"* was essentially the same as Field Ration B, packaged to furnish food for ten men for one day. *"The Five-in-One Ration"* contained the components of Field Ration B, packaged to furnish food for five men for one day.

There were also various emergency field rations. *"Field Ration C"* was a temporary ration of previously cooked or prepared food, packed in hermetically sealed cans, which could be eaten either hot (preferably) or cold, and consisted of six cans per ration— three cans containing a meat and vegetable component, and three cans containing crackers, sugar, soluble coffee and a confection. *"Field Ration D"* consisted of three four-ounce bars of concentrated chocolate. *"The K Ration"* was a pocket ration of concentrated foods for three meals, packed in cartons and consisting chiefly of a can of meat or cheese, biscuits, a confection, sugar and a beverage, including lemon powder. The latter ration was intended for occasions such as combat, and for special troops or missions where relatively light weight was desired.

Various other special rations, such as "jungle" and "mountain" rations, were devised, but their development and use were overshadowed by the usefulness and practicability of the 10-in-1 ration. As a consequence of the careful planning, research and organization carried on by the Quartermaster Corps with the cooperation and advice of the Medical Department, the American soldier got a good, wholesome diet which was as nearly perfect as modern science could make it.

The soldier was given regular supervised physical exercises as a part of his basic military training, and frequently that was augmented by participation in various outdoor sports. This factor alone played an important part in building up and maintaining

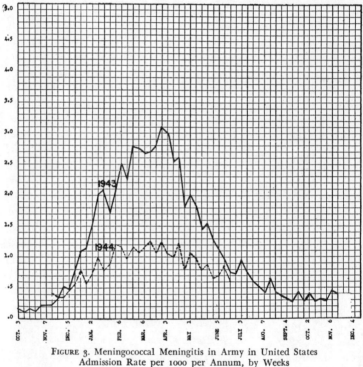

FIGURE 3. Meningococcal Meningitis in Army in United States
Admission Rate per 1000 per Annum, by Weeks

his general health and increasing his resistance to infectious diseases.

There is a marked contrast between the physical appearance of recruits and seasoned veterans; moreover, the admission rate for sickness is lower among trained troops. For example, the admission rates for such diseases as meningitis and other acute infections among military personnel have usually been much higher during the first six months of service than during subsequent periods of service. During 1942, 57 per cent of meningitis cases occurred in soldiers with less than three months' service and 82 per cent in those with not more than six months. (See Figures 3 and 4.)

Another important factor in the Army's health program was the intensive instruction and training in hygiene which the soldier received. He led an orderly life and his habits were regulated. He had to obtain adequate rest and sleep in carefully sanitated

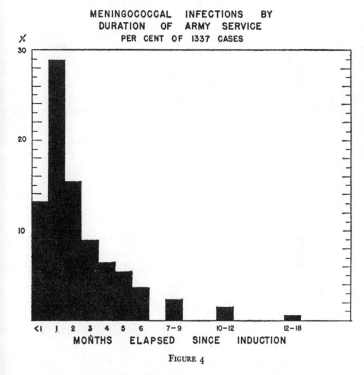

FIGURE 4

surroundings. He had to keep his clothes neat and his body clean. Every soldier who entered the Army was given formal instruction on how to keep well. This instruction included twenty hours of lectures stressing the importance of such subjects as personal cleanliness, care of the feet, the proper fitting of shoes and clothing, proper dietary habits, adequate rest practices, sex hygiene, the prevention of infectious diseases, and camp sanitation.

Clean, healthful surroundings are necessary to the welfare of troops, and the Army has always emphasized the importance of environmental sanitation. This function was intended to be carried out in all military installations in accordance with policies established by the Sanitation and Hygiene Division and the Division of Sanitary Engineering of the Surgeon General's Office. It included the practical application of the scientific measures required to provide at all times safe food and water supplies free from contamination and disease-producing organisms; the sanitary disposal of all wastes, including garbage and excreta; the elimination or control of the many insects and rodents which carry disease; and the correction of various other environmental defects which constitute a menace to troops both in permanent barracks and in the field.

Sanitation is primarily the responsibility of the commanding office of each installation. However, it is the duty of his surgeon, guided by the advice of the medical inspector, to recommend the proper sanitary procedures to be carried out. This makes it necessary for all military personnel, both medical and line, to have a working knowledge of the basic principles of sanitation, and for the medical inspectors, who are really military health officers, to be highly qualified in this specialty. Therefore, sanitation was emphasized in all courses of military training given in the Army, and extensive special training in the subject was given at the Army Field Medical School, Carlisle Barracks, Pennsylvania, to Medical Department officers when they entered military service.

In order to check on the manner in which sanitation was carried out, the surgeon of every unit in the Army was required to make routine monthly reports indicating the status of his organization and any defects that required correction. Special reports were made when required. These sanitary reports, with the proper recommendations, were sent to the commanding officer for action, after which they were forwarded to the War Department and analyzed in the Office of the Surgeon General.

Generally speaking, the sanitation program of the Army was efficiently carried out, especially in fixed installations, and this fact was reflected in the relatively low incidence of the food-borne and water-borne diseases in this country. However, certain organizations living under field conditions, especially overseas, had undesirable experiences with some of the filth-borne and insect-borne diseases because their commanders failed to enforce the necessary sanitary control, training and discipline.

In many instances, the health of troops is menaced by unsanitary conditions in near-by civilian communities. As the Army has no authority over such civilians, arrangements were made by the Surgeon General early in 1940 whereby in this country the United States Public Health Service, working through State and local health departments, assumed responsibility for environmental sanitation and disease control among the civilian populations within the vicinity of military reservations. Thus the sanitary work carried on by the Army inside reservations was supplemented and made more effective by the extra-military sanitation performed by civilian health agencies. The value of this useful arrangement was proved by the extremely low incidence of filth diseases among great numbers of troops that were trained and housed in this country. Similar arrangements were made abroad, when possible.

The Army's program of sanitation was being continuously improved by the development of new and more effective agents and methods which resulted from organized research initiated by the Sanitation and Hygiene Division in the Surgeon General's Office. Some of these agents, including the Army's newly developed insecticides and repellents, will be discussed in another place.

In addition to general health measures, the preventive medicine program included various other activities designed to protect the soldier against infection with specific diseases. The following divisions of the Surgeon General's Office dealt with this phase of the problem: Medical Intelligence, Epidemiology, Laboratories, Venereal Disease Control and Tropical Disease Control. These coordinated divisions were concerned with the collection of exact information concerning the diseases which might threaten our troops in all parts of the world, the analysis of current disease statistics for the Army, the maintenance of adequate laboratories for the identification of disease-producing organisms, the development of policies and the taking of immediate action to control outbreaks or threatened epidemics of disease, and the initiation of medical research in the laboratory and in the field in order to discover more effective control methods.

The innumerable infections which plague mankind vary greatly in their geographic distribution. It was essential to maintain exact, up-to-the-minute information concerning the disease hazards of all the countries where American troops were or might be stationed. This information was made available to the Army through the Medical Intelligence Division. It was collected from every available source, and after analysis it was used in preparing extensive detailed medical surveys by countries which were furnished to all officers and agencies responsible for the welfare of the troops sent to foreign regions. The medical survey for each country included recommendations for the special health precautions to be taken against local diseases. Similar information about current incidence of disease in the civil population of this country was obtained routinely from the highly efficient epidemiological staff of the United States Public Health Service.

Thus the Surgeon General was kept informed at all times of the exact status of disease and health conditions throughout the world, and was able to make intelligent plans for the protection of troops.

Current information concerning the diseases which occurred among American troops was reported routinely from each military unit to the Medical Statistics Division of the Surgeon General's Office, where it was analyzed and acted upon by the staff of the Epidemiology Division of the Preventive Medicine Service. Any unusual disease outbreak was reported directly to this Division by telegraph, radio or telephone.

The Epidemiology Division and the Divisions of Venereal and Tropical Disease Control were concerned with the investigation and correction of any unusual increase in disease prevalence. Assistance in the performance of this function was given by members of the Board for the Control of Influenza and Other Epidemic Diseases in the United States Army. This Board had two main functions. One of these was to investigate and control epidemics in the field; the other was to carry on research looking to the development of better control methods. The Board functioned effectively and contributed much to our fundamental knowledge of many diseases, including influenza, the pneumonias, streptococcus infections, rheumatic fever, meningitis, measles, mumps, epidemic hepatitis, the Rickettsial and neurotropic virus diseases, the tropical diseases including malaria, the dysenteries, sandfly fever and dengue, and the air-borne infections. Groups of experts from the Board were used repeatedly in the field in this country and in overseas theaters. The scope and effectiveness of the control program can be visualized by considering the immunization procedures employed and the plans for attack used against various broad groups of diseases.

Theoretically, vaccination would be the ideal method for control of all infectious diseases among troops. Unfortunately, however, only a limited number of immunizing agents have been discovered. Those which are available contributed richly to the health of our troops.

The Army's immunization program was briefly as follows: On induction, every soldier was actively immunized against smallpox, typhoid fever, the paratyphoid fevers A and B, and tetanus. Those sent to areas where they might be exposed to yellow fever, epidemic typhus fever, cholera and plague were immunized against these diseases. It is significant that none of these diseases occurred in threatening numbers. Other agents were available for local use if required to protect troops against diphtheria, scarlet fever, equine encephalomyelitis and Rocky Mountain spotted fever. Extensive experimental work has been done in the search for much needed protective vaccines against the bacillary dysenteries, gas gangrene, influenza and other infections. The results obtained with an influenza vaccine containing both A and B viruses look promising, but do not yet warrant their routine general use in the Army, as this is written.

The filth-borne gastro-intestinal diseases including typhoid fever, the paratyphoid fevers, the dysenteries and diarrheas, and cholera have long been the scourge of armies. However, none of these presented a serious problem except the dysenteries.

In 1911, vaccination against typhoid was made compulsory in the Army, and since then this disease has become so rare that it is a clinical curiosity. During World War I the paratyphoids A and B were added, making a "triple typhoid" vaccine, and consequently these diseases also became relatively unimportant. Various modifications and combinations of these vaccines were used during the period from 1920 to 1939, but throughout World War II the triple typhoid vaccine was given to all troops. This vaccine, which consists of a saline suspension of killed organisms, is injected subcutaneously in three doses of 0.5, 1.0 and 1.0 cc., respectively, at intervals of one week. Subsequently, a single stimulating dose of 0.5 cc. is given each year. There has been no increase in the low typhoid-paratyphoid admission rate among troops in this country, and most of the cases which did occur were in individuals who had not completed the initial vaccination. Overseas there were a few minor outbreaks of these diseases, due usually to gross, accidental contamination of water supplies. Apparently the protection afforded by vaccination will not always prevent typhoid under such circumstances. However, the incidence rate during the first two years of World War II was remarkably low—only 0.04 per 1,000 per annum as contrasted with 0.4 in the last war. (See Figure 5.)

The large group of disabling diarrheal diseases, including amebic dysentery, the various types of bacillary dysentery, and the

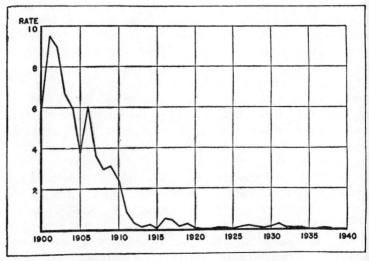

FIGURE 5. Typhoid and paratyphoid fevers, annual rates per 1,000 strength, white enlisted men in the United States since 1900. Typhoid vaccination was voluntary in 1909, compulsory a portion of 1910, and compulsory since 1911.

innumerable varieties of infectious diarrheas have constituted a serious military problem in our Army. There were rather extensive outbreaks of bacillary dysentery, chiefly among forces in tropical theaters where native sanitation was primitive and troops had to operate under field conditions. In many instances, these infections were derived from eating in unauthorized, filthy, unsanitated native establishments. Fortunately, many of the outbreaks were clinically mild and Shiga dysentery was rarely encountered. Amebic dysentery had been a comparatively minor problem but it was considered possible that latent infections might become manifest. Outbreaks of bacterial food poisoning due to staphylococci or members of the Salmonella group caused considerable annoyance, both in the United States and abroad. The cases probably outnumbered those caused by other diarrheal diseases in this country, but were relatively ineffective.

However, the admission rate for the total groups of dysenteries and diarrheas in the Army during the first year of the war was 35.9 per 1,000. This represents a moderate increase over the rate of 28.6 per 1,000 annually, from 1930 to 1940. It is also much higher than the rate of 22.4 during the last war. This failure to control adequately a group of diseases which are transmitted mainly by the ingestion of water or food contaminated with infective fecal material represented a weak point in our control program. In spite of the strenuous search for a prophylactic vaccine, no such agent was developed.

Therefore, the control of these diseases must depend on the provision of safe food and water for troops and the enforcement of sanitary discipline by the line officers who command them. It is obviously necessary that the medical inspectors of all units be physicians, well trained in preventive medicine, and that the commanding officers enforce the sanitary regulations required to protect their men against eating and drinking the contaminated materials which cause these diseases. It has become a truism that the incidence of enteric diseases is an index of the degree of civilization of a country. It might be added with equal truth that a high incidence of gastro-intestinal diseases in a military unit indicates inefficiency on the part of the commanding officer.

Relatively effective drugs are available for the treatment of the dysenteries. Good therapeutic results have been reported in bacillary dysentery with sulfadiazine, sulfaguanadine and sulfapyrazine. Sulfadiazine has been used for the prophylactic treatment of carriers of dysentery bacilli. (See Figure 6.)

Cholera did not occur in American troops during the war, although the disease is common in Asia and was epidemic among civilians in various parts of India. All our soldiers sent to that region were vaccinated against cholera, and special sanitary precautions were taken to protect them against exposure to the disease.

As already noted, the most dangerous diseases that attacked our Army during World War I were those which are transmitted through the respiratory tract discharges by personal contact. Certain of these, including the common cold, influenza, the pneumonias, measles, scarlet fever, mumps, diphtheria and meningitis occurred in epidemic proportions. Influenza, bronchitis, and pneumonia alone caused more than a million admissions to hospitals and 44,000 deaths. This represented one-third of the total admissions for disease and 80 per cent of the disease deaths. The

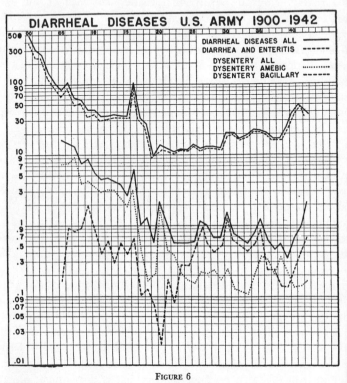

FIGURE 6

influenza epidemic alone was responsible for 800,000 admissions to hospitals and 24,600 deaths. This tragic experience left an indelible impression on the Medical Department. Consequently, great emphasis was placed on the control of respiratory diseases in wartime, and every effort was made to develop effective control procedures. With this in mind, intensive research on the respiratory infections was initiated through the Board for the Control of Influenza and Other Epidemic Diseases in the United States Army, and the Committee on Medical Research of the Office of Scientific Research and Development. (See Figure 7.)

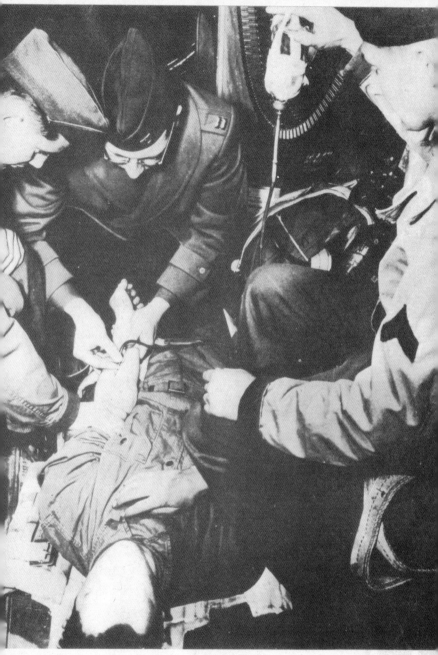

Administration of blood plasma in a combat plane. (SIGNAL CORPS PHOTO)

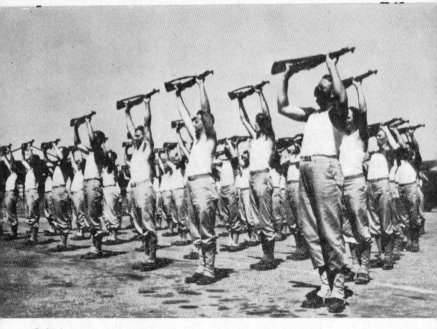

Calisthenics, a part of the Army's training program, taken by members of 163rd Sign Photo Company, Fort Sam Houston, Texas. (SIGNAL CORPS PHOTO)

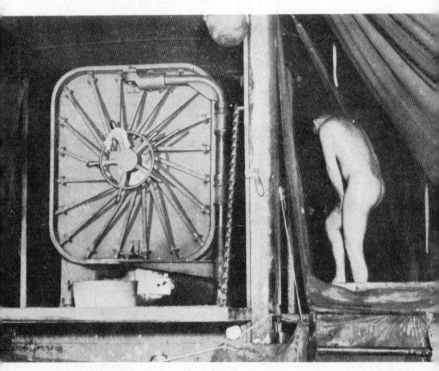

Portable field bath, complete with "delouser" — steam chamber in center.
(SIGNAL CORPS PHOTO)

During World War II, the prevalence of acute respiratory diseases, including the common ones, influenza and pneumonia in the United States were higher than during the peacetime years 1930–1940 inclusive, but lower than the rates for World War I. The admission rate per 1,000 per annum for the previous war was 440, as compared with 246 for the years 1942 and 1943. Two epidemic waves of mild influenza occurred; the first early in 1941 and the second in November and December, 1943. The latter accompanied an extensive civilian outbreak which struck heavily in the United States and the United Kingdom. In both these outbreaks the mortality was relatively insignificant. In only one month of the war did the maximum respiratory disease death rate reach the height of the lowest rate experienced during the last war. This maximum death rate of 0.24 per 1,000 per annum is about one five-hundredth of the maximum death rate of 100 reached at the peak of the 1918 epidemic of influenza.

During the last war the annual admission rate per 1,000 for all types of pneumonias among troops in this country was 21, as compared with a rate of 15 during the first two years of the present war. The corresponding annual death rates were 4.4 in World War I, as compared with 0.07 during the present conflict. During the present war, moreover, a new form of pneumonia designated as "primary atypical pneumonia" has been recognized and is now reportable in the Army. The incidence of this disease during the first two years of the war was 6 per 1,000 and the death rate was 0.01. Extensive investigations of this so-called primary atypical pneumonia have been carried on throughout the Army by the Board for the Control of Influenza and Other Epidemics in the Army and by other boards. Thus, it is apparent that the control of pneumonia during this war has been much more effective than in the past.

During the present war the admission rate for scarlet fever among troops in the continental United States has been only 2 per 1,000 per annum. as compared with 4 during World War I. Corresponding rates for the total Army were 1.6 during the present war, as compared with 2.8 during the First World War. Acute rheumatic fever has not occurred in sufficient numbers to constitute a serious problem numerically. It was not reported as such during the First World War; however, the admission rate from acute articular rheumatism was 7.6 among troops in the conti-

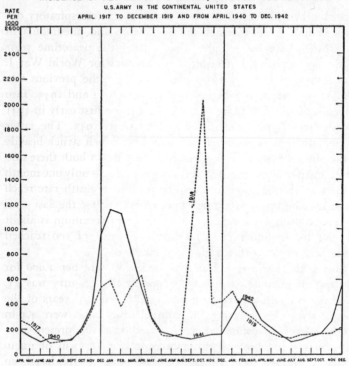

INCIDENCE OF RESPIRATORY DISEASES, RATE PER 1000 PER ANNUM

U.S. ARMY IN THE CONTINENTAL UNITED STATES

APRIL 1917 TO DECEMBER 1919 AND FROM APRIL 1940 TO DEC. 1942

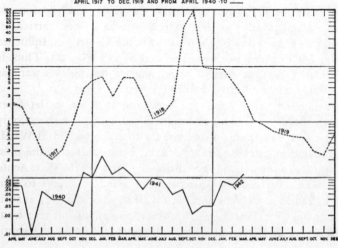

DEATHS, RESPIRATORY DISEASES, RATE PER 1000 PER ANNUM

U.S. ARMY IN THE CONTINENTAL UNITED STATES

APRIL 1917 TO DEC. 1919 AND FROM APRIL 1940 TO ____

FIGURE 7

nental United States. The admission rate among troops in the United States during 1942 and 1943 was 0.9 per 1,000 per annum. Streptococcal diseases and acute rheumatic fever, however, have shown an interesting geographical distribution. A few stations in the Rocky Mountain region, particularly in Colorado and Wyoming, have had cases of acute rheumatic fever with annoying frequency. The admission rate for this disease in the 7th Service Command during 1943 was 8, as compared with 1.2 for the Army in the United States.

Measles has long been recognized as an important military disease. During World War I, it was especially prevalent among recruits and in many instances was followed by secondary streptococcus pneumonia. There were almost 100,000 cases of this disease in the entire Army, and the fatality rate was unusually high. During World War II, measles did not present a serious problem. The admission rates were much lower and there were practically no deaths. These results were not due to the use of any specific prophylactic measures, so the low incidence of measles must be attributed either to general control factors which cannot be readily evaluated, or to the probability that a large proportion of inductees had been infected and had become immune prior to entering the service.

The Army has no agent for the active immunization of troops against measles. However, such passive agents as convalescent serum, placental extract and, more recently, gamma globulin were available for use in military situations requiring the temporary protection of men against this disease. For example, the production of a temporary immunity might be highly desirable in order to avoid delay in the shipment of troops overseas.

During the last World War, mumps was of great importance because of the long period of hospitalization required for the individual case. This disease ranked third as a cause of lost time. Mumps occurred much less frequently in the Second World War and was relatively unimportant. The mortality was negligible.

Diphtheria was not uncommon during World War I, but was of little importance during World War II. Only a few sporadic cases occurred and there were practically no deaths. The incidence was somewhat higher among troops overseas, particularly in certain tropical theaters, where cutaneous diphtheria was observed not infrequently.

The reduction in incidence from the figure of the First World War was not achieved through specific immunization in the Army although it may have been effected by the extensive anti-diphtheria campaign conducted in civilian populations during the last decade. Early in 1940, when the Army vaccination program was planned, it was decided not to adopt universal immunization against diphtheria but to make diphtheria toxoid available so that it might be used wherever required to meet local situations. Later, Schick test surveys among troops indicated that from 40 to 50 per cent of certain groups might be susceptible to diphtheria, and these observations again raised the question as to the advisability of general immunization, but the present policy was considered adequate.

The admission rates for meningococcal meningitis in the Army in the United States during World Wars I and II were 1.3 and 0.9 respectively. The corresponding admission rates for the total Army were 1.2 and 0.8, respectively. Meningitis no longer causes the serious problem that it did in World War I, because of the enormous reduction in its mortality. In the former war, the case fatality for troops in this country was 34 per cent. During the second war, the fatality was only 4 per cent. Complications and disabling sequelae were not common. This remarkable reduction appears to have been due chiefly to the use of sulfonamides, for there is little evidence that meningitis is any milder than it was formerly. The occurrence of meningitis continued to be characterized by the absence of any demonstrable connection between cases. The infection was usually distributed sporadically in different organizations. There is great need for further fundamental studies of the epidemiology of this disease.

Meningitis became epidemic in the winter and spring of 1943, coincidental with a rise in the civilian incidence to the highest rates ever recorded. The 1943 peak was, however, only about two thirds of that attained in January, 1918. A second season of increased prevalence followed in 1944, but the maximum incidence was less than half that of the previous year, in contradistinction to the civilian incidence, which was approximately the same in both years. The administration of sulfonamides to large bodies of troops upon the threat of an epidemic and to new recruits was practised extensively during the 1944 season and may have contributed to the lower incidence.

All our previous wars have been accompanied by an increase in venereal diseases among the troops and in the civil population. The chart which shows the incidence curve of these diseases in the United States Army for more than a century represents the most extensive record of venereal diseases available in this country. As indicated in this chart, voluntary prophylaxis and instruction in sex hygiene were introduced into the Army in 1909, compulsory prophylaxis, monthly physical inspection and forfeiture of pay in 1912, and official recognition of the responsibility of the unit commanders for venereal infections in 1922. In 1939, compulsory prophylaxis was abolished and greater emphasis placed on the education of troops and the elimination of unwholesome conditions in the vicinity of Army camps and stations. (See Figure 8.)

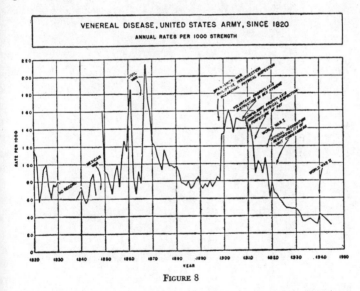

FIGURE 8

When mobilization began in 1940, it was expected that the Army would again experience a great increase in venereal diseases. Although more effective control measures had been applied in the civil population during the preceding decade, and knowledge concerning these diseases had greatly improved, no one with experience in this field believed that the Army could possibly escape a definite increase in its venereal disease rates. An increase did occur, but fortunately this increase was insignificant as compared with the records of the past. The annual rate for 1939 was 31 per thousand men, or the lowest incidence ever recorded in the United States Army up to that time. The annual rates from 1940 to 1943 inclusive were 42.5, 40.5, 37.7 and 26.3, respectively. It is estimated that from one-fourth to one-third of the cases reported during the first half of this period were acquired by selectees before induction.

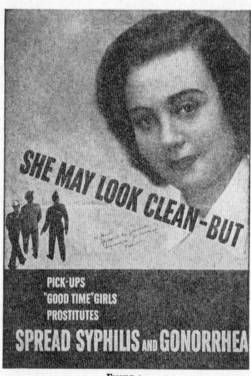

FIGURE 9

The rate for 1943 excludes those cases in which infection was acquired prior to induction. The syphilis rate in this country has consistently averaged slightly less than 5 per thousand men per annum, while the annual incidence of gonorrhea has varied from 20 to 23. The rate for the other venereal diseases, chancroid, lymphogranuloma venereum and granuloma inguinale, considered as a group, has been 2 per thousand per annum, and because of this low rate, they have not presented a serious problem to the Army. In no month of World War II was the annual venereal rate per thousand for troops in this country as high as the lowest monthly rate for the last war. By 1944, the incidence among troops was probably lower than among comparable civilian groups.

Many factors undoubtedly contributed to this excellent record. Specially trained venereal disease control officers were placed in key positions in this country and overseas. Close collaboration was developed with civil authorities in the suppression of prostitution and the discovery and treatment of sources of infection. An aggressive educational program was developed and all soldiers were instructed on the hazards of the venereal diseases and the methods of their prevention. An example of one of the posters issued monthly is illustrated in Figure 9. Recreational facilities were provided within the camps, and public-spirited civil agents provided healthful entertainment in cities. Finally, marked advances were made in the development of more effective agents for the prevention and treatment of venereal diseases in the Army. All troops throughout the Army were provided not only with materials for mechanical prophylaxis, but in 1943 a highly effective one-tube chemical prophylactic was developed and distributed. This tube contains an ointment made up of 15 per cent sulfathiazole and 30 per cent calomel. The use of sulfathiazole for therapy made it possible to treat gonorrhea on a duty status, and later experiments with penicillin showed that of the 40 per cent of cases which proved to be resistant to sulfathiazole, about 99 per cent could be cured with penicillin. As a result of lowering the rates and of advances in therapeutic methods, days lost from venereal disease dropped from 1,278 per 1,000 per annum in 1940 to less than 350 in 1944. (See Figure 10.)

The insect-borne diseases which assumed such great importance during World War II were of much less significance in World War I. This, of course, is because of differences in the geographic areas occupied by our troops during those two conflicts. Our experience during the First World War failed to indicate the potential military significance of the insect-borne tropical diseases. The admission rate for malarial fevers was only 3.7 per 1,000 per annum, with practically no deaths. There were no cases of yellow fever or plague, only two cases of epidemic typhus fever, and 17 of cholera. Since 1941, we have not been so fortunate. By 1944, practically all our serious fighting had been done in tropical countries where insect-borne diseases abounded. American troops were exposed in various parts of the world to yellow fever, dengue, filariasis, typhus, cholera, plague, trypanosomiasis, relapsing fever, tsutsugamushi and many other exotic infections.

Malaria is the most widespread of these diseases. It exists throughout the tropics and subtropics of the entire world and each year it causes more disability and deaths in native populations than any other infection. The Army established an enviable record in its peacetime control of malaria among troops living in

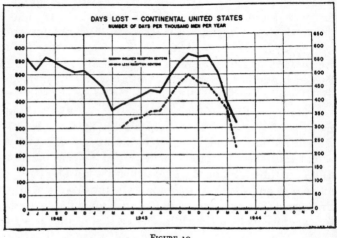

DAYS LOST — CONTINENTAL UNITED STATES
NUMBER OF DAYS PER THOUSAND MEN PER YEAR

FIGURE 10

permanent stations, even in our foreign tropical possessions. (See Figure 11.) By the execution of an extensive mosquito control campaign during the war, it was possible to maintain this good record in the continental United States. In 1941, the Army's mosquito control program in this country cost about $2,000,000 and the malarial admission rate per 1,000 was 1.8. In 1942, more than $3,000,000 was spent and the malaria rate was further reduced to 0.6 per 1,000. The rate for 1943 was 0.2 per 1,000, the lowest rate ever recorded in the United States Army. It should be noted that the highly successful anti-mosquito work done on our military reservations was supplemented by an equally effective campaign directed by the United States Public Health Service and extending for distances of approximately one mile outside the reservations.

Naturally it is much more difficult to protect troops fighting in active tropical theaters. In many such places permanent mosquito control measures could not be carried out and therefore it was necessary to resort to measures which would protect the individual soldier against infected mosquitoes. Briefly stated, the malaria control program for our troops overseas included the following:

(1) Individual protective measures, such as the use of bed nets and mosquito repellents, the wearing of protective clothing, the

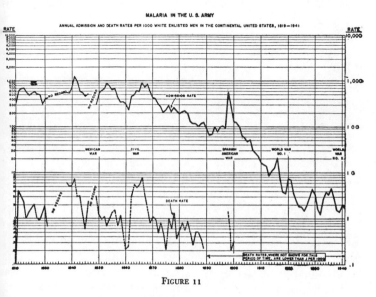

MALARIA IN THE U. S. ARMY

ANNUAL ADMISSION AND DEATH RATES PER 1000 WHITE ENLISTED MEN IN THE CONTINENTAL UNITED STATES, 1819—1941

FIGURE 11

spraying of dwellings and shelters with aerosol insecticides, and the taking of suppressive atabrine or quinine.

(2) Group control measures, including protection against adult mosquitoes by the proper selection of camp sites, by screening and spray-killing with aerosol insecticides and the elimination of mosquito breeding by draining, filling and the use of larvicides.

(3) The indoctrination of all personnel, both line and medical, concerning the importance of malaria control. The Medical Department supplied specialized malaria survey and control units to the overseas theaters. These units evaluated the malaria problem in newly occupied areas, planned and supervised control measures, and assisted field commanders in establishing and maintaining malaria discipline among troops. Four hours of special

training in malaria control measures were given to all soldiers in the Army. An anti-malaria detail, consisting of at least one non commissioned officer and one enlisted man, was required in each company, battery or similar unit. These details carried out the simpler procedure for malaria prevention in the area occupied by the unit.

Dengue fever, transmitted by *Aedes* mosquitoes, was a military problem in certain areas because of the non-effectiveness of explosive outbreaks. Since dengue is a disease of short duration and is practically never fatal, it does not approach malaria in importance. Personal protective measures against mosquitoes and control of breeding places of *Aedes* mosquitoes have been successfully employed in prevention.

Sandfly fever, or pappataci fever, a disease similar to dengue, was of some importance in the Mediterranean areas, where the vector, *Phlebotomus papatacii*, is abundant. Repellents and insecticides effective against mosquitoes also proved useful against sandflies. Nets of fine mesh (45 mesh or smaller) were required to exclude them. Treatment of the ground around buildings with petroleum oils prevented sandfly breeding.

Filariasis of the type caused by *Wuchereria bancrofti* is another mosquito-borne disease with widespread distribution in the tropics. It proved of military importance only in the South Pacific islands, where soldiers were quartered in close proximity to heavily infected natives. Mosquito control, screening of barracks, and individual protective measures against mosquitoes are the means of prevention. It was important also to segregate military personnel from the native population. A period of months is required before symptoms of infection become manifest. To prevent complications resulting from repeated infection, soldiers were evacuated from endemic areas when the diagnosis was made.

Tick-borne relapsing fever has widespread sporadic distribution throughout the world. Occasional cases were reported in Army personnel, and no specific preventive measures were available. Louse-borne relapsing fever was not a problem, except in Allied Oriental troops. Control measures for lice employed to prevent typhus also served to prevent the spread of this type of relapsing fever.

No case of plague had been reported in the Army up to 194. Vaccination was employed to protect individuals and units th might be particularly exposed to infection. Personnel trained in rodent control was available in the event that the disease should appear in military forces.

Rocky Mountain spotted fever occurred sporadically among troops in the United States, especially during maneuvers. Vaccination was not employed routinely for large units, but was used only in those individuals particularly exposed to tick bites in endemic areas.

Murine typhus (endemic typhus) occurs in many parts of the world, and occasional cases were reported in troops. The vaccine which immunizes against epidemic typhus is not effective against the murine type. Rat control to eliminate the rat flea vector was practised in places where infection of humans occurred.

For centuries a dreaded scourge of armies, epidemic typhus fever, was effectively prevented in our Army during World War II. Until early in 1944, less than 50 cases and no deaths had been reported in spite of the fact that large numbers of troops were fighting in endemic areas. An improved vaccine developed since the beginning of the war apparently afforded practical protection to the majority of immunized individuals. New methods of louse control, including methyl bromide fumigation and the individual and mass use of DDT louse powder, were further guarantees against epidemics in military forces. The United States of America Typhus Commission, established soon after the start of the war, was organized to investigate new problems which might arise and to lend assistance in combating epidemics among civilians in areas of military importance.

Although clinically similar to typhus and other Rickettsial infections, scrub typhus (tsutsugamushi) is a distinct disease. It is transmitted by larval mites (chiggers) belonging to the genus *Trombicula*. Scrub typhus was of considerable military importance in New Guinea, Burma and adjacent regions. No vaccine has been found which produces effective immunity. Repellents useful against mosquitoes act as lethal agents against the larval mite vector. Impregnation of clothing with repellents was thus an important preventive measure. Careful selection of camp sites and burning of grass and underbrush to destroy mite resting places decreased the risk of infection. In October, 1943, a research group formed under the auspices of the United States of America Typhus Commission and the Army Epidemiological Board was sent by the Surgeon General to investigate scrub typhus in New Guinea and recommend measures for prevention and treatment.

Leishmaniasis, trypanosomiasis and schistosomiasis, although of widespread occurrence in natives in areas where our forces operated, did not prove to be a military problem. Cutaneous leishmaniasis had a seasonal occurrence in the Middle East, but no case of the visceral type had yet been reported in the Army by 1944. Yellow fever did not occur in our Army.

Coccidioidomycosis received considerable attention owing to its presence in the arid regions of the southwestern United States selected for Army Air Force and Army Ground Force training areas. The incidence of primary infections in certain limited areas, particularly the San Joaquin Valley of California, was considerable, but disseminated fatal infections were fortunately very rare. Approximately 1,200 cases were reported in 1943, nearly all of which were of the benign primary variety. Owing to the difficulty in recognizing the disease, it is certain that the total was greater than this, and positive coccididoidin tests disclosed many non-apparent infections. As endemic regions were discovered, they were avoided as far as military requirements permitted. Since 1941, this disease has been studied intensively by the Board for the Control of Epidemics and other boards.

Particularly in the tropical theaters, mycotic dermatoses created a serious problem at times because of their interference with the efficiency of the command. While the feet were the usual site of such infections, mycotic otitis externa was observed frequently. Emphasis on simple hygienic measures in the care of the feet was always sufficient to bring the incidence of this form down to a satisfactory level.

While tropical ulcers were encountered with some frequency in certain areas, they were not an important factor in non-effectiveness and usually responded well to therapy. The finding of virulent bacilli in a considerable proportion of such ulcers was reported.

Infectious hepatitis was a vexing disease problem in certain overseas theaters. Although generally a mild disease with a low mortality, it was important to the Army because of its relatively prolonged convalescent period and resulting high non-effective rate. It was formerly thought that infectious hepatitis was spread solely through droplet dissemination from the upper respiratory tract of an infected individual, but studies conducted by commission members of the Army Epidemiological Board both in this country and overseas in close cooperation with Army medical officers have thrown further light on the hitherto obscure epidemiology of this disease, and while not completed, these studies suggest spread also through fecal contamination, and possibly by means of insect vectors.

III

The Medical Department of the Army has long recognized the need for scientific laboratory and field research in order to develop better methods for the control and prevention of disease. It is fortunate that during the period from 1893 to 1902, when so much progress was being made in the basic medical sciences, the Army had as its Surgeon General, George M. Sternberg, who was one of America's great pioneer bacteriologists.

General Sternberg established the Army Medical School, organized boards of medical officers to study the tropical diseases of Cuba, Puerto Rico and the Philippine Islands, and throughout his long service did everything possible to stimulate the spirit of laboratory research in officers of the Medical Department. His influence is reflected in the brilliant achievements of a host of Army officers, including Walter Reed, Gorgas, Ashford, Strong, Russell, Craig, Darnall, Vedder and others who have made many valuable contributions to medical science and especially to military preventive medicine.

Generally speaking, however, medical research in the Army has been limited by inadequate appropriations and personnel, and much of the fundamental investigative work done by medical officers has been carried on under difficult conditions and in spite of many handicaps. Recognizing these difficulties, the Surgeon General, as a part of his plans for World War II, initiated an enormously expanded medical research program, much of which has been executed through non-military agencies by civilian workers.

Early in 1940, when we were faced with the urgent need for better prophylactic and therapeutic agents for the prevention of disease, many of our involved problems were taken to the Division of Medical Sciences of the National Research Council for advice, and later to the Committee on Medical Research of the Office of Scientific Research and Development, which arranged for the necessary investigations. Since that time, the Committee on Medical Research has authorized, financed and supervised many projects for the Medical Department and has spent several million dollars in the search for answers to our problems. The actual investigations have been conducted by a host of civilian scientists working in the various laboratories and institutions of the country.

There have been hundreds of research projects dealing with different aspects of a wide variety of subjects, which include the control of infectious diseases; the discovery of new prophylactic and therapeutic agents against malaria and other tropical diseases; the discovery of effective insecticides and insect repellents; nutrition; fundamental studies of fitness and fatigue; transfusions and blood substitutes; shock; surgery; neuropsychiatry and aviation medicine. Extensive medical research is also being carried on through the Board for the Control of Epidemics, the Army Medical School and various laboratory and field installations of the Army.

This research program has already paid enormous dividends. Within a period of less than three years, the Committee on Medical Research produced three great contributions, any one of which would justify the cost of the entire research program. I refer first to the blood substitutes, particularly plasma, which was used so successfully to combat shock among our wounded soldiers overseas. Second, there was the rapid investigation and development of methods for the wholesale production of penicillin, which at the beginning of this war was little more than a laboratory curiosity. The third great achievement was the development of the Army's effective new insect repellents and insecticides, particularly DDT, which will no doubt prove to be one of the greatest contributions ever made to the future health of humanity.

The investigative work on insecticides and repellents, which had been initiated by the Preventive Medicine Service through the Committee on Medical Research, was done largely by the Bureau of Entomology of the United States Department of Agriculture. Too much credit cannot be given to the able, conscientious and productive labors of the scientists of the Department of Agriculture who worked so well in the experimental laboratory at Orlando, Florida, and produced for the armed forces new and potent weapons against the insect-borne diseases, especially malaria and typhus fever.

At the beginning of the war, the Army had available for the destruction of adult mosquitoes, only the well-known oil sprays containing pyrethrum. As an insect repellent, it had nothing better than oil of citronella, which was both ineffective and unpleasant to use. For the control of lice, it was dependent on the cumbersome and time-consuming methods employed during World War I. Since 1941, thanks to the cooperative research mentioned above, we acquired the most powerful agents ever developed for the control of the disease-bearing insects. These included the standard Army freon-pyrethrum bomb, which was used to destroy adult mosquitoes in barracks, tents and infested native villages, and the Army repellent, which, when applied to the soldiers' skin, repels for several hours the mosquito vectors of malaria, yellow fever, dengue and other serious diseases, and is similarly effective against the species of phlebotomus which transmit sandfly fever, aroya fever and leishmaniasis. It also protects soldiers against the mites which carry scrub typhus. New and revolutionary materials and methods, moreover, have been developed for the mass destruction of the larvae of anopheline mosquitoes.

Similar progress has been made in the production of new agents and methods for use in the destruction of lice, and the control of epidemic typhus fever. Methyl bromide gas was used for the delousing of clothing, employing methods which eliminated the necessity for the heavy, cumbersome sterilizing apparatus employed during World War I. The Army was also provided with a powerful new louse powder known as DDT. This powder was applied to the underclothes of infested individuals, keeping them free from lice for about a month. It can be applied by means of power sprayers inserted into the sleeves and other openings in the clothing, thus making it possible to delouse rapidly the populations of large cities without undressing the individuals. This method was applied practically during the outbreak of typhus in Naples when almost two million civilians were deloused with DDT powder within a period of two months and the epidemic was stopped. This episode is the most dramatic example of preventive medicine in action which occurred during the war.

When one considers the rapidity with which the research agencies of the country were mobilized and produced these new weapons for the prevention of wartime diseases, it is obviously important that plans be made to continue the emergency organizations which made this possible. It is considered essential to the future progress of military preventive medicine that the Office of Scientific Research and Development be continued during the postwar period or that some similar permanent organization be set up to assist the Medical Department in the solution of the important medical problems which remain. In this way the peacetime Army can further improve its preventive medicine program and be even better prepared to guard the health of our troops in any future war. Such an arrangement for directed cooperative medical research would also play an important role in strengthening the future health program of the nation.

Most of the diseases which occur among military personnel are derived from either direct or indirect contact with infected civilians. The Preventive Medicine Service therefore was actively concerned with the attempt to decrease the transfer of diseases to soldiers from such sources.

In this country the Army had the assistance of all Federal, State and local civilian health agencies. These agencies not only carried out the normal civilian health program for the the country, but they also participated actively by providing intensive extra-military sanitation and disease control in the areas surrounding all military camps, posts and stations. In certain foreign countries, where civilian health agencies were available and cooperative, similar arrangements were made locally. Naturally, close cooperation between the Army and the civilian health agencies was necessary in order to make such a program effective. For example, all cases of venereal disease contracted by soldiers in this country were reported to the civilian health authorities so that they could trace the sources of infection and treat the women responsible for spreading such diseases.

In order to guard the health of the great army of industrial workers who manufactured the munitions required by our troops, the Surgeon General, through the Division of Occupational Health, built up a special medical service to care for the civilian workers in Army-owned and operated industrial plants. This organization provided emergency medical care for the workers and maintained a group of industrial engineers who surveyed Army plants for occupational hazards and recommended the proper action to eliminate them. In this way the Army contributed to the health of more than a million civilian war workers.

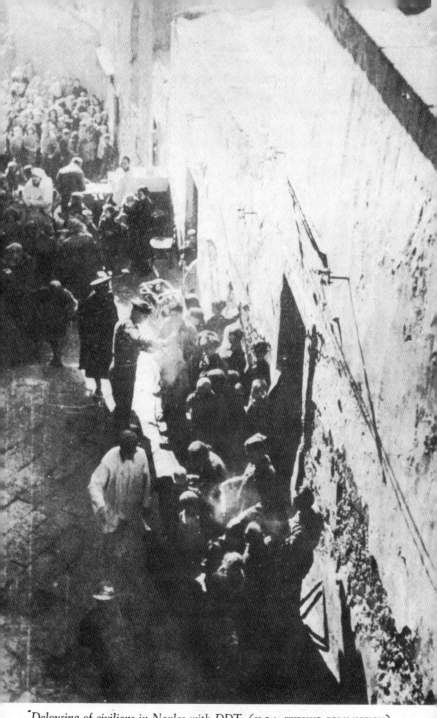

Delousing of civilians in Naples with DDT. (U.S.A. TYPHUS COMMISSION)

This native was suffering extreme malnutrition when he came into American hands as the Japanese were pushed back. He improved rapidly under the Army's careful diet. In this photo, he can scarcely stand. (SIGNAL CORPS PHOTO)

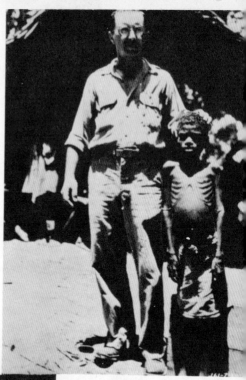

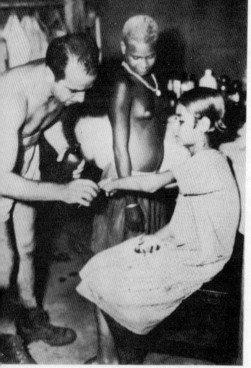

Native girl being treated for yaws by an Army medical soldier, Corporal Ralph Pierre, Wimber, Pennsylvania.

(U.S. ARMY AIR FORCES PHOTO)

Similar services for workers in contractor-owned and operated plants were provided by various civilian agencies with the assistance of industrial medical experts of the United States Public Health Service.

Through the Division of Civil Public Health of the Preventive Medicine Service, the Army undertook to provide a certain measure of health protection to the civilian populations of countries liberated or conquered during the war. This service is limited to the period of military occupation or government and includes such health activities as may be considered necessary in order to protect American troops in those countries or to assist in future military activities. For example, the health program of a liberated country might require intensive work to relieve starvation and to stamp out an epidemic such as the typhus outbreak in Naples, but it would probably not include a long-term program of tuberculosis control. The activities of the Civil Affairs Division include the preparation of detailed plans for the health programs of many countries throughout the world during the period of military government.

The primary purpose of the Army's health activities is the conservation of manpower during wartime. These activities, however, will ultimately exert a profound influence on the health of the civil population of this country. Millions of young men will return to civil life who are physically stronger, who have been immunized against various diseases, and, more important still, who have received training or orientation in the fundamentals of sanitation and hygiene. New therapeutic and prophylactic agents and procedures developed during the war will be available for civil use. The thousands of medical officers and men who have participated in the aspects of the Army's health program will return possessing new skills and interests. All these factors should contribute to the further strengthening of preventive medicine and stimulate the development of more effective objectives in civil public health. Thus it can be predicted with assurance that the Army's program of military preventive medicine will contribute richly to the further strengthening of the total health program of our nation.

Again and again doctors call attention with pride to the fact that anywhere from 9 to 15 per cent of men who were wounded in previous wars died of their wounds, whereas reports from various engagements in this war show a mortality among the wounded of only 1 to 3 per cent. Much of the amazing accomplishment in surgery in World War II is due to Brigadier General Fred W. Rankin, Chief Consulting Surgeon of the United States Army, a man who had already achieved the highest honors available to American physicians and who gave up his private practice, his hospital and his home to organize surgery for the benefit of our wounded.

For many years Fred Rankin was one of the leading physicians of the Mayo Clinic and a professor of surgery in the University of Minnesota School of Medicine. In World War I, he served as a major in the Medical Corps for seventeen months, attached to several divisions in France, as a commanding officer of a base hospital. He has been president of practical all the important surgical organizations in the United States and also of the American Medical Association. He is the author of half a dozen books dealing with surgery. In his chapter in "Doctors at War," he tells of the miracles wrought by surgery, the story of shock, plastic surgery, blood transfusion, transportation of the wounded, and all the other factors that have yielded such magnificent results.

CHAPTER VII

AMERICAN SURGEONS AT WAR

By

BRIGADIER GENERAL FRED W. RANKIN

Chief Consulting Surgeon, United States Army

I

THE TIRED LITTER-BEARERS entered the shock ward of the tented emergency hospital and gently placed the wounded soldier on wooden sawhorses. They had picked him up only a few hours previously after he was struck in the abdomen by a hand grenade fragment as he was attempting to flank a machine-gun nest which was finally destroyed by the soldiers he was leading.

The din of battle still raged not more than 1,500 yards away, but neither this nor the angry roaring of planes overhead interfered with the efficient, smoothly functioning teamwork of the hospital's personnel. The medical officer was already inserting a needle into the vein of the wounded soldier, and a medical corpsman was hanging up the bottle of plasma on a line slung across the tent, from which other bottles of this life-giving fluid were hanging opposite the row of wounded soldiers. From the soldier's finger another medical corpsman was taking a drop of blood which would be used to check the soldier's blood type and make certain that the right bottle of citrated whole blood from the blood bank would be used. The pale, wan face, the cold, clammy skin and the feeble, fluttering pulse made it evident that the soldier was in shock. But within a few minutes after the plasma started flowing into his veins, the color was flooding back into his face and the pulse began to slow down and become stronger.

Soon afterwards the medical officer gave the order to move him to the operating room, where the surgeon and his operating team were waiting. The soldier was placed on the operating table, and to the needle still inserted in the vein of his arm, which was now outstretched and supported by a board, a tube leading from a bottle of blood was attached. At the head of the table the anesthetist began administering the anesthetic, and in a few minutes the patient was ready. A medical corpsman removed the first-aid dressing and cleansed and prepared the area. The drapes were applied, the lights adjusted, the surgeon picked up the scalpel and the operation began.

Several weeks later, this wounded soldier, with the healthy smile of recovery on his face, was sitting up in bed in a cool, spotless ward in one of the Army's great general hospitals here at home, awaiting the second stage operation which would make him completely well and perfectly normal again.

This incident is not unique; thousands of similar experiences could be recounted, many of which are more dramatic. Had this soldier been similarly wounded in the last war, his chances of recovery would have been very slim. First, he probably would have died of shock; had he survived this, he would almost certainly have died of peritonitis. In the last war, of every ten men wounded in the abdomen, only about three or four recovered; in this war, we saved seven or eight. Even more striking is the difference between the survival rates of penetrating chest wounds in these two wars. In the last war, only about five out of every ten soldiers with such wounds lived, whereas in this war nine were saved. By 1944, the over-all mortality rate in the Army for wounded soldiers was only a little more than 3 per cent, which means that we saved 97 out of every 100 soldiers wounded in battle. This sets a record in military history, the significance of which may be better appreciated by comparison with the figure of more than 8 per cent in the last war, or with the figure of almost 14 per cent in the Civil War. Thus, despite the fact that the military agents used in this war were far more powerful and deadly than those employed in any previous war, the survival rate among our wounded was much higher than it had ever been.

There are a number of factors involved in the establishment and maintenance of this gratifying record. Essentially it was the result of a carefully planned and intensively applied program of medical care which extended from the front line of battle to the general hospitals here at home. Among the most important factors contributing to the success of the program were thorough training, careful organization and intelligent utilization of personnel; advancing hospital facilities as close to the line of battle as possible in order to provide prompt and specialized surgical treatment; the fullest use of the most modern developments and the most effective therapeutic measures of medical science; and the unexcelled functional performance of our young medical officers and medical corpsmen, whose proficient skill, devotion to duty, and high courage inspired everyone.

To return for a moment to the case of the wounded soldier already cited, observe how these factors were instrumental in saving his life. Only a few hours after being hit, this soldier was getting the type of surgical care that was absolutely essential in order to save his life. It is not sufficient to speak of early operation. Equally important are the judgment and technical skill employed in the operation. Never before in the history of warfare had battle casualties received such prompt surgical care by such highly skilled specialists. This was undoubtedly the most important consideration in the Army's program for the medical care of the wounded. It was made possible by a combination of two factors: first, the plan of medical service in the combat zone; and second, the availability and proper utilization of young, formally trained medical officers. The first factor was keynoted by the well-established principle that the sooner a wounded man gets proper surgical treatment, the more successful is the result.

The implementation and successful operation of this plan, however, were dependent upon the presence of formally trained young surgeons who were well qualified in their respective surgical specialties. The availability of these young surgeons was of paramount importance, and was a reflection of our carefully nurtured system of postgraduate medical education. It was the outward manifestation of the assiduous efforts of our civilian medical teaching centers during the past two decades to standardize and formulate more effective and suitable programs of postgraduate medical education. The result of these efforts was the production of a group of young professional men who were not only qualified to perform delicate operative procedures, but more important, were schooled and well grounded in the fundamental principles upon which good surgical practice depends.

These were the young medical officers who staffed our forward medical installations, and whose talents and skills yielded such high dividends in terms of lives saved. Just as their courage, their inspiring devotion to duty, and their ready adaptability to difficult situations were in every way worthy of their profession, so their proficient skill and excellent functional performance was a tribute to the American educational system which produced them.

It must be recognized, however, that the availability of these skillful and highly trained young surgeons became effective only if they were intelligently used. This was accomplished by the plan of medical services in the forward area, and particularly the organization of evacuation services. The plan of medical care in advanced battle zones was based upon the principle that the sooner a wounded man receives adequate first aid and subsequent definitive surgery, the more successful are the results. Accordingly, the formally trained, active, alert young surgeons went to the wounded while they were being evacuated toward centers where they could be properly treated. These surgeons, grouped in teams and working in portable surgical hospitals or in mobile field hospitals, were placed far forward, so that under favorable conditions wounded men were operated upon a very short time after injury. Even farther back, at the evacuation hospitals, the average time between receipt of injury and operation was often less than ten hours.

It is difficult to appreciate the full significance of this forward surgery plan or the problems and obstacles encountered in its practical realization. A global conflict, keynoted by a high degree of mechanization and mobility, with battlegrounds on terrain as varied as the face of nature, immediately posed numerous medico-military problems in the adequate care of the wounded. Certain types of engagements were characterized by a wide dispersal and rapid progression of troops which left the wounded scattered over a large area, and even a constantly moving first-aid station found it difficult to keep up with the advance. These wounded had to be sought on the battlefield where they lay after being hit, and in mountainous or jungle terrain the difficulties of their transportation were greatly increased, since this could often be accomplished only by litter carry. In some sections it required as many as eight teams of litter-bearers to transport one wounded soldier.

This is admittedly a fatiguing and time-consuming means of transportation, but in certain regions where the war carried us, it became absolutely necessary. In the dank, impenetrable jungles of New Guinea, there are no roadways, only indistinct native trails, and in some areas it was necessary literally to hack pathways through the jungle. Rivers and deep ravines could often be crossed only by rafts or by a suspension or hanging bridge. The time lag between the occurrence of the injury and the administration of proper surgical treatment was greatly increased by the difficulties of reaching and transporting the wounded in many battle areas.

The newer developments in the type and power of ordnance used in this war were also important considerations. Bombs, mines, booby-traps and mortar and shell fire were far more powerful and destructive than military agents used in previous wars. In this war, 80 per cent of the wounds were produced by such agents and only 20 per cent by bullets, whereas in the last great war it was 30 to 40 per cent, and in the Civil War 90 per cent of the wounds were caused by bullets, which are much less destructive agents. The change was reflected in this war by a higher incidence of severe injuries, with consequent increased tissue destruction and resultant shock, all of which emphasized further the need for reaching the wounded quickly, handling them gently and treating them promptly. In view of their condition and the impending state of shock, the removal of these wounded from the battlefield to a hospital far to the rear would have been highly undesirable even if it had been possible. It was better to advance the necessary facilities and bring adequate care as near these patients as possible.

Other serious problems in providing adequate care of the wounded, problems unique in this war, arose from amphibious operations. The assault of a well-fortified beach is an especially hazardous operation and considerably magnifies the difficulties of reaching and transporting the wounded and of rendering adequate treatment. Armed only with their first-aid packs, the medical units often landed on the beaches with the combat troops and carried out their mission of rendering first aid and evacuating the wounded in the face of withering enemy fire.

There were many difficulties encountered in this war which delayed treatment, imposed hardships and impeded the administration of adequate care of the wounded. The program of medical care in the forward area was designed to overcome these difficulties and to reduce to a minimum the period between injury and treatment by advancing and utilizing highly mobile installations, thus shortening the distance between first-aid stations and facilities having the personnel and equipment for emergency surgical treatment. These mobile units were staffed with well-trained surgeons who performed life-saving operations. The speed of evacuation was also increased constantly. All efforts were directed toward providing the wounded with a high level of professional care as early and as far forward as possible.

II

A brief description of the links in this chain of medical care in combat zones may provide better appreciation of the service. Treatment of the wounded in forward areas may be divided into two phases: the primary or urgent phase directed toward saving life and making the patient transportable, and the secondary or more definitive phase concerned with the performance of emergency surgical procedures. The former consists essentially of first-aid measures, arresting hemorrhage, applying occlusive dressings and splints, and administering sulfonamides to prevent infection, morphine to relieve pain, and plasma to combat shock. The medical units which perform these urgent functions are the battalion aid stations and the collecting and clearing companies. However, provision for the performance of emergency life-saving operations is made in these units by attaching to certain clearing stations surgical teams properly staffed and equipped to perform these procedures. All patients requiring surgical care whose condition permits transportation are sent to the evacuation hospital.

The procedure may best be described by following the wounded soldier from the time of injury until he is admitted to the evacuation hospital. All soldiers receive instruction in the principles of first aid, which they may apply in treating themselves or their comrades. The Medical Department also has company aid men who have been specially trained in rendering first aid. These men proceed immediately behind and, as prevously indicated, sometimes actually with fighting troops. It is their function to seek out the injured on the battlefield and to render first aid by applying dressing to the wounds and by relieving pain and making the wounded as comfortable as possible until litter-bearers can come up and take them to nearby battalion aid stations. Here their condition is carefully assessed by a medical officer, who, if he finds it necessary, may administer plasma to combat shock, redress the

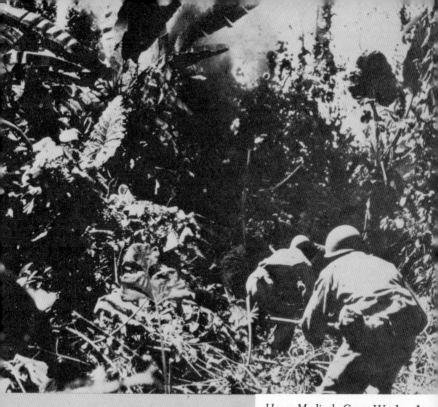

How Medical Care Works, I.—Patrol advances in a Southwest Pacific jungle. A Japanese mortar shell drops just ahead; enemy snipers are busy.
(SIGNAL CORPS PHOTO)

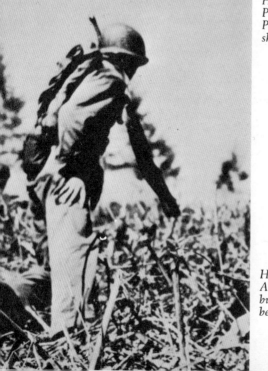

How Medical Care Works, II— A soldier is hit, grabs his hip where bullet entered, cries out that he has been hit. (SIGNAL CORPS PHOTO)

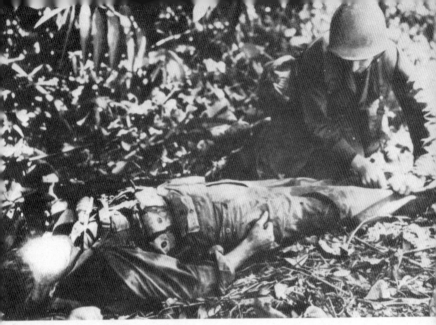

*How Medical Care Works, III.—Medical Corps aid man hears wounded man's cry,
finds him quickly, begins work.* (SIGNAL CORPS PHOTO)

How Medical Care Works, IV.—Soldier's wound is dressed. (SIGNAL CORPS PHOTO)

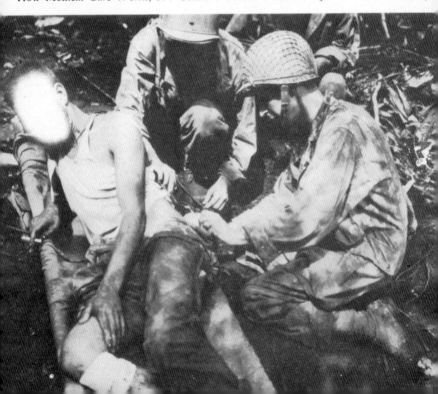

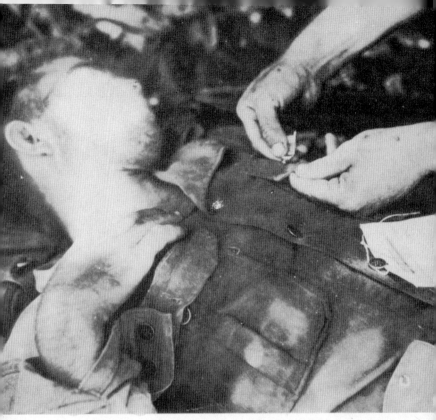

ow Medical Care Works, V.—First-aid man pins morphine syrette on jacket of ɪunded man. Tag on jacket button also shows he has been given morphine, contains other pertinent information. (SIGNAL CORPS PHOTO)

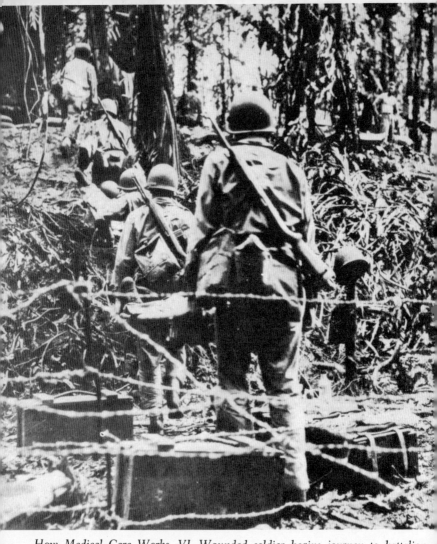

How Medical Care Works, VI—Wounded soldier begins journey to battalion station just behind front lines. Litter-bearers work carefully. (SIGNAL CORPS PHOT

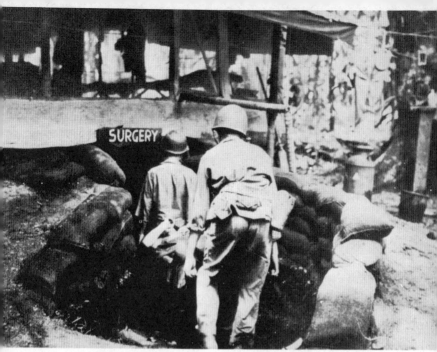

How Medical Care Works, VII.—From battalion aid station, soldier is taken by jeep to clearing station and carried to underground surgery room, which is protected from anything but direct hit. (SIGNAL CORPS PHOTO)

How Medical Care Works, VIII.—Soldier is made ready, anesthetic administered, and surgeons begin work. (SIGNAL CORPS PHOTO)

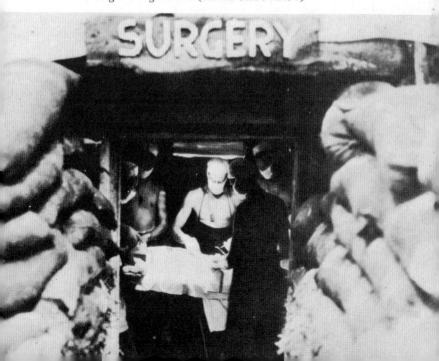

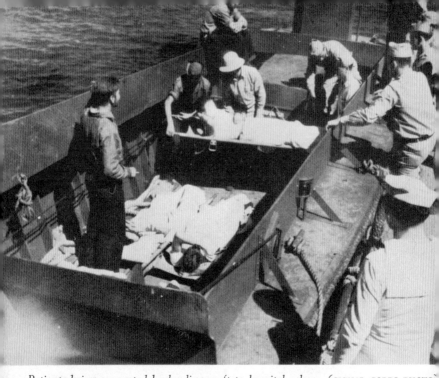

Patients being evacuated by landing craft to hospital ashore. (SIGNAL CORPS PHOTO)

Patients getting blood plasma in shock ward of a field hospital. (SIGNAL CORPS PHOTO)

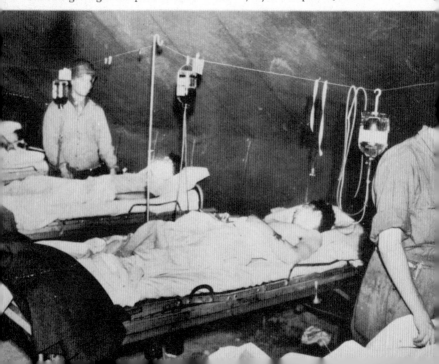

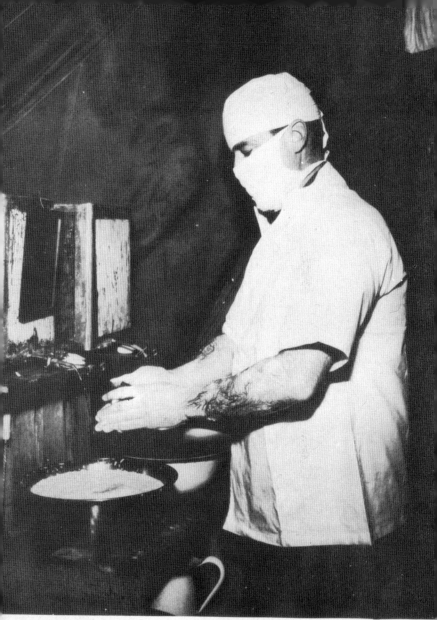

island base hospital, doctor washes hands in hot water from two five-gallon cans. Coal stove heats water. The scene is Alaska, 1942. (SIGNAL CORPS PHOTO)

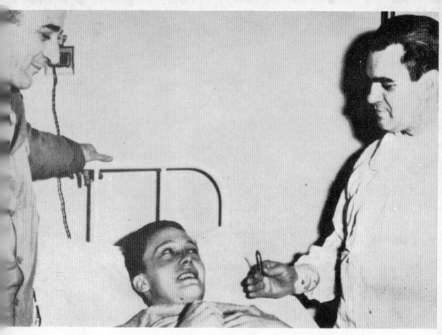

Lieutenant Paul R. Breeding, Hillsboro, Texas, Flying Fortress Pilot, sees armor-piercing bullet removed from his abdomen by Major Leslie G. Dodson, Owensboro, Kentucky, who holds the 2¼-inch steel missile. (U. S. ARMY AIR FORCES PHOTO)

Operating room of 94th Evacuation Hospital, while it was attached to the Fift in Italy, December, 1943. (MUSEUM AND MEDICAL ARTS SERVICE)

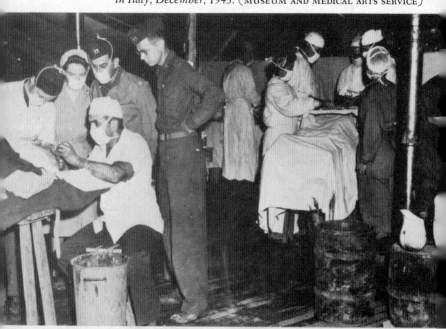

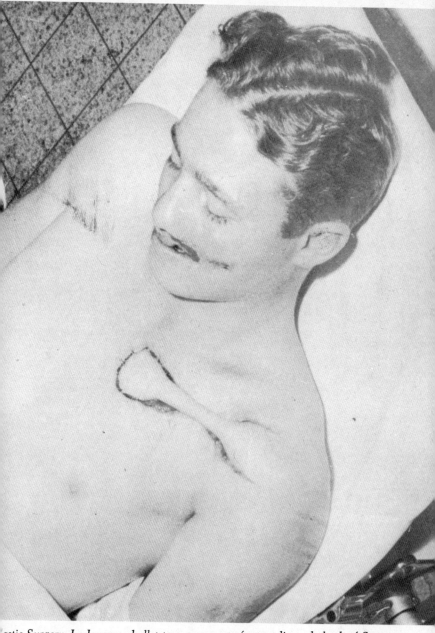

Plastic Surgery, I.—Japanese bullet tore away part of upper lip and cheek of Sergeant Carl W. McCracken, USMC, of Freedom, Pennsylvania, during Tulagi landings. Doctors at U. S. Naval Hospital, San Diego, prepared a flap from his shoulder preliminary to grafting new skin on his face. (OFFICIAL U. S. NAVY PHOTO)

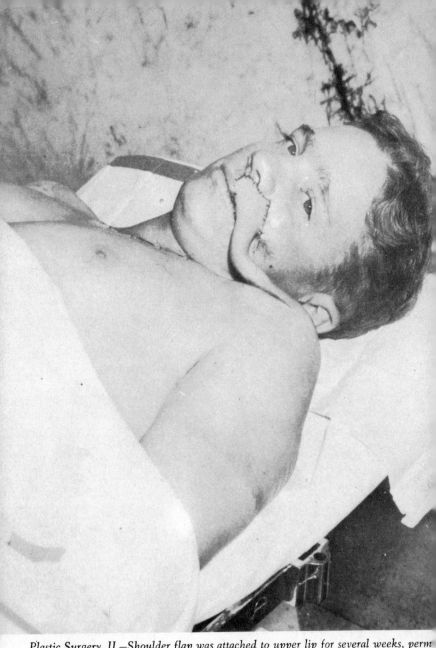

Plastic Surgery, II.—Shoulder flap was attached to upper lip for several weeks, permitting it to take hold and become a live part of face. (OFFICIAL U. S. NAVY PHOTO)

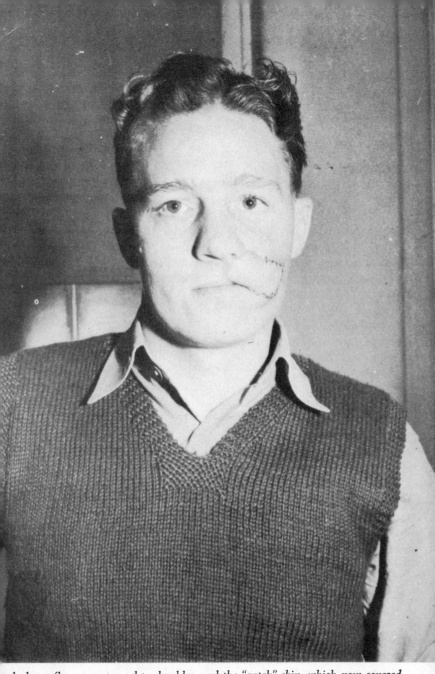

eeks later, flap was returned to shoulder, and the "patch" skin, which now covered the bullet hole, was prepared for trimming. (OFFICIAL U. S. NAVY PHOTO)

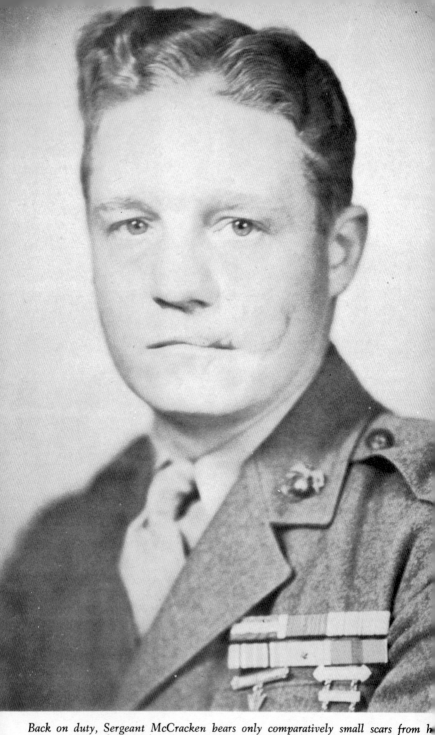

Back on duty, Sergeant McCracken bears only comparatively small scars from h[
wound. Even these traces will probably disappear in a few years.

wound, assure the arrest of hemorrhage, apply or adjust splints, administer sulfonamides and determine priority of evacuation.

As soon as the condition of the wounded man permits, he is evacuated, usually to the collecting station, by the most readily and suitably available method, which, depending upon regional circumstances, may be by litter-carriers, ambulance or converted jeeps. Since the condition of the wounded can be seriously affected by transportation, and a patient leaving the battalion aid station in a satisfactory condition may arrive at the collecting station in shock, all cases are rechecked here both as to general condition, and as to the condition of the dressing or splints. Further supportive treatment is given those who need it before they are sent to a clearing station, which is usually only a few miles farther to the rear.

The clearing station is equipped to give more elaborate treatment, and usually there is attached to it a mobile surgical unit or a field hospital platoon to care for cases with such desperate wounds that further removal to the rear without surgical treatment would endanger life. The wounded are critically examined and classified according to type of injury and required treatment. Patients in shock or impending shock are admitted to the shock section, where appropriate therapy can be instituted immediately. Those whose wounds need inspection or redressing or whose splints require adjustment are admitted to the surgical section for these purposes. All who require hospital care and can be moved are taken back to an evacuation or field hospital, where facilities and specialists are available to render this type of surgical treatment and the necessary post-operative care. Certain types of wounds, such as head wounds, some forms of chest wounds, and abdominal wounds are given priority in evacuation to the hospital, but as previously indicated, if the injury is such that immediate operation in order to save life is indicated, it may be done here by an attached surgical team. These cases also are sent back to the evacuation hospital as soon after surgery as the condition permits.

The time necessary for a wounded soldier to arrive at an evacuation hospital depends on his condition, the number of casualties, the availability of mobile transportation, the type of terrain, the activity of the enemy over the area, and the supply traffic on roads coming up to the front from the rear. Every effort is directed toward reducing this time, and the treatment of the wounded soldier prior to arrival at the evacuation hospital is designed to save life and limb, promote comfort and deliver him in a condition permitting emergency surgical treatment.

The evacuation hospital, although mobile in character, is fully equipped with all the modern facilities necessary for the performance of good surgery and is staffed by well-trained surgeons and specialists. Here the more definitive phase of emergency surgical treatment is performed. The patient's general condition is assessed, a careful examination is performed with particular attention to the region involved, roentgenographic studies are made according to indications, further supportive measures are applied in accordance with immediate and anticipated needs, and a decision of the type and extent of surgery is made as governed by the injury, the patient's condition, and other factors which may be imposed by the military situation. The surgical management of the wound itself is along well-established principles, and although these fundamental principles in the treatment of wounds are similar no matter how incurred, certain conditions in war preclude the use of some ideal measures and make modifications of certain others necessary.

These principles consist essentially in the prompt arrest of hemorrhage, the prevention and treatment of shock, the prevention of infection and additional trauma, the conversion of a contaminated wound into a clean wound with removal of devitalized tissue and foreign material, the anatomic approximation of the tissues, the splinting of the part to provide and promote local rest and improved circulation, and the furnishing of proper nutrients to permit the normal reparative process to occur without delay. Under ideal conditions and in wounds incurred in civil life, these principles can be rigidly followed, but in military practice there is one important exception. The civilian surgeon, after completing the surgical care of the wound, usually closes it by primary suture because he has operated within a short time following the injury, has had access to a well-appointed operating room, and can keep his patient in the same hospital for close supervision by him and his staff for as long as is necessary. Primary closure of the wound under these circumstances is desirable and proper.

In military practice, however, these ideal conditions rarely exist and the situation confronting the military surgeon is very different. Even under the best conditions, he can rarely operate on his patient as early as is possible in civil life. All war wounds are contaminated and many are badly contaminated. Although the operating room is well equipped, it may be in a tent or in an improvised shelter with a dirt floor. Except in unusual instances, the patient will not remain long under the constant supervision of the surgeon who operates on him in the forward hospital, since in order to make room for incoming casualties and to maintain mobility of such forward medical installations, the patient must be evacuated farther back. Under these circumstances, considerable danger from serious infection attends the primary closure of these wounds and experience has demonstrated that, except for a few special types, war wounds should never be closed immediately after débridement. Accordingly, the wound is allowed to remain open, vaseline gauze dressing is placed gently into the wound but not packed in tightly, and the part is splinted. A stimulating or "booster" dose of tetanus toxoid is routinely administered.

The efficacy of this procedure is shown by the fact that no case of tetanus occurred in American soldiers who had been properly immunized and had received those tetanus toxoid injections—a striking contrast to the last war, when tetanus was such a serious problem.

In many of these wounds, secondary closure can be performed safely within a week to ten days. Thus, in this method of leaving the wounds open at the first stage, immediately after the operation, and closing them at a second stage, when the danger of infection is past, the objective of good healing and early restoration of function is safely and soundly achieved. In addition to these principles in the surgical management of wounds of the soft parts, there are certain procedures applicable to special types of regional wounds, such as those of the head, face, chest, abdomen and the extremities. These are usually dealt with by surgeons well trained in the surgery of these special regions.

Up to this stage in the chain of medical care in the forward area, the wounded soldier has been brought from the very front line of battle, where he received first aid and the primary phases of treatment, to a hospital a few miles in the rear, where he was given emergency surgical treatment. By combining speed of evacuation with advancement of hospital facilities, it has been possible to apply life-saving surgery and minimize the grave complications that might otherwise develop.

This general plan of forward medical service is followed whenever possible, but it must not be regarded as a rigid but rather as a flexible plan which can be readily adapted to meet the varied demands which may be imposed by military strategy or terrain. In some situations it may be necessary for collecting stations to function as clearing stations and the latter as evacuation hospitals. This is readily done by attaching mobile surgical units or the auxiliary surgical groups, which are composed of specialized surgical teams including surgeons highly trained in neurosurgery, maxillo-facial and plastic surgery, orthopedic surgery, chest surgery and general surgery.

To meet this purpose and to cope with the limited transportation facilities characteristic of jungle warfare, portable surgical hospitals that can be transported by human carriers over jungle trails are used. These units consist of four medical officers and twenty-five enlisted men with special training in nursing, sanitation, jungle hygiene and other essential functions in the operation of such a compact hospital. They carry their own mess facilities, tentage, special jungle equipment and the medical supplies required in the performance of major surgical emergencies and other medical functions.

A medical officer described his experience in such a hospital as follows:

"The personnel and equipment were transported to the combat zone by air. Native carriers took the equipment and supplies the last few miles from the air strip to the site of operation, which was the only spot above water in an extensive area of swamp within 'litter-carry' of the battalion aid stations. It had the advantages of cover from overhead observation and the fact that many of the wounded reached it within one to three hours after injury. This schedule varied with the depth of the mud in the trail. The casualties were usually brought back in daylight, because of various hazards on the trail after dark, but a few seriously wounded were brought in at night, much to the credit of the members of the collecting company of the medical battalion.

"The organization relieved a similar one which had been on a long, exhausting march and utilized its tentage temporarily. The constant arrival of wounded allowed no time for expansion during the change-over. As equipment arrived by native carrier over the next two days, it was installed as time permitted. Rain and overflow of the nearby river produced mud six to ten inches deep over most of the hospital area. Both standard pyramidal tents and large wall tent flies were used to shelter patients. Tent flies were used for operating pavilions, since they gave more head space and caught what breeze there was—an important consideration. All tables, stands and other furniture were made by the detachment from the pandanus and bamboo in the vicinity. The detachment slept in individual 'jungle beds,' three feet off the ground with a roof of shelter halves. Army cots were available for the patients.

"A nearby stream supplied the water, which was double-chlorinated in Lister bags after standing to allow sedimentation. Four of these thirty-six-gallon containers were in constant use, including one for passing troops on the main trail, which ran through the hospital area. Latrine facilities comprised straddle trenches dug in series in a deserted native garden. The depth of the trenches was limited by the shallow ground water level.

"The food for patients and personnel consisted largely of C rations, to which a small amount of canned fruit or fruit juice was added for the patients when the air transport could spare cargo space. Heated in water in the cans, the rations were opened only just before eating, to avoid contamination by flies. This ration, thus used, was an important factor in the low incidence of gastro-enteritis which prevailed. All heating in the mess was done over gasoline burners. The lack of 'white' gasoline, however, resulted in rapid deterioration of the burners. Food spoiled rapidly after removal from the cans, and none could be preserved from meal to meal. All garbage was buried immediately. Incineration was impossible, because of lack of fuel and danger of detection of the smoke."

The difficulties encountered and the ingenuity and improvisations used in overcoming them in providing adequate care and evacuation of the wounded in other war sectors are thus described by another medical officer:

"The methods used during the offensive phase on Guadalcanal were as varied as the terrain and the situation. Hand-carrying, as previously stated, was usually the initial phase, and such hand-carrying was oftentimes of extremely great length over difficult terrain. Another complicating factor in this particular regard was brought about by the hostile force. Since the route of evacuation was often the route of supply for the combat troops, the litter-bearers were quite frequently subjected to sniper and machine-gun firing. As a result, on several occasions, patients who were being brought back by litter squads were wounded in transit by sniper fire. It also happened that quite frequently aid stations and collecting stations were subjected to all types of enemy fire. This particular factor made it necessary to arm the collecting personnel of the regiment. It was found that due to the hard physical labor imposed in carrying these patients, the litter-bearers were unable to carry rifles. It was obvious that the ideal weapon would have been the issue pistol, but unfortunately these were not available. To provide for the safety of the litter squads and the patients, a non-commissioned officer and one enlisted man were added to each litter-carrying party. The two additional personnel were equipped with a Thompson sub-machine gun and a rifle, respectively. This precaution proved quite satisfactory.

"Additional transportation of wounded could only be accomplished in many instances by having the litter-bearers carry along with them infantry entrenching tools and machetes. With the aid of these tools, footing could often be established where it would otherwise be impossible.

"Due to the absence of roads and the extremely difficult type of terrain, oftentimes the only vehicle that could be employed for the evacuation of patients was the converted one-quarter-ton reconnaissance-car ambulance. In these operations, two types of this vehicle were employed. One was a modification introduced by this regiment which carried three litter patients and one sitting patient, plus an orderly and driver. The other type was developed by Commander Moore, of the Navy Medical Department, and was accepted and operated by that service for use in forward evacuation. The work done by these vehicles was outstanding. Oftentimes they were driven to within 100 yards of the firing line and actually picked the patients up where they were hit and removed them from the field. At other times, where there was any suggestion of road net available, the reconnaissance-car ambulance was used to evacuate patients from the battalion aid station to the collecting station. There were very few situations under which this type of vehicle could not operate.

"In several instances, reconnaissance parties from the liaison section of the battalion found that many of the jungle trails could be by-passed and the streams running lateral to the coast could be used to great advantage to reduce the time required for evacuation. This was accomplished by the use of rubber boats furnished by the combat engineers, and capable of carrying an average of two litter patients or six sitting patients. These boats were manned by ambulance section personnel and were paddled downstream to an ambulance loading point. This system was improved by obtaining captured Japanese wooden collapsible assault boats and fitting them with outboard motors. When these were obtained, small numbers of patients were handled by the Japanese boats alone, and larger numbers were evacuated by towing rubber boats behind the Japanese boats.

"Another innovation was the use of tank lighters furnished by the Navy, and running these lighters along the coast and approximating as closely as possible a directing point just to the rear of the infantry front line. At these directing points, a collecting station or part of a station was set up to prepare patients for water transportation. Additional methods of evacuation required the use of motor torpedo boats from otherwise inaccessible points, and at times the use of Navy flying boats. In these particular cases, the rescue parties were officer and enlisted personnel from the collecting battalion. Plasma was always carried along with morphine, dressings and splints for these patients.

"An additional aid to evacuation was furnished on several occasions by the ingenuity of the enlisted personnel of the litter sections, working in conjunction with the combat engineers. Among these improvisations was the use of a steel cable to which a Stokes litter was attached on a pulley and a patient carried by this means from one ridge line to another in order to by-pass practically impassable ravines. Ropes were also used in some situations for the same purpose. Another improvisation was the use of a Stokes litter reinforced on the bottom with planks. This particular litter, attached to a rope, was slid down a long muddy slope, which was otherwise impassable for four days due to rain, and the litter was returned to the top of the hill by the use of the same rope after the patients were transferred at the bottom of the grade. This method proved very satisfactory and unusually safe, inasmuch as the mud formed a makeshift toboggan chute.

"Another method of evacuation was used in an attempt to keep up with the later phases of the offensive. At this time, the infantry troops were averaging two to three miles advance per day. The common method used was continually to advance companies through other companies which were already in line. The units which were passed through then took up the beach defense, protecting the rear of the advancing troops. To meet this situation, the common practice was to leapfrog either part or all of one collecting company through another, giving to one company the responsibility for evacuating the advancing troops and to the other company the responsibility for evacuating the beach defense section. Since the lack of transportation made it impossible for the clearing companies to follow this rapid advance, the collecting company which supported the beach defense also established a small hospital capable of performing life-saving surgical procedures and hospitalizing patients for periods up to 36 or 48 hours. This method proved quite satisfactory.

"Another problem of the collecting battalion was the necessity for providing evacuation for naval casualties and also ambulance and evacuation service for the airports. This was accomplished by placing an ambulance on 24-hour duty at each of the airports and by establishing in the vicinity of the naval operations section a small portion of one collecting company with sufficient equipment to provide for patients for periods up to three or four hours. This particular station was designated as an ambulance waiting station and was used to receive casualties brought in by litter, torpedo, or flying boats and served only to house and treat those patients until such time as ambulances were available."

Still other adaptations may be necessary, as, for example, in amphibious operations. Here, hospital ships that have as their primary function the transportation of the wounded can be converted to perform the function of an evacuation hospital. It may be observed, therefore, that even under the most adverse conditions and the most difficult and varied combat operations, it was possible by certain adaptations and modifications to advance hospital facilities and thus provide the prompt and highly trained surgical care of the wounded so essential in achieving successful results.

Following the receipt of emergency surgical treatment in the evacuation hospital, and as soon as is permitted by the patient's condition, the wounded soldier is evacuated to the general hospital, which is the next link in the chain of medical care. This is done by the most readily available means, including ambulances, converted jeeps, trucks or hospital trains. In some regions, especially in amphibious and insular operations, this is provided by the multipurpose hospital ships. In others, particularly in relatively inaccessible areas with limited and arduous transportation facilities, air transports have proved extremely useful and are playing an increasingly important role in the evacuation of the wounded.

The general hospitals are comparatively large installations of one thousand beds or more, usually located under more stable conditions well behind the line of combat. Possessing all the modern equipment and facilities for performing the most highly specialized surgical care, the professional staffs of many of these hospitals in this war came directly from the ranks of our medical universities and teaching centers and represented the most talented and experienced men of our profession. The medical schools of this country were extraordinarily liberal with their faculties in reincarnating these hospitals, which were staffed from their ranks in World War I. The establishment of these units was cheerfully done, in spite of the recognition by the affiliated institutions that the withdrawal from their faculties and staffs would seriously deplete their personnel and put a great strain on their functional capacities.

For contributing at least half their teaching strength, exerting every effort to obtain replacements from older or physically disqualified men or from women physicians, and for resolutely accepting greater responsibilities and accelerated curricula, the medical schools of this country deserve singular and unqualified commendation.

The function of these general hospitals in the care of the wounded consists essentially in the application of further and more definitive surgical treatment. Patients whose injury is such that further surgical treatment would permit their return to duty within a few months are treated accordingly. However, if the injury is such that return to duty within this specified period is not considered possible, or that prolonged hospitalization is required, as, for example, in the case of a fractured femur or of one requiring reconstructive plastic surgery, treatment is directed toward preparing the patient for evacuation to the general hospitals here at home.

The exceptionally well-qualified staffs of these hospitals and their highly trained specialists in all fields of surgery permit the performance of every type of definitive surgery. The steadily increasing numbers of wounded returned to duty in theaters of operation attested their high level of professional performance. This is an important military factor, since these are battle-tested, experienced soldiers whose return to the ranks of their combat crews adds strength to a fighting force.

Following their discharge from the general hospital, many of these patients are sent to nearby convalescent centers, where they are physically reconditioned in order to prepare them for combat duty. Other patients who require prolonged hospitalization or whose injuries preclude further military service are evacuated to the general hospitals here at home by transports, hospital ships and even air transport as soon as their condition permits.

The general hospitals here constitute the final link in this chain of medical care of the wounded. Arriving at ports of debarkation, wounded evacuees are immediately sent to nearby general hospitals, where a careful appraisal of their condition is made and appropriate supportive therapy given. Depending upon the type of injury and the locality of the home of the wounded soldier, the patients are sent in hospital trains to certain general hospitals in the interior. Specialized centers have been established for the treatment of certain types of injuries. Every effort is made to have the soldier sent to the hospital nearest his home.

In 1944, there were fifty-eight of these general hospitals strategically located in practically every part of the country. Equipped with all modern facilities and staffed by highly competent surgeons in all the specialized fields of surgery, these general hospitals provide soldiers with the best treatment known to medical science. For the treatment of certain conditions and types of injuries in which the highest degree of specialization is necessary, some of these hospitals have been designated as specialized centers. These include five centers for plastic and ophthalmologic surgery, six for chest surgery, eighteen for neurosurgery, three for vascular surgery, seven for amputations and two each for the rehabilitation of the blind and the deaf. Here the wounded soldier receives the final phases of definitive surgical care. All the resources available to medical science have been mobilized and focused here in an effort to restore the wounded so far as possible to a normal physical and functional capacity.

III

This description of the successive links in the chain of medical care of the wounded, extending from the front line of battle to the hospitals at home, may give the reader some conception of the magnitude of this problem and an appreciation of the manner in which it has been met. It is this plan and the intensive way it is being applied that have contributed so much to the gratifying record set in care of the wounded. In addition, the full use of certain modern developments in medical therapy has played an important role in the establishment of that record. Among the most important of these are blood plasma and blood transfusion in the control of shock, chemotherapeutic agents, such as the sulfonamides and penicillin, in combating infection, better and more effective methods in the repair of injured nerves and defects of the skull, more rational therapeutic measures in the treatment of burns, and improved technical developments in the immediate and subsequent treatment of chest wounds, abdominal wounds, vascular injuries, etc.

The development of blood plasma for use by the armed forces is undoubtedly one of the important contributions to military medicine. Sustaining life until adequate surgical treatment can be given, this truly vital agent has tipped the scales against death in more cases than we shall ever know. The military advantages of dried plasma lie in the fact that it can be preserved for long periods under all conditions, administered quickly without preliminary delaying compatibility tests, transported readily to the far corners of the fighting fronts, and thus made immediately available for emergency treatment in the field as well as in the hospital.

These advantages of plasma were quickly recognized and extensive preparations made for its provision even before the onset of war. Subsequent developments amply justified the soundness of this program. The work of the American Red Cross in the development and implementation of this program deserves much praise.

Although blood plasma has been of tremendous value in the control of shock, its limitations in the treatment of patients who have had extensive hemorrhage should be recognized. In such cases, whole blood transfusions are necessary, and the Army developed a plan to make whole blood available for these patients far forward in the combat zone. In these cases, plasma was used early in the front lines, at the first-aid stations, and during the evacuation to control shock and sustain life until they reached the forward hospitals, where emergency surgery could be done. There whole blood transfusions were used to supplement the extensive loss of blood. In this way, shock was controlled and life sustained until adequate treatment could be provided.

Chemotherapy also contributed materially to the exceptionally low mortality and morbidity rates in our Army. The value of the sulfonamides in controlling infections had already been hailed before the onset of war, and great confidence was placed in these drugs as a means of controlling infections in war wounds. At the same time, however, it was thought best to determine accurately the efficacy of these measures. Accordingly, extensive clinical studies on traumatic wounds were instituted through the medium of the National Research Council. On the basis of these investigations, which represented the largest and most carefully controlled experiment of its kind ever undertaken, it was concluded that while systemic administration of the sulfonamides would undoubtedly control the spread of infection, their ability to control local infection in a wound was minimal.

Although this may at first seem disappointing, it should be realized that it is an important observation. Since spreading infections are much more serious problems than local wound infections, the observation provides us with the heartening fact that here we have a means of adequately coping with spreading infections. Moreover, this has been amply confirmed by clinical experience in the field. Although many surgeons continued to frost the wound with sulfanilamide, the beneficial effects of the drug when applied locally, were questioned by careful observers and greater reliance was placed on their systemic effect following oral or parenteral administration to prevent general sepsis or spreading infection.

Another development in chemotherapy which appears to be of much greater importance is penicillin. Even before the war, preliminary observations by the relatively few workers in this field had revealed its highly promising therapeutic potentialities, but the difficulties involved in its large-scale production made widespread use prohibitively expensive.

However, in view of the encouraging reports of its efficacy, even in low concentrations, against a wide variety of important pathogenic organisms, many of which are resistant to the sulfonamides, the great value and military significance of penicillin became evident. Accordingly, strenuous efforts were immediately directed toward its development in increasing quantities so that extensive clinical studies might be undertaken with this preparation just as in the case of the sulfonamides. Despite the numerous obstacles to large-scale production of a penicillin which would meet all requirements of purity, this drug has been produced in quantities sufficient to permit not only clinical investigations necessary to determine its field of usefulness and the best methods of employing it, but also its widespread application in combat areas as well as at home.

When the initial supply of penicillin became available, the Army's allocation was devoted to a program of intensive and well-controlled investigations conducted in Army hospitals specially equipped for evaluating its therapeutic possibilities and ascertaining the most effective way to use it. The results of these studies were presented to the medical profession in a special report published in the *Journal of the American Medical Association*. Undoubtedly, with continuing studies, further significant observations in this field will be made, but it has already proved to be a real advance in military medicine, which can with pardonable pride claim credit for initiating the rapid progress in this chemotherapeutic endeavor that otherwise might have required several more years to reach its present stage of development.

In the United States alone, approximately 6,000 persons die annually of burns. In a war of intense mechanization and high explosives, it was expected that burns would constitute an important and serious form of injury. Fortunately, they represented less than 2 per cent of battle casualties, but because of their gravity and their crippling effects, they were none the less important forms of injury.

Recognizing the significance of burns and the varied and controversial forms of treatment, the Army early began concentrating its efforts on the prevention and treatment of this type of injury and evolved a therapeutic program which gave increasingly better results. This program was directed toward the early prevention and control of shock by the adequate use of plasma, the relief of pain with morphine, the prevention and control of infection by aseptic precautions and oral administration of sulfadiazine, and the prevention of contracture and excessive scarring by proper splinting and early skin grafting. Tannic acid and other escharotics were no longer employed. The burned area was treated by the application of sterile petrolatum and a firm pressure dressing. Cases with burns about the face, hand or other regions that caused contracture and disfigurements were sent, as soon as their condition permitted, to the special plastic surgery centers, where near-miracles were performed in the correction of those deformities. By these measures, both the mortality and the serious disabling complications of burns were greatly reduced.

Other advances in the repair of injured nerves and defects in the skull used by Army surgeons contributed greatly to the rapid recovery of the wounded. Wounds of the extremities made up the highest proportion of battle casualties, and 12 to 15 per cent of these were associated with injury to major peripheral nerves. The proper repair of these nerves was essential if the resultant crippling paralysis was to be minimized.

Under war conditions, primary anastomosis of several peripheral nerves is not generally feasible, although it is attempted whenever possible. In order to minimize the irreparable degenerative changes that occur if the condition is not repaired early, every effort was made to evacuate these patients as soon as possible to the neurosurgical centers in general hospitals in the United States, where the delicate operation and necessary post-operative care could be instituted. Later developments permitted operative repair within a week to ten days after the wound had healed, which is much earlier than was formerly thought possible. This is particularly desirable, since the earlier the operation can be performed, the better the end result is likely to be.

Certain technical advances in the operative repair of this type of injury permitted remarkable improvements in the results, and many men who formerly would have gone through life with a paralyzed hand or foot obtained normally functioning limbs. Similarly, in injuries with skull defects, the application of certain developments in their repair not only permitted physical restoration and correction of disfigurements, but also prevented subsequent serious complications.

Still other developments in the field of vascular surgery, chest surgery and abdominal surgery contributed to great saving in life and to the prevention and correction of many serious disablements which otherwise might have occurred. The Army Medical Department was alert to every new development and quick to seize upon any advance in medical science that could be utilized in bettering the treatment provided the sick and injured soldier. Moreover, methods which were found to be unsuitable or which did not give the desired results were quickly discarded, while others that were developed or perfected through adaptations were just as quickly adopted.

Finally, in addition to these developments in medical therapy and the plan of forward surgery, both of which undoubtedly contributed tremendously toward our gratifying record in the care of the wounded in this war, there was the much less heralded and perhaps insufficiently appreciated functional performance of the individual medical officers who formed the vanguard of Army Medical Service.

The indomitable resourcefulness, the moral courage, the physical stamina, the surgical proficiency and the efficient adaptability which these medical officers displayed in the skillful utilization of these new developments, and in the cheerful execution of their tasks under the most hazardous and adverse conditions, were the intangible factors most responsible for the unparalleled achievement in war surgery. These manifold attributes which our young physicians carried to the far-flung battlefields of a globe-encompassing war clearly reflected the best traditions of the medical profession as well as the distinctive and absolutely unquenchable spirit of America.

D-Day found the medical forces of the United States Army, which had been gradually assembled in England, completely ready for the invasion. Preparation had been a matter of years. The responsibility rested on Major General Paul R. Hawley, Chief Surgeon in the European Theater of Operations.

On July 9, 1943, he received the Legion of Merit for this work. The citation pointed out that, first as surgeon of the Special Army Observers Group in London, and later as Chief Surgeon of the European Theater of Operations, General Hawley had displayed remarkable professional ability, keen judgment and devotion to duty, and had rendered service of exceptional value to the government by planning all hospitalization and evacuation of the United States Army Forces in the United Kingdom and maintaining supervision over the medical situation in the European Theater of Operations.

General Hawley was graduated from the University of Cincinnati College of Medicine in 1914 and received the degree of doctor of public health from Johns Hopkins in 1923. In addition to the Legion of Merit, he has received the Presidential Medal of Merit of Nicaragua. His previous war service carried him all over the world.

There is an old saying that whenever three doctors get together they organize a medical society. General Hawley organized a medical society for the European Theater of Operations in June, 1943, and all officers of the United States Army Medical Corps are automatically made members of that society. Thus the men who were far removed from sources of medical information in the United States were enabled to keep abreast of scientific advancement.

General Hawley's account of the preparations for D-Day and the invasion is a record of which every American may well be proud.

CHAPTER VIII

HOW MEDICINE IN THE EUROPEAN THEATER OF OPERATIONS PREPARED FOR D-DAY

By
MAJOR GENERAL PAUL R. HAWLEY
Chief Surgeon, ETO

I

ON THE EVE of the greatest battle of history, the assault upon the steel cage of Europe, the service which was to give medical care to the invading troops was ready but relatively untried. The air onslaught from Britain had been unprecedented in weight and fury, yet, because of the nature of aerial warfare, wounded airmen needing medical care constituted a small fraction of losses sustained. Shiploads of battle casualties from the African Theater, which gave the surgeons of the European Theater some experience in war surgery, had been only occasional. There had been admissions to hospital for disease and non-battle injury from the great numbers of troops stationed in Britain, but military operations on the ground, wherein the Medical Service was to be tested and tried to the uttermost, had not yet begun.

Experience with battle casualties in the European Theater was limited at the time this chapter was written so the account given here must deal largely with the organization of the Medical Service, the preparations that were made for future operations, and the contributions to military medicine that were made by medical officers who occupied their time profitably during the months of waiting.

According to military doctrine, the area known as a theater of operations is divided into a "combat zone" and a "communications zone." The combat zone comprises the region required for the active operations of the combatant forces. The communications zone is contiguous to the combat zone and contains the lines of communication, establishments for supply and evacuation, and other agencies required for the immediate support and maintenance of the armies.

Medical Service is continuous. From the deepest thrust in the combat zone back to the rear of the communications zone, there must be personnel and installations to provide medical care for the troops, which entails not only organization for the treatment and evacuation of the sick and wounded but measures for the prevention of disease and, as an essential corollary, arrangements for the furnishing of medical supplies. Although the air forces had carried the attack deep into Germany, until the first troops landed on the Continent a combat zone on land did not exist. Concentrated in Great Britain were the armies waiting to invade, with their organic medical personnel mobile medical units, and fixed installations and agencies for their support.

The great responsibility of the Medical Service in a theater of operations is to provide for the care and evacuation of the sick and wounded. A description of the machinery prepared for the collection, transportation and hospitalization of casualties at each successive stage from front to rear will provide a picture of the Medical Service in the European Theater.

The forward terminus of a "chain of evacuation" is with the company aid men at the most advanced point of the combat zone; the rear terminus, at a general hospital in the communications zone. Starting from the front in the combat zone, there are small medical detachments as organic elements of all battalions and similar units of all branches of the Army. They serve with the infantry, artillery, engineers, with tanks, and jump with paratroopers. These battalion sections are the foundation of all field medical service. It is here that the sick or wounded soldier receives his first medical care, and his return to health often depends more upon the limited treatment given by these front-line units than upon the elaborate measures taken in well-equipped hospitals farther to the rear.

Each of the battalion sections consists of three functional groups, the company aid men, the litter-bearers and the battalion aid stations. (See Figure 1.) The company aid men actually live with their platoons, eat with them, sleep with them and play

with them, and when the fighting men go into battle, they know
that these friends of theirs, these trained medical soldiers, will
be right along with them, ready to give first aid and to help in
getting them to a sheltered place. The company aid men are
followed by the litter-bearer squads, who remove to the battalion
aid stations such casualties as are unable to walk. The aid station
is established as close as possible behind the firing line, and it is
moved whenever necessary to maintain close contact with the
combat elements of the battalion. It is here that the patient is
first seen, examined and treated by a medical officer, but only

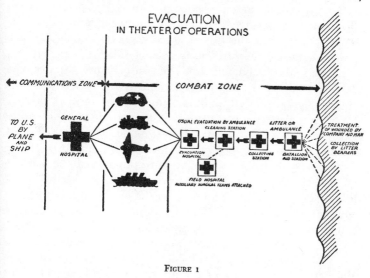

EVACUATION
IN THEATER OF OPERATIONS

FIGURE 1

emergency treatment can be undertaken in such an exposed position. This may consist of simple antishock measures, control of
hemorrhage, relief of pain, administration of blood plasma and
the fixation or immobilization of fractures.

Next in the "chain of evacuation" come the collecting station
and the clearing station, operated by medical units of the division. The Medical Service functions within the organization of
the tactical force, and each higher and larger group has definite
responsibilities suited to its location and facilities for movement
and protection. Litter-bearers and motor ambulances evacuate
casualties from the battalion aid station to the collecting station.
The collecting station may well be compared to the emergency

room of any large hospital. Here the casualty is again examined, dressings are adjusted or replaced, and such other emergency treatment is given as is necessary to save life or limb and to prepare the wounded soldier for further evacuation. From the collecting station he is taken to the clearing station by ambulance. The clearing station (normally one to each division) is established about four to seven or eight miles behind the front line. Here it is possible to employ somewhat more elaborate treatment measures than are practicable farther forward; however, treatment is still limited to such measures as are necessary at the time. There are better facilities here for shock treatment, and better fixation of fractures is possible, but little definitive treatment can be undertaken so near the front for several reasons, one of which is that definitive measures usually immobilize the patient for some time. Major abdominal or chest surgery usually precludes the movement of a patient for from four to seven days. So, in the clearing station as well as in the installations farther forward, the prime objectives of treatment are to save life or limb and to prepare the patient for further evacuation.

It must be remembered that many of the wounded will have only very slight injuries and after treatment will be able to rejoin their organization. This sorting out will occur all along the line of evacuation, depending on the degree of injury. Some may require a few days of hospitalization and rest, and facilities for this are provided at the clearing stations.

With the assembly of division casualties in the clearing station, and with their limited treatment completed, the task of the Division Medical Service ends and again responsibility passes to the next higher element, the Army. Here two types of hospitals are involved in the care and evacuation of the wounded, the evacuation hospital and the field hospital. The field hospital is a very mobile unit, sections of which, reinforced by highly qualified surgical teams, are established, when necessary, in the vicinity of clearing stations of the divisions, there to care for serious cases that cannot be evacuated immediately without grave danger, and cases that require immediate urgent surgery.

The primary principle of the evacuation system, as described so far, has been to bring the wounded speedily to a place where treatment by a skilled surgeon utilizing the most modern equipment is possible. Bringing the surgeon and his equipment, in the mobile surgical teams, to the wounded might seem to imply an opposing principle. Mobile surgical teams and field hospitals, in performing urgent surgery and providing hospitalization far up in the front line, will save many lives and facilitate increased mobility of the clearing station and other medical units, but their use is limited to certain situations. The basic principle of swift evacuation is still the most satisfactory and provides the widest use of highly trained specialists.

Evacuation hospitals are set up on rail or water lines, usually from 15 to 30 miles behind the front line. Army ambulances transfer the casualties from two or more division clearing stations to the evacuation hospital. This type of semi-mobile hospital is designed and equipped to undertake major surgical procedures, and it is the first installation that the casualty reaches where such treatment is really practicable. However, when these major procedures can *safely* be postponed, the patient is not operated upon until he reaches a general hospital. Since troops throughout the combat zone, and not only those in the most advanced sectors, are exposed to enemy fire by artillery or from the air, at every level there are aid stations and other agencies to care for the wounded and bring them into the chain of evacuation.

At the evacuation hospital the responsibility of the Army in the Medical Service ceases and passes to the communications zone, which transports the patient by boat, by airplane or by train to hospitals well outside the combat zone. It is in the communications zone that the patient first reaches the large fixed station and general hospitals. These installations are capable of giving complete medical care and are thoroughly equipped and staffed to undertake the most elaborate procedures in surgery. It is in these great hospitals that the largest part of the seriously wounded receive definitive treatment, but it must be realized that once the patient is in the hospital the problem is relatively simple. The real problem lies in the fields of organization and planning, in getting the patient to the hospital. How successful all our trained doctors, nurses and enlisted men are in caring for the wounded depends largely on how well the evacuation scheme works under the difficult conditions of battle.

What every American undoubtedly wants to know is what preparations were made in the European Theater for the task ahead. More than two years of planning and building preceded the day when blueprints were put to the test. It is no exaggeration to say that our Army has the finest Medical Service of any army in the world, and we feel that the European Theater lived up to this standard. One could not wish for finer doctors, dentists, nurses or other trained personnel of the Medical Department, and they were provided with excellent hospitals and equipment. The cream of the American medical profession served with our forces, and aiding them was a group of consultants, nationally known experts in their own fields.

In speaking of the activities of the Medical Service in Great Britain, it must be realized that these activities were twofold. On the one hand, there was for two years the continuous medical care given to troops massing in increasing numbers for the invasion, entailing measures to insure that their health was protected, that they had good food and living conditions, in addition to providing doctors, nurses and hospitals for the treatment of the sick and injured. On the other hand, there were the preparations for actual invasion: the integration of medical units into the tactical organization, their training in specific missions and the creation of a mechanism for evacuation and reception of the anticipated battle casualties. Essential also was the establishment of an effective organization for the furnishing of medical supplies.

Careful planning was essential. Nothing could be done haphazardly or left to chance; certain definite requirements had to be borne in mind. Study of the experience of the past furnished an idea of the number of soldiers who would become sick or be injured in the normal routine of an army not in battle. Similarly, past experience provided a fairly good indication of how many would be wounded in certain types of military operations. Careful evaluation of all these data and application to the number of our troops known to be involved enabled an estimate of the total number of hospital beds needed. This over-all figure then had to be broken down to provide the required number of beds in each type of hospital. The hospitals themselves had to be located so that they could serve their two functions: to care for the troops waiting to invade, and to be ready to receive battle casualties.

There were two types of these fixed hospitals, the smaller station hospitals for the more immediate treatment of troops in a permanent position, and the larger general hospitals where facilities and staff were provided for more thorough medical and surgical care. Station hospitals were sited, on paper, where large numbers of troops were to be congregated, while general hospitals were placed along lines of communication, so that they would be easily accessible to the station hospitals and would fit into the scheme of evacuation.

Of course hospitals were not simply to be had for the asking. The British also had military forces to provide for, as well as the injured expected from air raids. It might have been possible to bring materials and labor from the United States, but in the face of the critical shipping situation, this course was not practicable. Therefore a request was made to our British allies that they furnish us with the required hospitals, and this they agreed to do.

We realized that it would be a difficult job because of the shortage of labor and materials caused by the war, but fortunately the British had planned for the worst horrors of the German air blitz and had constructed or started construction on a number of large special hospitals under the Emergency Medical Service. Thanks to the magnificent victory of the Royal Air Force over the Luftwaffe in the Battle of Britain, not all these hospitals were needed and the British offered five of them to the Chief Surgeon.

These were fine, permanent structures, designed for use as county hospitals after the war. They had modern equipment and made ideal military hospitals. By invasion time, all five were in operation as typical general hospitals. In addition, a few British military hospitals were turned over for our use. However, Emergency Medical Service and military hospitals together met only a small part of our requirements. Later certain military camps would become available to provide for the increased load of battle casualties, but for immediate needs it was obvious that new construction was necessary. Plans for new hospitals were therefore drawn up by experts from the Medical Department and the Corps of Engineers, in collaboration with experts from British agencies. The layout and type of construction varied according to the location and the intended use. Although some hospitals were permanently constructed of brick, the majority utilized Nissen huts or buildings of hollow light brick and could be termed semi-permanent. All the hospitals, with but one or two exceptions, were built under contract by British labor and with British materials under Reciprocal Aid (Reverse Land-Lease). Most of the station hospitals and many of the general hospitals were of this type.

We believe that in both design and equipment it would be difficult to surpass these hospitals. Operating rooms were constructed according to the most modern plans; they were well equipped and lighted, being fitted in every instance with scialytic lights. Rooms fully equipped for the induction of anesthesia, treatment of shock and carrying out of resuscitation procedures were adjacent. Also adjacent, so that the patient could be transported to and from the operating room with the minimum of exposure and maximum of comfort, were the eye, ear, nose and throat and dental clinics and x-ray laboratories. In every hospital, at least two hundred beds were connected to the operating rooms by enclosed corridors, to prevent any exposure of the patient on his journey to the ward. The work in the special fields of medicine and surgery was, in each hospital, under the direction of the best-trained men in the medical profession.

Additional hospital beds were provided in military camps, which, before they could operate as hospitals, needed a certain amount of additional construction. These military camps were of three types, the militia camp, the dual-purpose camp and the conversion camp. The militia camp, built before the war, proved to be almost ideal for use as a hospital; the buildings were centrally heated, well lighted and well arranged; in fact, these militia camps made some of our best hospitals. The operating rooms, clinics and laboratories were of new construction. All were ready for rapid conversion into a hospital when the British or our troops moved out. The other two types of camps were built specially for eventual conversion into hospitals. One type, the dual-purpose camp, was built primarily as a hospital but so arranged that it could first be used as a barracks. The operating rooms, clinics and laboratories were constructed as part of the original plan, although they were not to be used while the installation functioned as a barracks. The third type, the conversion camp, was built as a barracks, but with the idea in mind that it could later be used as a hospital with certain constructional additions.

The hospital construction program reached its objective and we believe that the facilities provided were adequate in every way. Plants left little to be desired and our own fine doctors and nurses were ready in them, or ready to move in when needed. High praise has come from the Surgeon General of the United States Army, Major General Norman T. Kirk, who said, "British hospitals built here for United States troops and staffed by our Medical Department are better constructed and equipped than Army hospitals in the United States" (*Stars and Stripes*, April 4, 1944). It may be pointed out with pride, and with appreciation of splendid British cooperation, that the cost of the hospitals per bed was only about one-third of that for similar construction of military hospitals in the United States.

When our forces established themselves at some distance inside the Continent, fixed general hospitals were needed nearer to the combat zone to permit speedy evacuation of the wounded to them. Some type of fairly permanent buildings had to be provided, since we could not often expect to find buildings still standing in a battle area. A plan was worked out by which these buildings could be made available with the minimum waste of time. In cooperation with the Engineers, a detailed program was evolved by which a complete general hospital could begin taking care of patients on a new site within a few days.

The construction took place in phases. At first the hospital was entirely tented. The Engineers laid out roads and put down the concrete floors for the tents; the hospital unit moved in, pitched its own tents, installed its equipment and was soon ready to receive patients. While the hospital continued to operate, more permanent structures were provided by the Engineers. Starting with the operating rooms, they erected Nissen huts to replace the tents throughout the hospital. New patients were taken to the most recently constructed wards, so that eventually every tent was replaced, and in the last phase the whole hospital was housed in semi-permanent buildings, the entire construction having taken place without interruption to the operation of the hospital. Throughout, the principle was that the patient must receive the same care and material comfort as he was given in normal fixed installations.

Since this was a new departure in hospital construction and organization, it was vital that it be tried out so that we could see how well the general plan worked in practice and correct any faults of detail. Accordingly approval was obtained by the Chief Surgeon and the Chief Engineer from the British War Office to construct such a hospital on an experimental and operational basis. A site was chosen which we felt would provide a good test. The conditions proved to be ideal in that they were very bad! As the hospital unit came in, a period of rainy weather started and the whole area became a sea of mud. This situation brought out all the difficulties inherent in the original plan and disclosed certain technical errors. However, the plan as a whole was shown to be practicable. All mistakes and errors of design and problems of construction were carefully noted, and corrections were embodied in the final policy and plan. Other experimental units were set up in Great Britain and soon everything was ready for their use overseas. The officers assigned to command such units were trained in the program to be followed. Each had a complete set of plans and instructions and had gone over the experimental set-up, so that he could visualize the problems to be faced in the field. Special Engineer units were assigned to this specific task, and materials for building the huts were packed, ready to be shipped when the time came.

The rule that the success of an operation depends, to an extent greater in this war than ever before, on the availability of supplies of the right quality and quantity at the right time and place, is of particular importance to the Medical Service. Any account of the Medical Service in the European Theater must make mention of the preparations made for the procurement, storage and issue of medical supplies.

In this theater supplies were procured, in accordance with supply levels established by the War Department, from two sources: the United States, and from the British by Reciprocal Aid. In the early days of the theater, when the shipping situation was critical and when production in the United States had not got fully into its stride, the Medical Service aimed at procuring as much as possible in Great Britain and as little as possible in the United States, thus saving valuable shipping space and increasing the volume of supplies that could be dispatched from the United States to other theaters. But with victory in the Battle of the Atlantic and an unprecedented increase in the volume of production at home, it was possible to obtain more supplies from the United States and thus reduce the tremendous burden placed on British manufacturers, who not only had to meet the demands of their own forces but also had to contend with the menace of air attack.

The procurement of supplies is, however, but one part of the problem of making them available at the right time and place to all elements of the fighting forces. It is the fundamental principle in supplying an army that the impetus of supply is from the rear to the front. A "chain of supply" must be established, and each element in this chain must push supplies forward within reach of elements in front.

In order to insure the swift and unbroken flow of supplies from the rear to the front line units, a chain of supply agencies was established in this theater. The chain began with depots in the communications zone, from which supplies flowed to fixed installations within the zone, and also to Army depots and to Air Force supply points for redistribution.

In Great Britain, medical supplies were stored in and issued from medical branch depots and medical sections of general depots. A function of certain medical branch depots was to service equipment, particularly technical items such as x-ray and optical equipment. One depot was set aside for the receipt of all supplies procured from the British.

The equipment authorized by tables of equipment for fixed medical installations of the communications zone was assembled in depots and issued to the units when they occupied the completed plants.

Upon arrival at the port of debarkation, the medical officer of each unit of the Field Forces having a medical detachment received medical supplies sufficient to enable him to give any emergency medical care needed until his unit arrived at its station. Upon reaching it, the unit received its full equipment, previously assembled and shipped to a neighboring depot.

The levels of supply to be maintained by units were prescribed and, having received their initial equipment and supplies, units thereafter made known their own requirements, within authorized allowances, to issuing agencies. Ultimately, units were notified of the depot situated most conveniently, from which they could draw supplies directly upon request. These depots supplied fixed installations of the communications zone and in addition the Army depots and Air Force medical supply points, which in turn made further distribution.

In order to insure that stocks were so distributed that the speedy and effective supply of all needs was certain, some form of central control was necessary. The Supply Division of the Chief Surgeon's Office exercised this control, effecting the equitable distribution of stocks among depots. There was in effect a system of stock control through which, by means of periodic inventories from all depots, the central office knew the exact status of stocks within each one and could therefore distribute incoming supplies intelligently and maintain adequate stocks throughout the chain of supply agencies.

There was not an equally plentiful supply of all items, and a key depot system was established to effect economy of items in short supply. By this system, key depots were given priority on incoming shipments of certain items in short supply, and maintained a stock of these items, to meet any need for them that might arise. It was in effect a rationing of shortage items by centralization of stocks rather than dispersal into small lots.

Too extensive a dispersal of supplies into small lots is uneconomic, but because of the constant threat of air attacks every effort was made to effect a distribution which was consistent with effective operation but which would at the same time insure that bombing attacks at particular points did not menace the entire stock of any item.

To meet the particular problem of the invasion of the Continent, in which supplies would probably have to withstand immersion in water, a form of amphibious packing was designed. Equipment exposed to immersion was specially packed in strong, light, waterproof boxes, which not only protected the contents but could be used later for storage purposes.

Medical maintenance units were shipped automatically to the armies in the early phases of the operation, before the military situation became stabilized sufficiently to permit units to draw supplies direct from depots. Each of these medical maintenance units contained the quantity of supplies which it was estimated would fill the requirements of 10,000 men for thirty days.

No effort was spared to obtain equipment and supplies of the highest standard. The supply system kept abreast of the most recent scientific discoveries. Stocks of blood plasma, sulfa drugs and penicillin were maintained in quantities sufficient for both prophylaxis and treatment and to assist in the successful performance of surgery, although we realized that drugs never lessen the need for the good surgeon but merely help him in his job

In short, the most highly qualified doctors cooperated with the most skilled technicians to make certain that the best type of equipment for the particular job was available wherever needed, from the company aid men in the firing line to the general hospital in the rear.

During the preceding months, it had not been easy to obtain great quantities of medical supplies of the desired quality needed for the coming operations and to establish an organization whereby these supplies would be made available at the right time and place wherever needed. In the end, however, each soldier could go forward confident that should he be wounded or fall sick, the drugs and instruments necessary to aid his return to health would be at hand.

When large groups of people are congregated closely together, as in the concentration of an army in the field, there is an ever-present danger of epidemic disease. It is a primary concern of the commander to prevent the spread of such epidemic disease as wrought havoc among armies in other wars.

From the moment our troops began to arrive in the European Theater, there was a continuous program of preventive measures. Many of these diseases were caused by faulty sanitation and could be controlled. Fortunately, this theater differed from many others in that there was no significant problem of insect-borne disease, such as malaria or yellow fever. However, other diseases almost equally crippling to an army can be transmitted in food and water.

In general, the water supply of Great Britain was excellent, but with the building of camps and hospitals, it was necessary to develop new sources. Americans, known to be great users of water, made heavy demands on the British distribution system. In many instances, water had to be brought considerable distances and purification systems installed and supervised. Sanitary engineers of the Medical Department checked continually on all aspects of the supply system to insure that the water was potable. The problem, of course, was greatly complicated when our Field Forces went into battle. Every source of water was doubly suspect, for in addition to the ordinary hazards, there was the possibility of deliberate contamination by the enemy. Our men were trained to appreciate the dangers of contaminated water and carried individual equipment for its purification, while to make certain that the water supply system as a whole was satisfactory, there were trained groups with special equipment.

Since the effect of food on the health of the troops is of primary importance, the content of the Army ration and its preparation was of great concern to the Medical Service. Nutritional experts worked with the Quartermaster Corps in improving the rations supplied in this theater, both that for permanent camps and the more compact types to be used in the field. Some of these compact rations, while adequate in calories, essential food elements and vitamins, are not appetizing over a prolonged period. Therefore supplements were planned which not only added to the nutritive value but also gave variety and thus provided a diet which was both balanced and appetizing.

In the early days of the theater, food products, along with many other supplies, had to be procured in England. The ration supplied to British troops was found to be not completely satisfactory for American soldiers, largely because of the difference in national tastes. Extensive studies were made, and the result was the successful incorporation of British foodstuffs in the American ration, thereby permitting a considerable saving of shipping space.

Meat and dairy products were brought from the United States and had to be carefully inspected before distribution. The Veterinary Corps conducted inspections at ports and food storage plants in order to see that the products were satisfactory for consumption and that proper provision had been made for refrigerated storage on incoming transports, in depots and on inland transport.

These safeguards were useless unless the food was cooked and served under the highest standards of sanitation. Epidemics of dysentery and other diarrheal diseases quickly arise if kitchens, mess halls, cooking utensils and other mess equipment are not kept scrupulously clean. The high standard of mess sanitation maintained in this theater, with the enforcement of rigid rules and frequent inspections, was indicated by the fact that there were no large outbreaks of any diarrheal disease.

Modern science, through the perfection of immunization, has almost entirely eliminated the dangers from certain diseases which in past wars have taken a tremendous toll of life. In the Spanish-American War, a great many more soldiers died from typhoid than from battle injuries. In the First World War, inoculation completely changed this picture, but typhus and tetanus were still menaces. Newly developed methods of immunization are now available to combat these diseases. All our troops in this theater were immunized against typhoid, smallpox, typhus and tetanus.

The medical officers with the Air Forces, under Brigadier General Malcolm C. Grow, did a splendid job in caring for our fliers, not only in treating their injuries but also in developing means for their protection when in the air. Enemy fighters and anti-aircraft fire were not the only hazards the airmen had to face; the deadly effects of altitude and extreme cold also had to be guarded against.

The flight surgeons lived and flew with their men and came to know them intimately, and to appreciate their problems. Knowing them so well, they were quick to see any signs of fatigue, a serious matter among combat crews, and to suggest steps to prevent and alleviate it. Special recreational resorts were established where the airman could relax in pleasant surroundings, play games and get a complete rest. This recreation was a great help in keeping our Air Force men in fighting trim.

The arrangements for the treatment of Air Force casualties were carefully organized. A returning plane signaled to the airfield that it had wounded men aboard, and was given priority to land. Ambulances rushed to the plane, where trained helpers removed the wounded, placed them in the ambulance and took them to the field dispensary, where everything was ready for immediate treatment. A special litter was devised to facilitate removal of the wounded from the cramped spaces of a bomber. Sometimes, however, the nature of the injury made it inadvisable to try to remove the wounded man from the plane immediately, and special personnel and equipment were prepared to take care of him while he was still in the plane. Emergency surgical procedures could be performed, transfusions given and other measures taken to prevent shock. A patient could thus be treated and kept comfortable for hours, until it was safe to move him. If the patient's condition required more elaborate therapy than could be given at the field, he was taken to a nearby station hospital. A chain of these were located in proximity to the air fields of bomber commands.

From study of the injuries received by airmen, medical officers were able to work out means of protection. For instance, it was noticed that many wounds were caused by missiles of low velocity, and it was felt that some sort of body armor would prevent a large percentage of these wounds. After extensive research, an "anti-flak" suit and helmet were developed. The suit, which was quite light, was built up of a great number of small, very strong steel plates, placed in little pockets in the material of the suit. Tests showed that these plates would stop all but projectiles with a high velocity. For instance, the suit stopped bullets from a .45-caliber pistol fired only a few feet away. A rip-cord device released the suit in an instant. Many fliers owe their lives to this suit, developed by the Medical Service of the Air Force under General Grow.

Frostbite is a constant menace to airmen. Owing to the extremely low degrees of temperature met with at high altitudes, sometimes as low as 65° below zero Fahrenheit, and exaggerated by the terrific blasts of air when there is any opening to the outside, the briefest exposure of any part of the body will cause serious damage, much more pronounced than the usual frostbite. Pilots wore electrically heated clothing plugged into the electrical system of the plane, but even with this there were occasions when a part would be exposed. Research by medical officers developed new methods of treatment, a scientific advance of major importance.

However, experimental studies in cold chambers and under actual flying conditions showed that only proper clothing could prevent freezing and that no extraneous substances, such as drugs or protective ointments, were of any use as preventive agents. Therefore every effort was made to improve flying clothing, particularly shoes and gloves. In order to help to prevent freezing of the hands when gloves had to be removed in an emergency, electrically heated muffs were available in different parts of the aircraft. The development of an electrically heated blanket in which the wounded could be wrapped in the plane proved of great value. All this work was a good example of how physiology and medicine aided in the development of aviation.

Another example of the Medical Service's contribution to aviation was the improvement made in the oxygen mask. For flying at high altitudes, beginning at 10,000 feet, oxygen must be breathed and there must be an uninterrupted flow of it, supplied through a mask. Great difficulty has been caused by freezing

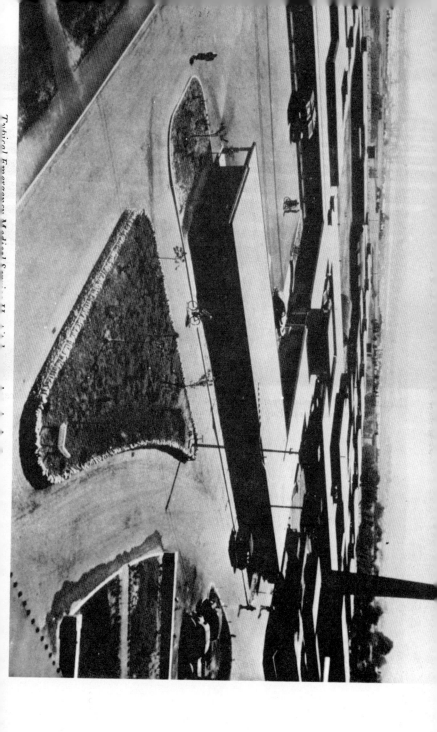

Typical Emergency Medical Service Holding Area and stocked ward area.

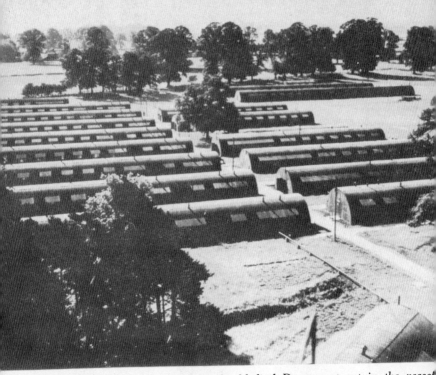

*Nissen hutted hospital operated by the Medical Department, set in the peacef[ul]
surroundings of English countryside.* (U. S. ARMY PICTORIAL SERVICE)

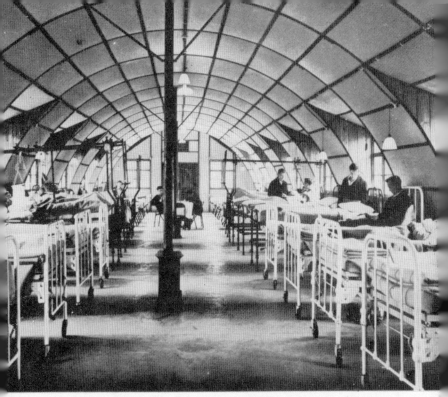

Surgical ward of a Nissen hutted hospital. (U. S. ARMY PICTORIAL SERVICE)

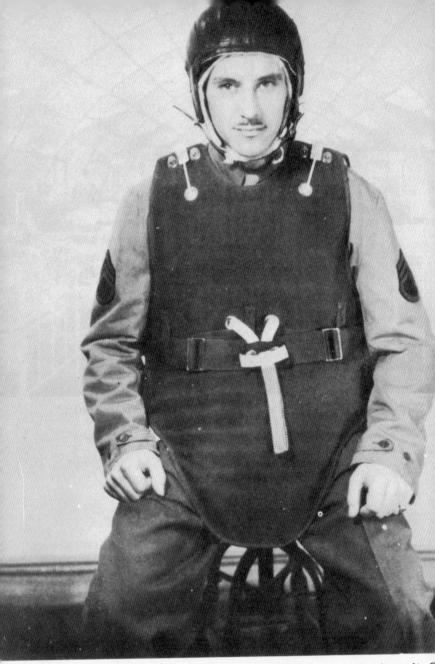

Anti-flak suit and helmet designed by Medical Department of the Army Air C worn by flight personnel over regular clothes. (ARMY AIR FORCES PHOTO)

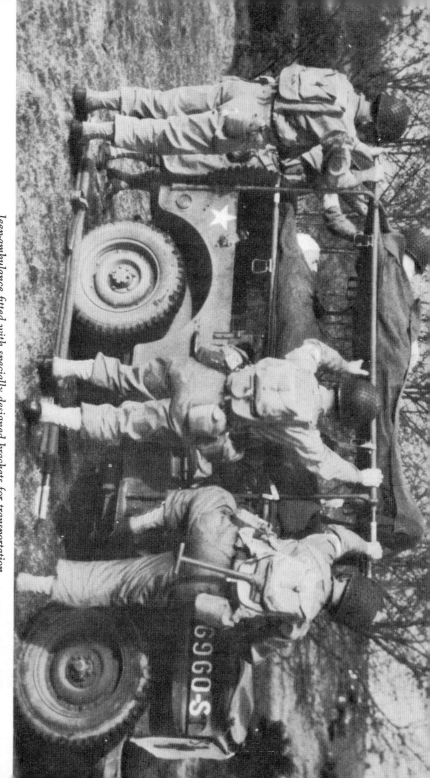

Jeep-ambulance fitted with specially designed brackets for transportation

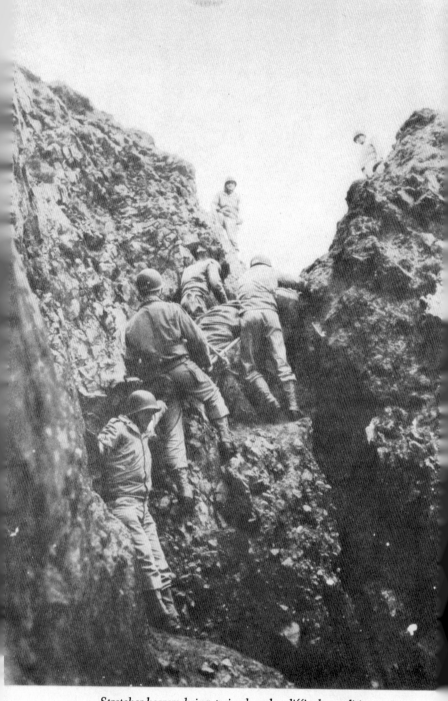

Stretcher-bearers being trained under difficult conditions.
(U. S. ARMY PICTORIAL SERVICE)

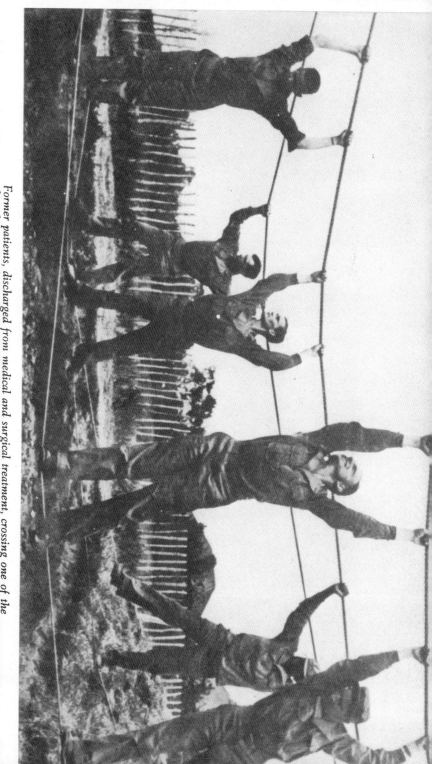

Former patients, discharged from medical and surgical treatment, crossing one of the

of the mask and the consequent block in the vital oxygen line, but medical scientists, working at the Central Medical Establishment of the Eighth Air Force, after months of research developed a mask in which this tendency to freeze up was effectively reduced. This was a positive contribution of medicine to the great success of our air war against Germany.

II

So far we have discussed those activities, continuous since the theater opened, which took place in fixed installations, the agencies which back up invading armies. These activities continued at an increased tempo with invasion. Throughout the period, other preparations were under way which were utilized when our forces moved into battle. These included facilities for evacuation of the wounded, both in the combat zone and in the communications zone, and the preparations made by medical units of the Field Forces.

When the landing was made on the shores of Europe, the evacuation plan outlined earlier was put into practice. The fact that part of the route was over water was of necessity an important factor. Many different facilities were used to transport the wounded, ranging from hand-carried litters to hospital trains and large ships. In the front lines, the wounded were picked up by trained litter-bearers. These men were carefully instructed in their task, since the wounded man is greatly affected by the way in which the litter is carried and placed in the ambulance. The litter-bearers had to be continuously on the alert to note any change in the condition of the wounded. Sometimes the carry was over considerable distances, but wherever possible, ambulances worked their way forward to take over the evacuation. When there were no roads fit for ambulances, the ubiquitous jeep was used. A large number were fitted with special frames to carry litters. Great fleets of various types of ambulances were used. The majority of these were built on the chassis of a one-and-a-half-ton truck and carried four litters. There were also smaller ambulances and some with half-tracks.

At the beachhead, the control of transportation was in the hands of the Navy. Cooperation between the Army and the Navy was excellent. Every detail was worked out in conferences between surgeons of the two services, who worked together on the evacuation craft. Special hospital carriers and LSTs (Landing Ship Tanks) were used to carry the wounded back to Great Britain. All kinds of small craft, including specially modified DUKWs, took them out to the large ships. The LSTs had special apparatus for holding litters, which were made ready as soon as the tanks went ashore.

Air evacuation was also utilized. As soon as possible, airfields were established on the far shore and ambulance airplanes brought into operation. These flew back to airfields in England, located near certain general hospitals. Trained groups of doctors and nurses performed this service, prepared the wounded for air travel, and cared for them en route. The aim was to utilize air evacuation of casualties to the maximum extent made possible by release of planes for Medical Department use.

When the wounded reached Great Britain, everything was ready for their reception. Special treatment groups waited at the ports to give them immediate attention and to arrange for their transportation to general hospitals by ambulance and by hospital trains. These trains were built for us, to our plans, by the British from British rolling stock. They were equipped with all necessities for the care and comfort of the wounded. Hospital trains were also constructed for use on the Continent.

The final step in evacuation back to the United States was taken by those men unfit to return to duty in this theater who were able to stand the journey. They were transported by hospital ship and in some cases by aircraft. They embarked on this voyage only after they had had definitive treatment at general hospitals and had been made ready for the journey. Travel to the ports or airfields was by hospital train.

When the ground assault on Europe began and the full fighting strength of the United States and its Allies—infantry, artillery, tanks, air-borne divisions and all the supporting troops—was thrown against the Germans, the mobile medical units and hospitals of these field forces had their first real test. A few of the personnel had already had battle experience in North Africa and Sicily, but for most of them this was a new adventure. The long months of waiting had been well spent in learning to work with their combatant colleagues, and in seeing that every item of equipment, from trucks and tents to surgical instruments, was ready.

Some of this equipment had been developed in this theater on the basis of experience gleaned from other war areas. For instance, it had been found that modern mechanized warfare had so lengthened the lines of communication that greater mobility had to be provided for the auxiliary surgical teams and their equipment if they were to be of maximum usefulness. The first thought was to put an operating room on wheels in a specially constructed truck. However, this plan presented immediate difficulties. It would have required special construction, a decided disadvantage when supplies were short and time at a premium. And with everything concentrated in one vehicle, a single hit by enemy fire might pin down the whole unit. It was decided to devise a unit from standard equipment that could carry in trucks the doctors and all the equipment necessary for extensive field surgery, but so assembled that it could be set up and dismantled quickly and efficiently. The surgical consultants of the Office of the Chief Surgeon and officers of medical field units studied the problem from every angle, selecting the supplies that would be necessary and working out on paper all the steps of packing and assembly. Then they tried out their ideas in the field, pitching the tents, setting up the surgical apparatus, and even performing surgical operations. Only when every phase appeared perfect was the plan considered ready to be put into general use. The unit, which became standard in the ETO, carried in two trucks sufficient personnel and equipment to perform a total of one hundred operations, with two operating tables working simultaneously. Materials were available for applying plaster casts and for treating shock. It could travel three hundred miles on its own gasoline, and be set up ready to treat patients within an hour of arrival at its location.

Similarly, in order to get x-ray apparatus up to the forward installations, a mobile x-ray unit was developed. This unit, also transported by truck, was capable of giving complete x-ray service. It was particularly useful in the treatment of fractures, and in the localization of foreign bodies.

Another important phase of supply to field units was that of whole blood. Everyone is familiar with the remarkable results achieved in the treatment of shock by the use of human blood plasma, but there are certain injuries in which there has been a serious loss of blood, where plasma must be supplemented by transfusions of whole blood. There were great difficulties in supplying this fresh blood, since it could not be packed and shipped as easily as dried plasma. After many months of research, a program was put into effect which assured that our wounded would have the means for life-saving transfusions when necessary. A medical general laboratory was the center for this research, as well as for many other important studies on the prevention and treatment of disease. Here scientists worked out the methods for the storage and transportation of blood. This laboratory acted as a central depot and was responsible for collection, storage and delivery. The blood was obtained from soldier volunteers, a panel having been set up in every unit. About four-fifths of a pint was taken from each donor. This amount of bleeding has no ill effect and neither reduces physical capacity nor predisposes to illness. The blood was collected by mobile bleeding teams that took it back in refrigerated trucks to the depot. There it was tested and typed and a preservative added. It was then stored in refrigerators until needed. It was sent forward in refrigerated containers. Arrangements were made to transport it by air wherever possible.

Of course, there were times when it was not possible to get blood up from the blood bank; to meet the needs under these conditions, an emergency transfusion kit was designed. With this, blood could be taken from donors right in the field and given immediately. It must be emphasized that this program in no way did away with the great need for plasma, the supply of which remained as essential as ever, and for which we continued to depend upon the people at home.

It is sometimes hard for those at home to understand why medical men should need further training when they are in the Army, since they have already spent so many years of study preparing for their professional careers. But the appreciation of the many new and peculiar problems to be faced by them, particularly those in which they must work within the framework of a huge fighting force in battle, furnishes the explanation. They are compelled to be soldiers as well as doctors, and this is especially true of the officers of the field units.

A medical field service school similar to that at Carlisle, Pennsylvania, was established in England, and one of its primary functions was to train these officers in the aspects of military medical practice not ordinarily familiar to civilian physicians. The curriculum covered not only the treatment of war wounds and unusual diseases, and the application of military sanitation to the prevention of disease, but also the relationship of military organization to the practical application of the medical art.

The nurses also had to have such training in the field aspects of their work; it was really wonderful to see how they adapted themselves to conditions so far removed from their usual life. They became good soldiers. This emphasis on the military side is not something superimposed, but represents an attitude that is vital to the successful accomplishment of the unusual task of taking care of the sick and injured under the trying and dangerous circumstances of battle.

The other aspect of training in ETO was that of teamwork. The entire medical unit had to practise together until every step was second nature, and finally, in tactical exercises, it coordinated its functions with those of all the other arms and services with which it had to work in combat. Thus, those units which were in the spearhead of the assault had gone over and over again, under simulated conditions, every detail of handling of the wounded during the landing on the beaches and cliffs of Europe. They had practised with the equipment they were to use, had loaded jeeps and DUKWs and, working with the Navy, had gone over each step in loading and unloading hospital carriers and LSTs. Other units had gone on maneuvers with paratroopers, the doctors jumping with the rest. Still other medical units, with air-borne divisions, had been carried by gliders with all their equipment and, on landing, had set up their aid stations. Units which played their part all along the chain of evacuation had been perfecting their technique by continual practice from the loading and unloading of ambulances and hospital trains to the complete installation of an evacuation hospital under tents, ready to receive two or three hundred patients.

The work of the Medical Service is not over when the sick or injured soldier is pronounced well according to usual medical standards. A rehabilitation and reconditioning program was started which aimed to return the soldier to his full strength and spirit as soon as possible so that he could go back to his duties with confidence in his ability to perform them. The program was to begin in the general or station hospital, while the patient was still convalescent. Carefully graduated exercises can do much to decrease the physical deterioration so often seen in patients who have had a long period of hospitalization. An important feature of this phase of the program was the effort to get the patient away from the hospital atmosphere and to get him back to living and acting like a soldier. Special wards were set aside for the training, and an educational and recreational program was planned to occupy the patient's leisure time.

When the patient no longer needed medical or surgical treatment, he was sent either to a reconditioning camp or to a rehabilitation center. The purpose of the reconditioning camp was to recondition physically the medical or surgical patient who no longer required active hospital treatment and who needed no remedial exercise or special training, but who did require general physical hardening before he was fit for full duty.

The rehabilitation centers had as their aim the physical rehabilitation of the medical or surgical patient who was ambulatory and required no further medical or surgical care other than certain remedial exercises and special training to restore to normal functioning certain abnormal parts of the body. The remedial exercises, as well as specific and general physical training, were under close supervision of medical officers. At these centers, certain technical training was given which not only kept the trainees active in their former occupations, but trained men in new activities in cases where their disability prevented return to their former assignment.

The officers and enlisted men who conducted these courses had specialized training as physical instructors in remedial exercises. Special obstacle courses were constructed, and when the once sick or injured man completed this course, he was fully confident that he was physically and mentally ready for his job.

The governing policy for all these activities was directed by the Office of the Chief Surgeon, each phase being the scope of one of the divisions of the office. These divisions covered both the administrative and professional aspects of military medicine, and in each were experts in their fields who planned and coordinated the various programs, which were then put into effect through regular military channels. The divisions of the office were as follows: Administrative; Operations, covering planning and evacuation; Hospitalization; Personnel; Supply; Medical Records; Preventive Medicine; Professional Services; Gas Casualties; Dental; Nursing; Veterinary; Rehabilitation; Historical.

The Professional Services Division was concerned with maintaining high standards of medical practice in hospitals and throughout the Medical Service. In order that the best scientific advice might be available, a group of consultants was appointed. These physicians and surgeons were the foremost experts in their respective fields, and in civilian life were professors in our leading medical schools. They represented all the specialties of medicine, surgery and dentistry. Their function was to keep our doctors abreast of the latest advances in scientific medicine, and to see that the caliber of professional work was of the highest.

Most of the research in the theater was under the supervision of the consultants. Mention has already been made of many of these studies, such as the highly important contributions to aviation physiology and medicine from the Air Forces, the development of new equipment and procedures, mobile surgical and x-ray units, and the blood bank. Behind all these were intensive scientific study, experimental work in laboratories and practical trials in the field. In addition to the medical general laboratory, the laboratories of our many hospitals took part in the research program.

All this research was undertaken with the idea of immediate application to the current military situation, but many of the findings will be of permanent significance. This is particularly true of the studies on war wounds and on the prevention and treatment of various diseases. An elaborate research program has been under way on the use of the various sulfonamide drugs and of penicillin in the prevention of wound infection. A number of important scientific articles have been published as a result of this study. Much work has been done on the newer methods for the treatment of venereal diseases, including intensive arsenotherapy, the sulfonamides and penicillin. The medical scientists in our service recognized the great opportunity and made good use of their time.

The physical condition and the general health of the United States Army in the European Theater were consistently good, judged by the relatively few days lost owing to injury or illness. This time-loss was about three-fourths of that experienced by the Army in the Continental United States, which was the most comparable group. The communicable disease record was excellent. There were no serious epidemics. This record indicates not only that the preventive measures had generally been successful, but also that our men had become acclimatized and that their hard training had toughened them. They were ready for the task.

Vice Admiral Ross T. McIntire, who is also Surgeon General of the United States Navy, has received the highest rank ever accorded a medical officer in the military service of our country. He has been, incidentally, physician to the White House since 1933.

After graduation in medicine and some years of medical practice, Dr. McIntire entered the Navy in 1917. He specialized in diseases of the eye, ear, nose and throat, and his competence in that field was recognized. However, his efficiency in the field of administration and his genial personality were equally important with his medical achievements in gaining for him the position he holds.

Under his administration, the Navy Medical Department has undergone the greatest expansion in its history—an expansion which is likely to be maintained because of the immense growth of our Navy during this war.

Admiral McIntire's duties as physician to the President of the United States have taken him to all the great conferences that have been held by President Roosevelt in the North Atlantic, in Teheran, in Africa and in the Pacific. No one could describe more authoritatively than does Admiral McIntire the service rendered by the physicians of our Navy in the war.

CHAPTER IX

THE NAVY DOCTOR AT WAR

By
VICE ADMIRAL ROSS T. MCINTIRE
The Surgeon General, United States Navy

IT IS NO longer a new story that the size of the Medical Department of the United States Navy in 1944 exceeded the strength of the entire Navy as it existed at the outbreak of World War II in September, 1939. We grew accustomed to counting our medical and dental officers and our nurses in the thousands, and our hospital corpsmen in the scores of thousands, although it was only a few years ago that they ran only into the hundreds.

In the late 1930's, during the early part of my first term as Surgeon General, I knew practically every one of our doctors by name and face. By 1944, there were about 17,000 members of the Navy Medical and Dental Corps on active duty, and I had to realize that to most of them I was just an impersonal name rather than a co-worker.

My purpose in launching these remarks with a few words about the expansion of this particular branch of America's Naval Service is not to indulge in nostalgic reminiscence of a day that is gone, probably forever. True, there is a certain charm in smallness. With mounting size, whether it be in a business establishment, a city or a ship, the familial bond is strained. Without denying this, I am still convinced that the manifold increase in the strength of the Medical Department of the Navy was not merely essential in the interest of national defense, but that there will be resultant benefits long after the guns are spiked.

These gains will be shared by the Navy, by the doctors and, most important, by the population at large. Our service has profited abundantly by the 10,000 physicians and surgeons who came to us from civil life, bringing into the Corps a leavening factor which had a most salutary influence. They were assigned everywhere—to warships and hospital ships, to the Marines, to our hospitals ashore, to research laboratories, as flight surgeons and teachers and epidemiologists—and everywhere they were assimilated and made the grade. Examine a roster of naval medical heroes who distinguished themselves in action against the enemy, or note who made up the teams from whose labors came one life-saving discovery after another, and you will invariably find the names of Reserves scattered literally through the lists. It was our hope that many of them would choose to remain with us after victory, but even if every one returned to his home, the Navy would still benefit for years to come by what they contributed in knowledge and in sacrifice.

What these men gave may be said to be its own reward. But there is also more tangible compensation than the expression of gratitude conferred upon his doctor by a wounded man whose pain has been relieved, however sufficient that silently eloquent demonstration of thanks may be to the doctor who lives his Hippocratic oath. Beyond this, there was the incalculable value of having the opportunity both to practise a specialty and yet to have a hand in everything from diphtheria to battle surgery. There was the soul-filling spirit with which all members of a fighting team were imbued when they realized that as a group they could be no stronger than their weakest cog. There was the satisfaction, tempered by sober appreciation of their responsibility, of working with chemotherapeutic agents still withheld from the civilian practitioner because of wartime exigencies; the inner thrill accompanying the performance of a service that was indispensable if this nation and its institutions were to be preserved; and, not least, the character-ennobling influences of camaraderie and mutual aid within a self-contained unit, whether it was a ship's company or an advance base on a tiny island, which are an inseparable part of Navy life.

Perhaps the most forceful manner in which doctors' appreciation of these facts was demonstrated was the rush to volunteer, ever since Pearl Harbor, by middle-aged and elderly practitioners who served in the last war. Mustered out in 1919 and 1920, they returned to their home communities, some to resume interrupted practices and the younger ones to embark upon careers which were scarcely begun when they answered their country's call in 1917 and 1918. Nearly a quarter of a century later, you found them making tracks toward our Officer Procurement offices, eager to get back into uniform. Many got their wish. Some, because of age or physical disqualification, were disappointed. Of the latter group, I am happy to say that a large number served the Navy, notwithstanding, as teachers in the medical and premedical schools, preparing for naval service many hundreds of young men and women.

War itself is fatal, destructive. But the measures which a people take to fight a war are not necessarily without a constructive side. Into the struggle we poured our energy. We had to exercise our ingenuity, calling upon the final measure of inventiveness and enterprise not only for the perfection of offensive weapons but also for the protection and maintenance of the men who operated those weapons.

Under such circumstances, it was inevitable that we should develop methods and instruments to prevent and cure disease, restore the wounded, promote sound hygiene, and rehabilitate the maimed. A great many gains were achieved and the treasury of medical knowledge was being constantly enriched. Late in 1944 there had been made available to the civilian population only a comparatively few of the advances gained by military medicine, and these only on a limited scale. For there was no disagreement on the point that where the supplies were not sufficient for universal application, whether they consisted of penicillin, stainless steel or physicians themselves, the needs of the fighting forces had to be met first.

But we knew that eventually the child wasting away from a fever in some Middle Western town, and the aged woman down South who was bedfast with a fractured hip, would be benefiting from the innumerable improvements which were put to the test on land and sea. Necessarily, there had to be an interval during which the public received only meager direct benefits from the things which had to be conserved for the welfare of our soldiers and sailors, but this waiting period was not without its compensations.

As I have observed, the new drugs, new surgical techniques, immunizing agents, biologicals and prospective life-preserving aids without number all had to be proved effective without the slightest shadow of a doubt before they could be adopted. The Army and the Navy, with their millions of men, furnished that proving ground, paving the way toward universal application with no loss of time. And the men responsible for the successful execution of these tests were the personnel of our Medical Department, about 85 per cent of whom—speaking of the Navy—were Reserves who had come from private practice.

In dedicating the National Naval Medical Center, situated in Bethesda, Maryland, on the outskirts of Washington, on August 31, 1942, President Franklin D. Roosevelt said:

"Let this hospital, then, stand, for all men to see throughout the years, as a monument to our determination to work and to fight until the time comes when the human race shall have that true health in body and mind and spirit which can be realized only in a climate of equity and faith."

The rugged stone and sentry-like tower of this great Center stand, indeed, as a symbol of the aspiration expressed in such stirring words by the President. I like to view them, and the pulsating activity that goes on ceaselessly within the walls, as a proud example of cooperative enterprise and joint endeavor.

Here, on a 242-acre tract, are a 2,500-bed hospital, the Naval Medical School, the Naval Dental School, the Naval Medical Research Institute and, most recently established, the Navy's only school for training members of the Women's Reserve for service in the Hospital Corps.

As this was written, in 1944, thirty-two hundred men and women constituted the crew—medical officers, dental officers, nursing officers, enlisted personnel and officers of the Hospital Corps, specialists in bacteriology, entomology, biochemistry, nutrition and kindred sciences who were members of the Naval Reserve (both men and women), and civilians. The research unit worked in close relationship with the hospital and the schools. The Medical School performed the hospital's laboratory work, the Dental School its prosthetic work. Medical and dental officers collaborated in maxillofacial surgery and on other problems of mutual interest. All units shared the medical and crew libraries, the ship's service department, the mess halls. The Hospital Corps Waves in training served rotating duties throughout the interlocked commands of the Center. The Regulars and the Reserves bent over operating tables together, were instructed together and tackled abstruse research problems together on identically the same terms. From their teamwork there has come, and will continue to come, an accretion of knowledge whose future benefits are incalculable.

You would find a department devoted to study of one of the Navy's major worries—tropical diseases. Malaria and filariasis, to name the most troublesome blights, were far from vanquished in 1944, although they were not the dire threats they had been in 1942 and 1943. In the hospital also you would find scientific specialization in neuropsychiatric disorders, which accounted for altogether too large a percentage of admissions to the sick list. Fortunately, only a very small proportion of these patients were found to have true psychoses and, in the Navy, all who were so diagnosed were routed to Bethesda for survey prior to their transfer to a Federal hospital for mental illness.

Although the specialties of tropical medicine, neuropsychiatry and neurosurgery were stressed at the Bethesda Naval Hospital, all types of cases were accepted and a most liberal variety could be found there at all times, because it was not only a referral hospital but also a reception center for patients from the Potomac River Naval Command. Wards were dispersed through the floors of the tower, which rises 558 feet above sea level, and through several one-story temporary buildings which were added in recognition of wartime necessity. The seventeenth and eighteenth floors were equipped with lounges and solariums for the use of patients. All wards in the main building were provided with sunrooms.

The principal functions of the Naval Medical and Dental Schools were to indoctrinate newly commissioned officers, to offer special instruction in malariology, epidemiology, neurosurgery and certain other fields, and to give advanced training to men and women of the Hospital Corps in such diversified subjects as clinical laboratory technic, property and accounting, roentgenology, medical art and oral hygiene. Applicants for commission in the Medical and Dental Corps of the United States Navy received their entrance examinations here.

Housed in buildings of its own on the National Naval Medical Center reservation is the Naval Medical Research Institute. This unit was commissioned in October, 1942, and given the unenviable responsibility of solving myriad problems:

Find an effective insect repellent!

Improve atmospheric conditions in submarines!
Reduce occupational hazards in naval industry!
Provide better emergency rations!
Develop a flash-burn preventive!
Give the aviator better oxygenation equipment!
Minimize the pressure peril confronting the deep-sea diver!
Look into nutritional problems!

I am extremely gratified to report that marked progress was made all along the line, not only in the projects enumerated but in other avenues of research far too many to list. No leads were left unchecked. Given the most modern equipment, much of it ingeniously invented or improvised by staff personnel, and a heroic complement of men and women, officers and ratings, Regulars and Reserves, the Naval Medical Research Institute has long since justified the great expectations held at the time of its conception.

Any discussion, however skeletonized it may be, of the work being done at the National Naval Medical Center leads logically to consideration of naval medical performance in the field. Some writer termed Bethesda the hub of medicine in the United States Navy. If this metaphor is appropriate, then the spokes in the wheel were the sick bays in our ships, the more than two score naval hospitals within the continental limits, the mobile and advance base hospitals overseas, whose number I am not at liberty to divulge at this writing, the dispensary of every naval activity at home and abroad, every medical unit with our Fleet Marine Force, the special investigation units, whose geographical locations and assignments I must also withhold from mention, and, last but certainly not least, our busy hospital ships and evacuation transports.

Even before President Roosevelt's declaration of a state of national emergency in 1940, the Medical Department had begun to gear itself for any eventuality. One year earlier, the Naval Mobile Hospital had been visualized on the blueprint table and, within a matter of months, tried out at Guantanamo Bay. To quote the officer who was placed in command, Captain Lucius W. Johnson:

"Naval Mobile Hospital No. 1, familiarly known as Mob. 1, was the experimental unit, sent out as a guinea pig to determine by trial and error the best type of housing, equipment and administration for hospitals at advance bases. Our experiment developed a thousand gremlins, griggetts, goblins and other jinxes that took a grim humor in complicating our work and increasing our problems. These have been almost completely eliminated in the later mobile hospitals."

Mobile Hospital No. 2 was having the finishing touches applied to its construction at Pearl Harbor when the Japanese attacked on December 7, 1941. Overcoming every handicap, the staff turned to with such efficiency and courage that a unit commendation was bestowed upon its men and women by the Commander in Chief of the Pacific Fleet. Late in 1943, with the new Naval Hospital at Aiea Heights in commission and the security of Hawaii more firmly established, plucky Mob. 2 was decommissioned and its worthy complement assigned to other activities for duty.

The first of our Mobile Hospitals to be set up in the South Pacific was No. 4, established at Auckland, New Zealand, in the summer of 1942, with a strength of eighteen medical officers, two dental officers and some 300 enlisted men, chiefly hospital corpsmen. Most of the men and all the officers except the commander and his executive were Reserves embarked upon their first naval duty. The doctors were specialists in their various fields but for the first few weeks following the arrival of their ship with its strange cargo—a prefabricated hospital—they were grease-stained mechanics.

"The brain surgeon put on the roof, the dental officer the ventilators, the psychiatrist put up the side walls, the eye man put in the windows, one surgeon laid the decks, and another surgeon and the skin man put in the floor beams, while the obstetrician dug the holes and put in the footings for the foundations."

That was the description given by Captain J. H. Robbins, who had been placed in command of Mob. 4 when it was commissioned several weeks earlier in Brooklyn.

"None of our personnel had ever seen any of our equipment, including the buildings, except in the crated form. The buildings themselves consisted of steel panels which could be bolted together and contained the necessary windows and doors, and the only thing we had to work from was blueprints. During the building period, the weather was of the vilest type imaginable, with a heavy, cold rain falling most of the time. It is probably a mistake to say that it was falling, as, owing to the wind, it was more in a horizontal direction. Native labor was hired to assist in digging sewer and water lines and install certain plumbing fixtures, but remember the actual work of construction was done by the medical officers and enlisted personnel. To their credit be it said they did a wonderful job, for despite the handicaps of inexperience, bad weather, etc., this hospital was erected, equipped and handling 400 battle casualties in exactly 28 working days.

"In the first year of operation, approximately 16,000 patients from the battle area passed through this hospital with a total of only ten deaths."

The experiences of Mob. 4, both its tribulations and its high performance standard, were duplicated by many of our hospitals in the Pacific, where the great majority of our naval casualties occurred. When our first advance base hospital was established in the South Pacific early in 1942, medical officers unloaded equipment shoulder to shoulder with Seabees and hospital corpsmen. Despite the inexperience of most of the personnel in this kind of work, more than 40,000 tons of cargo were taken off without a man injured. Inventory of the first year's operation, during which period the hospital grew from 400 beds to 1,500, showed a mortality rate of less than one-third of one per cent.

The obstacles which the men and, later the women—Navy nurses were attached to virtually all our hospital overseas—who made up the staffs of these oases successfully overcame are almost unbelievable. To name a few: procurement of necessary equipment and supplies, climatic problems (some of the hospitals were situated where the heat would melt a miser's heart, and others were in frigid regions), racial differences with the surrounding population, insects, homesickness.

Hospital ships? Same story. One of them, during an eight-month period, traveled a distance the equivalent of twice around the earth—more than 50,000 miles—in performing twenty major evacuation missions. Among the first 10,000 patients treated and transported by this ship, beginning on December 7, 1941, there was a grand total of sixteen deaths. That is a mortality rate of 0.16 per cent.

The same ship evacuated many wounded from the amphibious operations in the Gilbert and Marshall Islands. Some patients were brought directly to the vessel from the beach, others were transferred from transports. Many were fished out of the water.

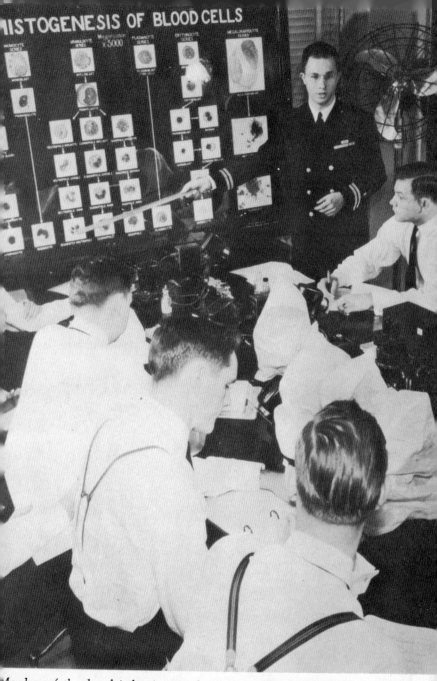

Members of the dental indoctrination class at the Naval Dental School, National Naval Medical Center, Bethesda, Maryland, listen to Lieutenant William Umiker (MC), USN, deliver a lecture on hematology. (OFFICIAL U. S. NAVY PHOTOGRAPH)

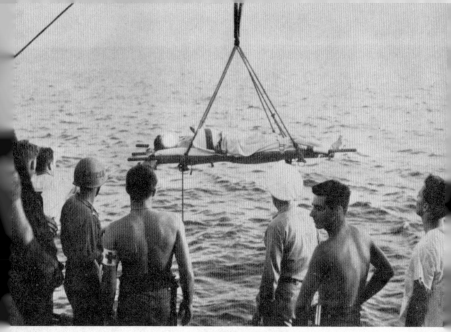

Battle casualty coming aboard a transport. Litter is secured in crane hook.
(OFFICIAL U. S. NAVY PHOTOGRAPH)

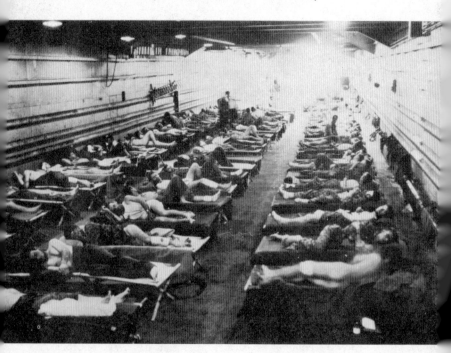

*With long rows of cots set up in its hold, this LST transports scores of wounde
Marines and other servicemen back from front lines to a base hospital.*
(OFFICIAL U. S. MARINE CORPS PHOTO)

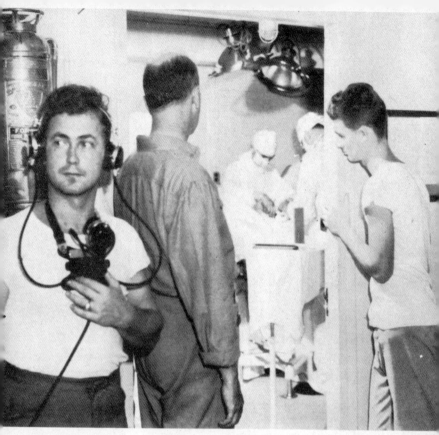

Lieutenant Alexander S. Angel (MC), USN, removes appendix from Private Harold
S. Smith, Army Air Corps, aboard a transport carrying Army troops to the South
Pacific. Lieutenant Angel had his own appendix removed later that day.
(OFFICIAL U. S. MARINE CORPS PHOTO)

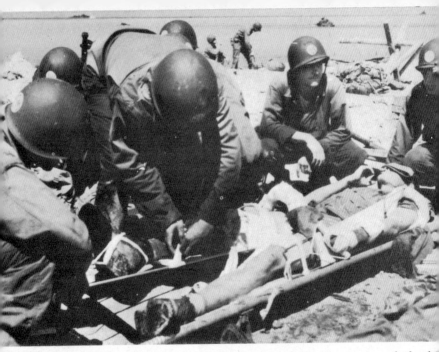

Wounded Marine at Tarawa dressing station smokes calmly as traction is applied to his fractured leg by Navy medical corpsmen. (OFFICIAL U. S. MARINE CORPS PHOTO)

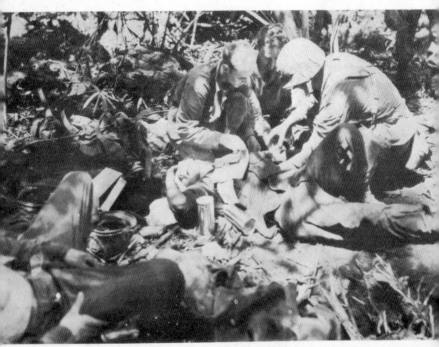

Wounded Marine gets treatment from Navy corpsmen at a jungle aid station behind the lines on New Britain. (OFFICIAL U. S. MARINE CORPS PHOTO)

Soldiers, as well as sailors and marines, were represented among the casualties. Almost every type of wound imaginable was treated. From the moment that every casual was taken aboard, thorough treatment was begun. It was not simply a matter of stanch the blood, control shock, apply a bandage and where's the next patient? Fractures were promptly immobilized in plaster. At Eniwetok alone, 414 units of plasma and 112 whole blood transfusions were administered. Chemotherapy was deliberately instituted and rigidly supervised. The laboratories kept busy making blood counts and doing various analyses. Penicillin was used in a number of cases and found to be effective both prophylactically and therapeutically.

Thirty per cent of all the serious casualties at Eniwetok were evacuated to this hospital ship, but only 5 per cent of the total who succumbed as a result of this action died aboard. To illustrate her splendid record with another figure, she had a mortality rate of 1.3 per cent, not counting the men who were moribund when brought aboard the vessel.

But what happened in an emergency aboard one of our smaller warships, say, with its solitary medical officer and a few hospital corpsmen? Here the equipment and supplies were stripped to essentials, with all the handsome implements to be found in our hospital ships and even the larger warships conspicuously absent. Not long ago I received a report that bolstered my pride in having as my associates men who so genuinely merit the Navy accolade: Well Done.

"Seven prisoners were brought aboard this vessel [a destroyer escort], five of whom were wounded," wrote young Dr. X, a Lieutenant (junior grade) in the Medical Corps of the United States Naval Reserve. "There were two serious cases. One, a chief engineer's mate, suffered a compound fracture of both tibia and fibula of the left leg. The right leg below the knee was badly lacerated with the loss of a great amount of blood. He also had a deep laceration of the dorsal aspect of the left hand and many minor abrasions and lacerations about the limbs and torso. Treatment consisted of ½ grain morphine syrette and two grams sulfathiazole stat and controlling hemorrhage and shock, Thomas splints were applied to both legs, 1,500 cc. of plasma administered before amputation of right leg above the knee. When the blood pressure was stabilized, the man was moved to the wardroom, which had previously been rigged up for an emergency operating room. It was thought wise not to transport the patient down a hatch to the sick bay for operation because of his unstable blood pressure.

"The operation was successful in spite of difficulties that arise on a small vessel of this type. One thousand cc. of normal saline with glucose, 500 cc. of plasma and several injections of adrenalin were administered during the operation. The man responded well to first administration of plasma and was talkative and had complete presence of mind. His condition at the end of the operation was fair. Two days later, he was given 200 cc. of whole blood by multiple syringe method, and he continued to improve.

"The other serious case was a seaman who suffered a wound of right foot, with all small toes shot away, the great toe hanging by a shred of tissue, and a large wound of the right buttock. He was given two grams of sulfathiazole and treated for hemorrhage and shock, then transported to wardroom when shock was controlled. Five hundred cc. of plasma and 1,000 cc. normal saline with glucose was given during the amputation of the right foot at the metatarsal level. Then the buttock wound was débrided and 'salted' with sulfanilamide crystals and bandaged. Many minor punctures, abrasions, lacerations were dressed with tincture of merthiolate and 'salted' with sulfanilamide.

"The three minor cases were dressed with tincture of merthiolate and 'salted' with sulfanilamide and dressed. . . . All wounds were examined daily and their progress was quite gratifying. Upon evacuation in a foreign port for further disposition, all patients were vastly improved. From the comments by the prisoners we conceived that they were surprised at the professional ability of the corpsmen and the humane treatment rendered them by everyone. The comfortable bunks, the quality of the food, real coffee and American cigarettes were prized by them."

The restraint, the almost casual overtone of that report, notwithstanding the fact that it dealt with two major amputations under trying circumstances, by a young Reservist who probably was on his first battle cruise, may give the reader some idea of the quality of skill and resourcefulness possessed by the men into whose hands your fighting sons have been entrusted. There need be no worry or concern about the care which wounded members of any combat unit received, when the medics of that unit are capable of such a performance as that turned in by Dr. X and his assistants—working on enemy prisoners!

But it is not my intention to imply that one must look to the sea, or to foreign shores, for commendable examples of medical and hospital care. Right at home, in the United States, the Navy in 1944 was administering 60,000 beds—all on dry land. Looking after the patients in these beds were physicians, surgeons, dentists, nurses, corpsmen and technicians who, from the standpoint of essentiality of the job at hand, were surpassed by none. The motto, "To keep as many men at as many guns as many days as possible," was no less meaningful to them than to the senior medical officer of a battleship or cruiser. Indeed, a great proportion of this personnel had been on sea and foreign duty earlier in the war. Not infrequently they encountered, in Key West or Seattle or Boston, patients whom they had attended in Kula Gulf, New Hebrides or at Salerno.

The point I wish to make, however, is that these men and women of the Navy's Medical Department were fulfilling not solely a humane mission. They were putting fighting men back into action. Remember, when a wounded sailor or Marine was evacuated to the mainland, it did not mean necessarily that his days of active duty were over. From the moment of admittance to a Naval Hospital, it was the prime objective to restore the patient to condition for full, unlimited duty or, if this was impossible, to a form of duty which, though limited, was essential. Finally, if persevering treatment and hospitalization were unable to make the man fit for retention in the service, he was rehabilitated with the purpose in view of ultimate discharge to civilian life, equipped physically and psychologically to pursue a useful career.

Adherence to this precept of rehabilitation was universal in all our naval hospitals. Certain ones, however, were selected for special services. Worthy of mention are the amputation centers at Mare Island, California, and in Philadelphia; the rheumatic fever and tuberculosis departments at Corona, California; neurosurgery at Bethesda, Maryland, and Chelsea, Massachusetts; vision and hearing cases in Philadelphia; neuropsychiatry at Mare Island and Bethesda; plastic surgery at San Diego and Oakland, California; tropical diseases at Bethesda and Treasure Island, San Francisco, and the cancer pavilion in Brooklyn.

The great disparity between Navy-Marine casualties in World War I and World War II makes any comparison invidious. Nevertheless, one may observe that the mortality rate of wounded in 1917–1918 was 12 per cent; in 1943, 2.2 per cent. As of March 31, 1944, more than 55 per cent of all sailors and Marines wounded since Pearl Harbor—including the large number of casualties of that infamous day—had returned to active duty. Forty per cent were still under treatment, and a large proportion of these could be expected to resume their regular duties in the near future. It was necessary to invalid less than 2 per cent from the service. Only three out of every hundred succumbed to their wounds.

The observations set forth here do not presume to do more than touch upon a few highlights. A more lengthy exposition of the responsibilities and activities of the Medical Department would tell of the strides taken in aviation medicine. It would have something to say of the valuable contributions made by women in uniform: nurses, medical officers, dental officers, the Waves in our Hospital Corps. There would be garlands for the aviators, crewmen, doctors and corpsmen of South Pacific Combat Air Transport—better known as "Scat"—for the enormous part they played in reducing mortality of the wounded through speedy evacuation by air. And more of the same for our gallant representatives in the submarine service.

There is, finally, a certain specialized field that merits something more than a perfunctory notice, even if there were no reason other than a general lack of appreciation of its very existence, not to mention its value. One rarely hears of it because its province is not within the realm of the spectacular. It is something usually taken for granted, though without it the efficiency of the Navy would be disastrously impaired. One might call it, to borrow a phrase from our submariners, the Medical Department's own little "silent service." I refer to the industrial hygiene program.

Early in 1941, when we were well embarked upon a policy of planning, research, development and expansion in preparation for whatever might befall, when our mobile hospitals and blood substitutes and other pioneering ventures were just beginning to show faint signs of promise, in this tense pre-Pearl Harbor period, an industrial medicine section was established in the Bureau of Medicine and Surgery. Founded upon the premise that any mechanical job can be performed safely if proper precautions are observed and careful study given in advance to all possible hazards, the section and its field personnel were dedicated to protection of the hundreds of thousands of men and women—principally civilians—employed in Navy Yards, Naval Air Stations, Naval Ordnance Plants and other shore establishments.

Medical officers were sent away for postgraduate instruction in industrial hygiene. Chemical engineers, sanitary engineers, mechanical engineers, chemists and other specialists were assigned to the section. All necessary laboratory and field equipment for study and analysis of dust, fumes, illumination, noise and ventilation was procured. Close liaison was set up with the Shore Establishments Division of the Navy Department.

Dividends were liberal. On the one hand, the health, safety, earning power and efficiency of the worker were protected. On the other, maximum production of vital material was promoted by lowering incidence of disease, minimizing exposure to death or disabling injury and reducing absenteeism. Prospective employees received physical examinations by naval medical officers, whose findings had a large bearing upon the type of job to which the applicant was assigned, if any. For example, a man found to have an organic condition which disqualified him for a Navy Yard's iron foundry might be perfectly acceptable for some lighter, but equally essential, duty.

Once hired, all workers were physically examined at intervals, the periodicity depending upon the job. Whereas an annual checkup was deemed adequate for locomotive operators, welders of painted or coated materials were examined four times a year. Industrial hygiene laboratories were maintained in the big yards and plants, and reports were filed on all accidents, injuries and industrial illness, whether time was lost from work or not.

Here again, in the behind-the-scenes field of industrial medicine, it was demonstrated that teamwork can do wonders. A handful of medical and line officers of the Navy, given the cooperation of the workers whose welfare they served, and of the interested civil authorities in the various localities where the industrial centers were situated, have done an untold amount of good in helping to launch ships on schedule and in furnishing them with all the guns they required. Teamwork is the key to success, in peace as in war.

Anyone who has seen the motion pictures of the invasion of Guadalcanal and Tarawa will realize the hell of fire and devastation endured by our soldiers, sailors and Marines in those engagements. Our record of men killed was great. The number of wounded, considering the total size of the invading forces, was tremendous. That so many men recovered was largely due to Captain French Robert Moore of the United States Navy Medical Corps, who was in charge of the medical service in those battles.

Captain Moore was graduated from the University of Oregon Medical School in 1926. His career has been that of the typical American physician who enters on medical practice and then, when the nation needs him, volunteers his services and becomes a military physician almost overnight.

Captain Moore's account of the invasion recites dramatically the amazing exploits of the men who participated in it, and indicates why many of the physicians in these battles were decorated by our government for conspicuous bravery.

CHAPTER X

THE DOCTOR AT GUADALCANAL AND TARAWA

By
CAPTAIN FRENCH R. MOORE
Medical Corps, United States Navy

I

IN THE BATTLES for Guadalcanal and Tarawa, I found that the alert American mind, with its talent for inventiveness, could handle satisfactorily the most unexpected and surprising situations.

This special quality was backed by the thorough indoctrination of all hands, from the highest ranking officer down to the enlisted man, in the care of their own wounds. Medical personnel were taught to give plasma, to perform proper splinting, to clamp large bleeders and to include the clamp in the dressing, to avoid the use of tourniquets, and to apply sulfanilamide powder thoroughly to all parts of the wound.

In addition—and this was most important—we insisted that no patient be evacuated to the rear until the shock was counteracted by plasma. Abdominal wounds were given priority in evacuation, next came chest wounds, then the head, neck and extremities, in that order. Plasma was given in company aid stations, which might be in a hole, behind a tree stump, or in any place that afforded some protection. In order to provide the best care for the wounded, all personnel connected with the chain of evacuation were instructed thoroughly in the treatment of all types of wounds, so that they could function as one team.

Hospital corpsmen were drilled not to expose themselves to fire. At Tarawa, many wounded were rescued from dangerous positions by a corpsman crawling along behind whatever protection he could find, pushing a flat litter in front of him until, protected by machine-gun fire, he could roll the patient onto the litter and drag it out after him. These corpsmen were the real heroes of our organization. They were the first to see the casualties, and by their skillful use of sulfa drugs, control of hemorrhage, bandaging, splinting, giving plasma to control shock, and rapid evacuation, many lives were saved.

More decorations and letters of commendation were given hospital corpsmen, in proportion to their number, than to any other group in combat. Their exceptional courage, resourcefulness and determination in rescuing wounded men under fire were truly remarkable. Here are a few of the men's stories, with their decorations noted:

ANDREW P. CHITWOOD, JR., Pharmacist's Mate First Class, USN, Silver Star Medal. Chitwood was serving with Marine Aircraft Wing during an attack by Japanese air and surface forces at Guadalcanal on the night of October 13–14, 1942. When the Japanese made a vicious attack on Henderson Field, and salvos from hostile warships fell short and exploded in the bivouac area, Chitwood voluntarily left his place of safety at the height of the action and helped to extricate wounded officers from their shelter, which was buried under a mass of fallen debris. Then he assisted in carrying the injured on litters to the sick bay bomb shelter.

WILLIAM LOUIS GORMAN, Pharmacist's Mate Second Class, USNR. Silver Star Medal. Gorman was attached to the Second Marine Raider Battalion during an attack on Japanese forces along the Numa Numa-Piva Trail, at Bougainville, on November 8, 1943. Courageously, he exposed himself to withering enemy rifle and machine-gun fire on numerous occasions while he accompanied assault troops into combat. He made his way to wounded men on the firing line, where he administered effective first aid before he removed them to a place of safety.

PAUL STANLEY FRAMENT, Pharmacist's Mate Third Class, USNR. Silver Star Medal, awarded posthumously. In action against Japanese forces in the Solomon Islands from November 3 to 13, 1942, Frament served with a battalion of Marines, and with utter disregard for his own safety, worked his way to a point where he was dangerously exposed to hostile sniper fire while he was treating a wounded comrade. Later, he ran unhesitatingly into a heavy mortar barrage and continued to give aid to the injured until he was knocked unconscious by an exploding shell. Evacuated to a hospital in the rear, he got an immediate release the following morning, and on his own initiative, returned to his unit. On November 10, while working in another sector under heavy fire, he collapsed from extreme exhaustion and again had to be evacuated. Returning two days later, he was injured by naval gunfire after his unit had been withdrawn to a reserve area.

DANIEL A. JOY, Pharmacist's Mate Second Class, USNR. Navy Cross, awarded posthumously. At the height of a Guadalcanal battle on October 5, 1942, Joy unhesitatingly braved enemy fire and made his way through to the front lines to remove the wounded and carry them to safety. He went on with this hazardous task, above and beyond the call of duty, until he was killed by Japanese gunfire.

THADDEUS PARKER, Pharmacist's Mate Third Class, USN. Navy Cross. Parker was a corpsman with the First Marine Raider Battalion during an engagement with enemy forces on Guadalcanal, on the night of September 13–14, 1942. With his company almost completely surrounded and under attack from all directions, Parker constantly exposed himself to enemy fire to care for and evacuate the wounded. He undoubtedly saved the lives of many injured men who otherwise would have perished.

EUGENE E. BAXTER, Pharmacist's Mate First Class, USN. Navy Cross, awarded posthumously. While he was serving with the First Battalion, Second Marines, during the campaign in the Solomon Islands from August 7 to November 3, 1942, Baxter risked his life on October 9 when he spent more than an hour in the shark-infested waters of Lengo Channel to effect the rescue of ten survivors after a personnel boat had capsized off Guadalcanal. Later, he deliberately exposed himself to terrific enemy fire during an offensive against the Japanese beyond the Matanikau River, Guadalcanal, on November 3, and lost his life while he was carrying a wounded Marine from the battle line to a place of safety.

JAMES DUDLEY BARKER, Pharmacist's Mate Second Class, USNR. Navy Cross, awarded posthumously. Attached to a rifle company during the action at Tarawa on November 20, 1943, Barker was seriously wounded while he was disembarking from an amphibious tractor on the strongly fortified Japanese beachhead. He refused medical attention and cared for his own wound. Undaunted by a constant hail of enemy machine-gun and mortar fire, he administered first aid to wounded comrades on the beach in spite of his own intense pain. Barker was urged to seek protection in a nearby dugout with other casualties, but he remained at his post until he was mortally wounded by an enemy sniper. His gallant conduct and devotion to duty directly contributed to the saving of many lives.

JOHN ELLIS HARDY, Pharmacist's Mate Third Class, USNR. Silver Star Medal, awarded posthumously. Hardy was attached to the Second Marine Division during the landing on Tarawa, November 20, 1943. Injured severely in the right arm while he was disembarking from an amphibious tractor, Hardy none the less administered first aid to the wounded on the beach and rescued four others from the water. Under intense enemy fire, he continued to care for his comrades and carried on for more than five hours in spite of his own wounds, until he was killed by a Japanese hand grenade.

Medical officers with battalion and regimental aid stations were most exposed to enemy fire, and were frequently given citations, decorations and letters of commendation for their courage and skill. Here are a few examples which tell the story:

LIEUTENANT STEPHEN L. STIGLER, Medical Corps, USNR. Navy Cross. Lieutenant Stigler was Junior Medical Officer of the Marine Raider Expedition's landing force against Makin Island, on August 17–18, 1942. He braved intense enemy fire to evacuate the helpless and injured on the front lines, and during evacuation operations, he swam into the surf and rescued those unable to help themselves. After returning to his ship, he conducted several major operations under most difficult circumstances and, as a result of his skillful and tireless efforts, succeeded in bringing all his cases back to the base line in excellent condition.

LIEUTENANT COMMANDER ROBERT W. SKINNER, III, Medical Corps, USNR. Navy Cross. Lieutenant Commander Skinner was attached to the First Marine Raider Battalion during an action in the Solomon Islands from August 7 to October 10, 1942. In the fierce battle for possession of Tulagi, he distinguished himself by his expert professional skill and courage, often in positions exposed to heavy enemy fire, in administering aid to the wounded and supervising the evacuation of casualties. As a result of his work, there were no cases of infection, and practically all the wounded recovered. Later, when his battalion was fighting on Lunga Ridge, he voluntarily made at least three trips from the forward to the rear dressing station, traversing several hundred yards of exposed terrain which was swept frequently by hostile fire. Subsequently, he accompanied our forces in the second and third Matanikau River battles, and in the latter moved forward with his battalion despite a badly injured knee.

LIEUTENANT COMMANDER THEODORE C. PRATT, Medical Corps, USNR. Navy Cross. Lieutenant Commander Pratt was Chief Surgeon of a Division Field Hospital on Guadalcanal from August 7 to September 24, 1942. While enemy planes bombed the area repeatedly and surface craft shelled the hospital, he coolly and courageously attended the daily casualties which came under his care, operating on the wounded and supervising their treatment with a high standard of efficiency.

LIEUTENANT COMMANDER EMIL E. NAPP, Medical Corps, USNR. Navy and Marine Corps Medal. As Regimental Surgeon during operations of the First Marines, First Marine Division, on Guadalcanal from August 7 to December 22, 1942, Lieutenant Commander Napp displayed exceptional courage and loyalty in attending wounded personnel on numerous occasions. At the battle of the Tenaru, he repeatedly exposed himself to terrific hostile fire in order to evacuate his injured comrades. On the night of October 13–14, when Japanese warships shelled the regimental command post and struck a dugout in the area, he abandoned his shelter voluntarily at the height of the bombardment and worked his way through an intense barrage of enemy fire to administer prompt medical attention and first aid.

LIEUTENANT (jg) JACQUES C. SAPHIER, Medical Corps, USNR. Silver Star Medal, awarded posthumously. Lieutenant Saphier was attached to the First Marines during an action against a Japanese landing force of about 700 men which launched an attack at the mouth of the Tenaru River, Guadalcanal, in the early morning of August 21, 1942. With cool courage, he proceeded to the front lines and persisted in giving medical aid to wounded personnel in the face of heavy and accurate Japanese fire. He gave up his life in the service of his country.

LIEUTENANT HENRY R. RINGNESS, Medical Corps, USN. Navy Cross, awarded posthumously. Lieutenant Ringness was Flight Surgeon of a Marine Aircraft Group during action against enemy

Japanese forces on Guadalcanal on the night of Ocober 13–14, 1942. When a hostile task force moved in off our beachhead and began a vigorous bombardment of the island airfield, Lieutenant Ringness, trapped in a foxhole in the camp area by the sporadic bursting of shells, was mortally wounded by a near miss which killed four of his companions and wounded four others. Completely paralyzed in the lower half of his body and suffering great pain, he nevertheless persisted in giving morphine and blood plasma to wounded personnel until he was finally evacuated to a base hospital. Even then, with unselfish devotion, he tried to minimize his own critical condition in order that others might be given preference in medical treatment. He died three days later as a result of his injuries.

The medical officers with combat field units had the finest opportunity of any group in the battle zone to do surgery. It is with combat units that abdominal wounds must be operated on if the patient is to survive. Wounds of the head, face, neck, chest, extremities, amputations and spinal injuries must be properly treated and prepared for evacuation. Therefore, medical officials assigned to combat units had the chance to perform a greater variety of surgical procedures than those attached to the hospitals in the rear areas. Because of this, a medical officer had to have a clear conception of how to treat the many types of war wounds encountered.

Doctors in the battalion and regimental aid stations were the first medical officers to treat the casualties received from the front line. They gave plasma to the seriously wounded and checked splints and dressings. They also ligated blood vessels so that tourniquets could be removed. However, surprisingly few tourniquets were used. Bleeding was always controlled by a ligature as soon as possible, so that prolonged use of the tourniquet was avoided. Then they selected the patients to be evacuated to the field hosp't.l. The aid stations in a defensive or stabilized position could be made quite comfortable and fairly secure.

Jeep ambulances were first used on Guadalcanal. By using the rugged jeep in this manner, we were able to go far forward and to evacuate casualties rapidly to the aid stations and back to the field hospitals. One jeep type, converted to carry two stretchers and two sitting wounded men, was received and used in the last part of the Guadalcanal campaign, and again at Tarawa, with great success.

The field hospitals were staffed with exceptionally well-trained groups of surgeons. Wherever we were, the best of the captured buildings were used for hospitals, with tentage furnishing additional bed space. At one of three buildings used as a division field hospital, once a Japanese barracks, the four-way infusion was first used. The medical officers who developed this infusion, on duty at the hospital, were Commander J. K. Patterson (MC), USNR, Santa Barbara, California; Lieutenant R. H. Jones (MC), USNR, Norfolk, Virginia; Lieutenant Commander F. G. Simpson (MC), USNR, Milwaukee, Wisconsin; Lieutenant E. R. Crews (MC), USN, Andrews, Texas; and Lieutenant K. N. Roberts (MC), USN, Keota, Oklahoma.

In the receiving operating room of another field hospital on Guadalcanal, the surgery was built by the doctors and corpsmen from any kind of lumber they could beg, borrow or steal. Commander L. G. Sussex (MC), USNR, of Harve, Montana, who commanded this hospital, was an exceptionally well-trained surgeon, and many wounded men are alive today as the result of his fine surgery.

At Tarawa, the field hospitals remained aboard the transports where, working with the medical officers attached to the ships, they treated two thousand wounded men in four days. Evacuation of the wounded at Tarawa during the first twenty-four hours was particularly difficult because of the heavy enemy fire. After the island was practically secured, one hospital came ashore and set up an emergency black-out surgery in the only building that was left. It wasn't much, but it was the only shelter remaining on the island.

In spite of mud, heat, rain and mosquitoes, and a good many other difficulties, excellent surgery was performed. The death rate from wounds was less than 3 per cent. In World War I, 8 per cent died from their wounds.

The main factors in producing this low death rate were sulfa drugs; plasma and other blood derivatives, such as serum albumin; the use of whole blood near the front; rapid evacuation from jeep ambulances to field hospitals, from air ambulances to base hospitals, and from hospital ships to base hospitals; bringing the treatment to the patient by the use of mobile surgical units closely following the advance of troops; and coordinated treatment of the casualty from the front line to the base hospital.

Jeep ambulances were used far forward, and when the front line was on a ridge, they could be driven within a few yards of the casualties and thus saved much time in evacuation. For the severely wounded, plasma was continued in the jeep ambulance. By counteracting shock, if possible before evacuation, it enabled the patient to reach the field hospital in good condition, and not in irreversible shock. Hence plasma was used in considerable amounts before the patient ever arrived at the hospital. It was really "the life-saving fluid."

Combat wounds most frequently encountered were classified as follows:

1. Extremities.
    (a) Flesh wounds.
    (b) Compound fractures.
    (c) Large wounds involving bone and blood vessels requiring amputation.
    (d) Traumatic amputation.
        (1) Large caliber missile (artillery, mortars).
        (2) Shell fragments.
        (3) Hand grenades.
        (4) Bombs.
2. Head, face and neck.
3. Chest.
4. Abdomen, or combination chest and abdominal.
5. Pelvic.
6. G.U. tract (kidneys and bladder).
7. Spinal wounds.
8. Burns. In a large number of naval casualties we treated at various times, burns often headed the list in combination with other types of wounds.

II

Out of our experience, we were able to list these basic principles in the treatment of war wounds:

1. Remove unattached bone, loose bodies, such as bullets, shrapnel fragments, clothing and any foreign material, such as splinters, pebbles, coral.

2. No débridement is done except badly devitalized tissue. *Use sharp scissors for this.*

3. Cleanse wound with soap and water or saline and glucose.

4. Ligate all bleeders, both above and below, and divide the vessel. This prevents secondary hemorrhage by vessels retracting.

5. Nerve injuries. Approximate ends of nerve with black silk. Most nerve injuries occur in wounds of the extremities, in which there is a compound fracture, with tissue loss. These wounds are immobilized by plaster or splinting to include the joints above and below the wound, in a position of maximum relaxation.

6. Sulfanilamide powder is applied to war wounds after cleansing, using a gloved finger or instrument to spread the powder into every part of the wound. In a deep penetrating or through-and-through wound of the soft tissue of the thigh or buttocks, use a catheter to instill a 2½ per cent sulfathiazole solution. In deep, open wounds, lightly pack base and side walls with gauze saturated in 5 per cent sulfathiazole ointment.

7. *Do not suture wounds except to control hemorrhage.* Small, clean face wounds are the only exception.

8. Immobilize all extensive soft tissue wounds, even without fracture.

9. Give morphine in adequate doses but do not give it in ½-grain dose to the slightly wounded, as this may make them stretcher cases.

10. Shock. Plasma, blood, and saline and glucose are used in large amounts. If necessary, give four-way infusion. Blood must be used after plasma in the severely wounded, because of the large loss of blood. Four-way infusion in severe shock is life-saving. In this four-way infusion, plasma is given in each arm and one leg, with saline and glucose in the other leg. While this is going on, get the blood ready. In severe gunshot wounds, involving kidneys, liver, chest and abdomen, as much as 12 units of plasma, 1,000 cc. of saline and glucose and 10 to 12 pints of blood were given in a period of 2 to 3 hours.

11. Sulfonamides were given to all with severe wounds, either orally, intravenously or rectally.

Gunshot wounds of the extremities were the most frequent type of wound. The bones were shattered and there was a large tissue loss, particularly at the exit of the missiles. The patients were first treated near the front line by a corpsman, who gave morphine, sulfanilamide powder in the wound, applied dressing and splint and gave plasma. During evacuation to the field hospital, additional plasma was often given and the splint and dressing checked.

A casualty arrives at the field hospital one to three hours later, where a medical officer, wearing a mask, examines the wound, does a cleansing débridement, ligates vessels, approximates nerve ends and, using a gloved finger, makes an emulsion of the sulfa drug with blood and serum, which is applied to all parts of the wound and ends of bone, and then dresses the wound. Reduction and alignment are easily accomplished because of the paralyzing effect on the extremity of the high velocity bullets. Casts are applied—first a posterior splint, followed by circular plaster. When a large number of wounded are being received, Thomas splints are used only for immobilization; reduction and casts come later. In using Thomas splints, only light traction is applied, because an overtight glove may cause a severe ulceration of the foot. All casts applied to arm or leg are split down the center to the stockinet. If numbness or cyanosis appears, the cast is immediately separated.

In amputation, the guillotine procedure was used. We saved as much soft tissue and bone as possible. Vessels were ligated, sulfanilamide powder was used freely, and the wound covered by 5 per cent sulfathiazole ointment gauze. All amputations were supported by splinting or cast extending beyond the stump a few inches.

Gunshot wounds of the head, both penetrating and compound types, were seen. Here is the treatment: Cleanse wound with saline and/or soap and water. *Do not apply alcohol or iodine.* Remove loose bone fragments or shell fragments, but be careful of hemorrhage in doing so. Dust wound with sulfanilamide powder and apply a sulfanilamide ointment gauze dressing. Elevate head and start sulfa drugs by any method possible.

In wounds of the face, the usual cleansing débridement is done, followed by sulfa powder locally. Then, if the wound is clean, the edges are approximated with dermol or silk. *Do not close these wounds under tension.* In wounds opening into the mouth, mucous membrane is stitched to the skin. When the mandible is involved, the dental surgeon comes into his own. All tissue and bone possible must be preserved and the face contour maintained.

Laceration of the scalp by gunshot wounds was more frequent than imagined. Because of the excellence of the helmets, the bullet was often deflected so that the bullet, instead of penetrating the skull, merely grooved the scalp. These wounds were cleansed with soap and water, sulfa powder applied, and the wound edges, if widely separated, were approximated only. The rule is: *Do not close;* in all wounds of the scalp, investigate the skull to see whether it has been damaged.

Neck wounds were not uncommon. The anterior-posterior wounds, if not too near the mid-line, seldom struck vital structures, and caused little trouble. The transverse and mid-line wounds are usually fatal because large vessels are struck. Tracheotomy tubes were used frequently in these cases and proved invaluable.

In wounds of the chest, if the gunshot wound is centrally located, the patient usually dies. If the bullet's entrance is near the outer border of the chest, he will probably recover. At the front line, these wounds were immediately sealed with gauze and adhesive. If respiratory embarrassment occurred, aspiration was done immediately. This embarrassment was usually caused by hemothorax and rarely by pneumothorax. Aspirations of the chest were frequently done in battalion or regimental aid stations. Only enough blood or air was removed to relieve the immediate situation. These cases were then treated for shock in the usual manner and kept quiet for a week or ten days, if possible, before evacuation to a base hospital.

Wounds of the abdomen were seen less often than chest wounds, because a man in combat is usually bent forward. Because of this position, the bullet may enter the lower chest, strike a rib and be deflected down, where it may damage the liver, spleen, kidneys or any of the abdominal organs. Of course, in some wounds of the chest or abdomen, a large vessel was hit, and the man died before anything could be done for him. But this was not always the case, and by the use of plasma from the front line back to the field hospital, these patients arrived in fairly good condition. Then, if necessary, the four-way infusion was used, and in some cases 10 to 12 units of plasma followed by 8 to 12 pints of blood were given in a period of 2 to 3 hours, after which the patient was ready for surgery. If we had not had plasma in large amounts to give these patients while blood was being collected and matched, many of these severely wounded men would not have survived.

Here are two cases we encountered:

CASE 1. A Marine was wounded in the lower chest. The bullet was deflected down through the liver, shattered the right kidney, struck the fourth lumbar vertebra, and left by a large wound in the right flank. By the use of plasma from the front line to the field hospital, the patient arrived still alive, but nearly pulseless. The four-way transfusion was immediately started. In all, the patient received twelve units of plasma, eleven pints of blood and 1,000 cc. of saline and glucose in two and a half hours. After the blood pressure stabilized, a right nephrectomy was done, a strip of muscle was cut from the flank and placed in the liver wound, and the liver wound and diaphragm closed by mattress suture, a handful of sulfanilamide powder was then placed in all parts of the wound, and the wound closed with a drain. Three units of plasma and two pints of blood were given post-operatively, and the patient had an uneventful convalescence.

CASE 2. An aviator whose plane was damaged landed in the water just off the beach from one of our field hospitals. Some sharp object cut a large, ragged wound extending on the left side from the spine nearly to the navel. He arrived at the hospital twenty minutes later with a shirt jammed in the wound. He was nearly pulseless. The four-way infusion was started and the patient received twelve units of plasma and ten pints of blood within a period of two hours. A hemi-nephrectomy was done, as the lower pole of the kidney was nearly torn off. The descending colon was cut nearly half in two. This was brought up and extraperitonealized. By the use of plasma and blood post-operatively, the patient made a good convalescence.

Simple perforations of the small intestines were merely closed. When two or more perforations were found in the same area, an end-to-end anastomosis was performed and the intestine extraperitonealized.

Wounds involving the sigmoid, bladder and small intestine were the most difficult type encountered. In these cases the bullet usually entered the buttocks region, and striking the pelvis, flattened out, tearing a large opening in the sigmoid and bladder, and occasionally involving the small intestine. Fortunately, these cases were few. In most wounds of the intestinal tract, except single perforations of the small intestine, the intestine is extraperitonealized. The skin and subcutaneous tissues were left open about the incision. At first, the usual type of colostomy or ileostomy was performed, but a few subcutaneous abscesses developed, which endangered the fixation of the intestine. We overcame that by leaving the skin and subcutaneous tissue open and suturing the intestine to the deep fascia.

Post-operatively, a Levine tube was used in all abdominal cases. In the serious cases, plasma and blood were given in liberal amounts. All blood for transfusions came from corpsmen, Marines and occasionally a doctor.

Wounds involving the bladder, genitalia and lower urinary tract were rare. Suprapubic cystotomy was performed in most wounds of the lower urinary tract. Injuries to the ureter are the rarest of all, and were found only once in a wound involving the sigmoid, bladder and ureter. The patient received a colostomy and a cystotomy, and the ureter was transplanted to the skin, because a large portion had been destroyed. This patient failed to survive.

Spinal wounds occurred rarely without damage to the kidneys or other abdominal contents. We had three spinal wounds that involved no other structures; one of the fourth dorsal, one of the tenth dorsal and another of the second lumbar. Laminectomies were done in each case. Two of the patients had contusions of the cord with local hemorrhage, and both made good recoveries. The third case, that involving the fourth dorsal, had a complete laceration of the cord and a hemothorax. This case terminated fatally on the fourth day.

Burns are rarely encountered in land warfare. The most frequent cause of burns in forces operating ashore came from gasoline being thrown on a fire around the galley. We did, however, receive a large number of naval casualties. In one group of these casualties, there were 67 burn cases involving 20 to 40 per cent of the skin surface. Each of these 67 patients received an average of 5,000 cc. of plasma within 48 hours, plus enough saline and glucose to maintain a urinary output of more than 1,000 cc. daily. Nearly all these patients received their plasma via the femoral vein, because burns on the arms and legs made the usual veins inaccessible. Locally, the burns were treated with 5 per cent sulfanilamide ointment saturated in gauze with compress dressings. Many of these patients had other wounds, but all were saved. We had these cases nearly three weeks, and by keeping the burns of the face thoroughly covered with sulfanilamide ointment, there was no contracture of the eyelids or the other soft tissue of the face.

Blast injuries to the abdomen, resulting from underwater depth charge explosions in the vicinity of survivors from sinking ships, were not infrequently seen. These injuries have been termed "hydraulic abdominal concussion" and frequently cause intestinal perforations, similar to a blow-out seen in an automobile tire. All these patients must be operated on if they are to survive. Patients without perforation of the gut are treated conservatively. Blast injuries from bombs usually involve the lungs more than the abdomen. All such patients are treated conservatively, oxygen being used to ease the air hunger.

Three types of anesthesia were used. Spinal anesthesia was used in all abdominal cases, and amputations of the lower extremities; local anesthesia and intravenous sodium pentothal were used in all other types of wounds. Intravenous anesthesia, plus local, was used more and more in doing abdominal surgery. The dental officers gave a great deal of our intravenous anesthesia in addition to taking care of wounds involving the upper and lower jaws.

The advances in surgical technic since the last war, as taught in our medical and dental schools and postgraduate centers, have been responsible for saving hundreds of lives. By bringing these skilled surgeons to the patient, through the intelligent use of plasma, whole blood and sulfa drugs near the front line, plus the rapid evacuation to the field hospitals, the mortality rate of the wounded was reduced to less than 3 per cent.

The corpsmen, dental and medical officers with whom I served in the Pacific campaign are the finest group, both personally and professionally, that I have ever known. Their loyalty, courage and skillful surgery were a constant inspiration.

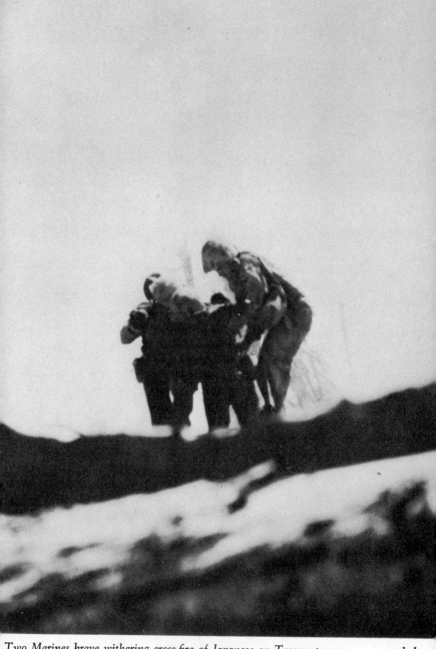

Two Marines brave withering cross-fire of Japanese on Tarawa to rescue a wounded buddy. (OFFICIAL U.S. MARINE CORPS PHOTO)

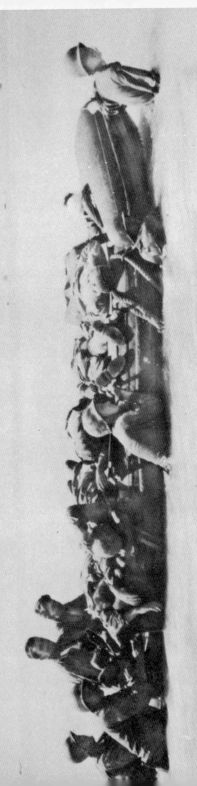

Marines wounded in Tarawa landing are towed out to larger craft on a rubber landing boat. Larger vessels took them to base hospitals. (OFFICIAL U. S. MARINE CORPS PHOTO)

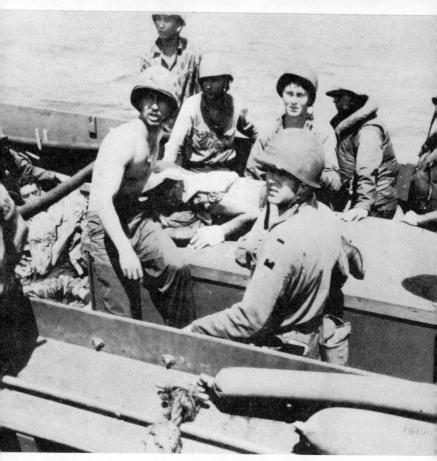

Wounded Marines at Tarawa are taken back to troopship in a landing barge. One Marine (left) lies in bottom of boat, while man on hatch cover is covered with towel to keep flies out of wounds. (OFFICIAL U. S. MARINE CORPS PHOTO)

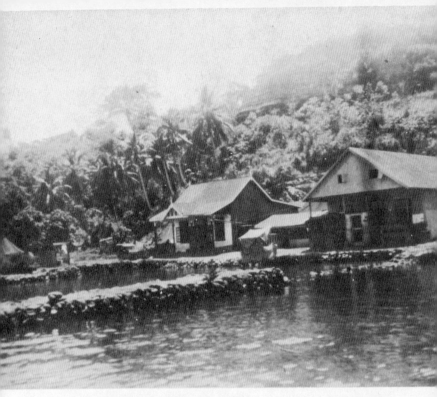

Part of "D" Medical Company hospital on Tulagi, December, 1942. Buildings were originally stores. At left, tents have been erected and camouflaged.
(PHOTO COURTESY DR. JUSTIN J. STERN, SAN DIEGO, CALIFORNIA)

THE UNITED STATES PUBLIC HEALTH
SERVICE IN THE WAR

This total war in which we have been engaged mobilized every medical force in the United States, and especially the United States Public Health Service. On that service rested the prevention of epidemic disease, the control of venereal disease in and around camps, the prevention of industrial disease, and the assurance of the health of the American people at large. Surgeon General Thomas Parran has earned for himself a repute among the people of America so great that today his name is familiar to almost every American.

After serving notably as health officer of the State of New York, he was called to Washington by President Roosevelt, and under Dr. Parran's leadership there has been a great expansion of the work of the United States Public Health Service. No doubt he is best known for the campaign against venereal disease and for the removal of the mystery long associated with its prevalence. To the medical profession, however, he is known as a leader in the expansion of health service in general. As a member of every leading medical organization in the country, he has received decorations from many colleges and universities and several medals of distinction for scientific achievement as well as decorations from foreign countries.

A review such as is offered in Dr. Parran's article on "The United States Public Health Service in the War" will inform many readers for the first time of the quiet and efficient way in which our lives are protected by this agency of the United States government.

CHAPTER XI

THE UNITED STATES PUBLIC HEALTH SERVICE IN THE WAR

By
THOMAS PARRAN, M.D.
The Surgeon General, United States Public Health Service

I

IN TOTAL WAR, the health of civilians is second in importance only to the health of the armed forces. The work of the United States Public Health Service during the war has reflected the effectiveness of the nation's total health forces, as well as concurrent advances in the sciences and the acceptance of governmental responsibility for the well-being of the citizens of a democracy.

When President Roosevelt in June, 1940, declared a state of emergency, Federal, State and local health services were in a more advanced position for the prevention of disease than at any previous time in our history. The United States Public Health Service had been strengthened, cooperation with State and local health organizations had matured and extended, and the foundation had been laid for a health service truly national in scope. Without such a foundation, organized health services in the United States would have been ill prepared to meet the enormous demands of war.

The operation of title VI of the Social Security Act for five and a half years had produced a sound and steady growth of basic health services throughout the country. By 1940, nearly 1,700 counties were served by health units under the direction of a full-time medical officer. About 6,000 professional employees of health departments had received formal training in public health at leading universities. The National Venereal Disease Control Act of 1938 had established strong programs in every State and in every city of 500,000 population and over. Existing services of all types had been strengthened. All along the public health front there had been marked progress.

This hardy growth, however, had not been sufficient to meet the emergency demands. Military and industrial expansion, with its attendant disruption of the civilian population and community life, was certain to intensify the health programs of the nation. No great amount of public health foresight was needed to realize that, in many areas, local authorities would not be prepared to cope with their new burdens. Basic sanitary facilities and communicable disease control were inadequate for increased populations. Shortages of medical and health personnel of all types and of hospital facilities were bound to occur. Since the conduct of the defense program—and subsequently the prosecution of the war —was clearly a responsibility of the Federal Government, the States needed, and reasonably looked to the government to provide, additional help in meeting their public health responsibilities.

In the summer of 1939, the Public Health Service undertook sanitary reconnaissance in Army maneuver areas and later extended it to areas of mobilization and industrial expansion. Teams consisting of a medical officer and an engineer surveyed the public health, housing, hospital and medical facilities of some 250 areas, securing first-hand information on the health status of communities and needs for Federal assistance. Subsequently, this work was taken over by the district offices of the Service, and in the end more than 400 areas, or ten times the number originally surveyed, had been studied with respect to health problems and facilities.

A special conference of the State and Territorial health officers with the Public Health Service was convened in September, 1940, to discuss these problems. This interchange of information between the Service and the State health authorities disclosed that certain areas of public health activity would need to be strengthened and that the most critical needs of the States would be for personnel, equipment and facilities. Stronger control measures would be needed against venereal diseases, tuberculosis and malaria; protection of sanitary facilities and food supplies would become more difficult. In addition, the resources of the Public Health Service would be taxed to the utmost in conducting essential research, in providing medical and hospital service for its beneficiaries, and in administering the national quarantine laws under war conditions. Shortages of medical and nursing personnel in civilian health services would create critical situations in many parts of the country, and might seriously impede the war effort, if the needs of the Army and the Navy could not be met.

In the four succeeding years, the work of the Public Health Service was entirely directed toward meeting these war needs, in so far as it was possible within the limitations of governmental authorization of activities and funds. The growth of the Service during the war is reflected by the increases of personnel employed and of appropriations made to the Service. The total appropriations to the Public Health Service for the fiscal year 1940 were $19,594,320, and 9,592 persons in its employ were on active duty. The total appropriations for the fiscal year 1944 were $108,698,680, and 16,000 employees, including 2,202 commissioned officers, were on active duty.

The first appropriation, authorizing the Public Health Service to assist States in war areas, was made by Congress in March, 1941, when $525,000 was appropriated for a three months' period. As needs increased, Congress increased the appropriations for aid in critical areas. The appropriations for Emergency Health and Sanitation Activities for the fiscal years 1942 to 1944 were as follows:

1942	$ 4,470,000
1943	9,273,700
1944	11,679,000

The Emergency Health and Sanitation appropriations were expended for the following purposes: (1) assistance to States; (2) administration; (3) malaria control in war areas; (4) *Aedes aegypti* mosquito control; (5) industrial hygiene; (6) milk and food sanitation; (7) tuberculosis control; (8) emergency medical care; (9) cooperation with other agencies; (10) laboratory services; and (11) typhus control.

To augment inadequate staffs of health departments in defense areas, the Public Health Service undertook to recruit qualified physicians and other professional health workers for assignment to critical areas. Intensive orientation courses, scheduled monthly through the first half of 1941, were established and held at the National Institute of Health, Bethesda, Maryland. From April, 1941, to April, 1944, there was a total of 15 orientation classes.

Of the 936 trainees, 327 were medical officers and dentists; 324

were sanitary engineers, veterinarians and sanitarians; 230 were public health nurses; 34 were laboratory workers; and 45 were health educators and others. These workers were not recruited from the ranks of those already engaged in public health work.

A medical officer, a sanitary engineer and a public health nurse of the Service devoted the major portion of their time to recruiting new public health personnel. Notices in medical, nursing and sanitary engineering journals were helpful; engineering schools were visited; and letters were sent to recent medical and nurse graduates. Many interns in United States Marine Hospitals and recent graduates of engineering schools were recruited.

Emergency Health and Sanitation personnel were assigned to those State health departments in which the needs were greatest. It was urgent that this policy be adopted because imperative requests for personnel outnumbered the supply from the beginning. For example, at times only 75 or 80 recruits were available, while requests totaled 300.

Although the PHS has never been able to meet the personnel needs of the States, the recruitment and training program adopted by the Service showed the States the value of setting up training programs of their own. By the close of 1942, there was an urgent need for 2,000 or more sub-professional workers in local health departments. In 1943, North Carolina, Oklahoma, Louisiana and West Virginia set up orientation courses and training programs of their own. In 1944, a three months' war training course for sanitarians was established at the University of North Carolina, to operate throughout the year, for the duration.

Thus, under the Emergency Health and Sanitation program, the Public Health Service furnished many booming or undeveloped communities with at least a nucleus of health organization. The physicians, engineers and nurses assigned to these localities often had to start from scratch, providing services which more advanced communities had been furnishing as a matter of course for 25 or 50 years. The Service also sent its mobile laboratory units into critical areas to assist in the analysis of milk and water supplies, and in the appraisal of restaurant sanitation.

The need for public health education was re-emphasized by the many problems which arose in war communities. In 1941, the Public Health Service assigned two health educators to the North Carolina State Board of Health to develop intensive community health education programs, as a demonstration. Later, as the effectiveness of the demonstration was recognized, additional health education personnel were employed to organize programs in other States. The demonstrations served also to inspire State health officers to initiate similar programs.

In 1943, the Kellogg Foundation made available to the Public Health Service funds for the establishment of training fellowships in community health education. The training courses were developed first at the University of North Carolina and later at Yale and the University of Michigan. At the close of the school year 1944, 36 students had completed their training. Nineteen more students had been trained with funds provided by State health departments.

In the summers of 1942 to 1944, local school teachers were employed in each of 100 Southern counties to conduct intensive malaria education programs in their communities.

On June 28, 1941, the President signed Public Law 137, 77th Congress, known as the Lanham Act (Community Facilities). This law authorized the Federal Works Agency to allot Federal funds for the construction of sewerage, waterworks, schools, hospitals and other community facilities where the absence or inadequacy of such facilities would impede the war effort and where the community itself could not provide them without unreasonable financial burden. Shortly thereafter, the Federal Works Agency was directed by the President to utilize the resources of the Federal Security Agency and other Federal departments in administering the Lanham program. This directive was recognition of the fact that these agencies not only had data on the facility needs of war areas, but had established working relationships with official State agencies.

It was agreed that the Federal Works Agency would depend upon the Public Health Service for surveys and recommendations of need for health projects. Consultation with the Federal Works Agency was provided by the Public Health Service. The Sanitary Engineering Division covered facilities for water supply and distribution, sewerage, and garbage disposal; and the Hospital Facilities Section of the States Relations Division covered public health centers, hospitals, nurses' homes and training facilities.

The major activities of the Service in the Lanham program have been: (1) recommendation of need; and (2) development of basic designs for medical facilities, and provision of architectural consultation on individual projects.

Prior to the war, no standards had been set for the buildings which housed State and local health departments, although some experimentation had been done by private foundations. Designs for modern public health centers, developed by the Hospital Facilities Section, were first released in the fall of 1941. A description of the program and the designs were published in the *Architectural Record* for July, 1942, and later appeared in the January 22, 1944, issue of the English medical journal, *The Lancet.*

Early in 1942, war production priorities made it necessary to restrict construction of community facilities, and many projects had to be redesigned. Hospitals and architects had been accustomed to multistory structures. Now, because of the impossibility of securing steel, it became necessary to develop single-story types. The functional designs developed by the Hospital Facilities Section were distributed early in 1942, and appeared in the August, 1942, issue of the *Architectural Record.* In July, 1943, they were published in *Hospitals,* under the title "Planning Suggestions and Demonstration Plans for Acute General Hospitals."

Consultation on the architectural plans for individual projects was provided by the Section whenever requested. The Service also was consultant to the War Production Board on the need for construction of non-Federally financed facilities.

As of March 1, 1944, the following projects recommended and approved by the Public Health Service had been constructed or were in progress: (1) general hospitals—162 new hospitals and 409 additions; (2) 377 facilities for schools of nursing; (3) 254 health centers; and (4) 139 venereal disease treatment facilities (for the most part, old structures in need of renovation and reconstruction). These figures do not include the health facilities made available by other means than new construction—rental, reconditioning, etc.

The Public Health Service in 1941 transformed its plague-investigation forces on the West Coast into a control organization and affected working agreements for more extensive rodent control with the Fish and Wild Life Service, Department of the Interior. In 1942, the number of mobile plague-investigation laboratories was increased from 4 to 10. Six of the units made a survey from the Rio Grande to the Canadian border, between the 100th and 105th longitude meridians, to determine the eastern limits to which plague infection in wild rodents had spread.

Between 1942 and 1944, plague infection was reported in rats, wild rodents, or ectoparasites from rodents in Hawaii and nine Western States—California, Colorado, Idaho, Montana, Nevada, New Mexico, North Dakota, Washington and Oregon. The control program included extensive field surveys, extermination of rodents in and around military cantonments and maneuver areas in endemic regions, and assistance to State and local health authorities. A laboratory was maintained in San Francisco for the examination of animal tissues and fleas, identification of animal and insect vectors, and determination of epidemiologic factors related to the disease.

Typhus fever is more widespread than plague in the United States. It has been endemic throughout the South and seems to be spreading to other areas. For example, since 1939, typhus infection in rats and cases of typhus fever have been reported in the Southern part of California.

In May, 1942, the Public Health Service established an office of Typhus Fever Control, with headquarters in Atlanta, Georgia, to help civilian and military authorities to cope with the problem of rat infestation in war areas. Technical assistance was given to States and cities in the form of trained personnel, equipment and materials, and consultation service was given to the Army.

Control measures were designed to reduce the rat population. Surveys of rat harborages were made, one district at a time attacked, and all buildings ratproofed and rats destroyed. Work was concentrated in the business sections of communities, and procedures included protection of food in storage, proper collection and disposal of garbage, exterior ratproofing of buildings, and extermination of rats by trapping, poisoning and fumigation.

The projects served to demonstrate that rat infestation can be permanently controlled at a relatively low cost. Personnel of local health departments were trained in all aspects of rodent control so that the work could be continued after the withdrawal of Public Health Service personnel.

All phases of the national venereal disease control program have steadily expanded since June 30, 1941. This expansion has been tangibly reflected by the increasing amounts of Federal, State and local funds made available for control activities.

During the fiscal year 1941, a total of approximately $13,153,000 from all sources was budgeted for the control program, $6,362,000 of this amount being Federal funds. In 1942, the total budget was about $15,433,000, including Federal appropriations of $8,448,000. The total expenditures for 1943 were $18,053,000, of which $10,596,000 were Federal funds. The State and Federal budgets for the fiscal year 1944 totaled about $20,237,000, of which $10,-953,000 were Federal funds.

Of all Federal funds appropriated for venereal disease control, approximately 80 per cent was allotted to the State and Territorial health departments as grants-in-aid. In 1942, $1,727,000 of the Federal grants to States and Territories was earmarked for cooperation with the armed forces and other war needs, and in 1943, this earmarked fund was increased to $3,229,000.

In May, 1940, an *Eight-Point Agreement* on measures for the control of venereal disease was adopted by the Federal Security Agency, the War and Navy Departments, the Selective Service System, and the State and Territorial health departments. The serological examination for syphilis of all volunteers and Selective Service candidates which grew out of this cooperative program resulted in the largest case-finding survey in the history of public health. Among the first 15,000,000 men examined, 726,000 were found to have evidence of syphilis.

Follow-up and treatment provided by civilian health service and the armed forces rendered non-infectious a large proportion of those in the early stages of infection and enabled them to take their places in the armed services. A most valuable by-product of this mass blood-testing program was the compilation of data which provided for the first time a reasonably accurate measure of the prevalence of syphilis in the nation's male population, by State and by counties.

An outstanding development has been the establishment of national network of special hospitals for the intensive treatment of syphilis and gonorrhea. Most of these rapid treatment centers have been operated by State health departments, in cooperation with the Public Health Service and the Federal Works Agency. As of June, 1944, more than fifty rapid treatment centers had been placed in operation and a number of others had been planned.

In addition to providing for actual quarantine of persons with infectious syphilis or gonorrhea in wartime, the rapid treatment center plan has made possible research in the newer methods of treatment for both diseases.

Research in venereal disease control was completely oriented to war needs. The more important research projects included: (1) rapid evaluation of sulfonamide drugs; (2) retrospective study of intensive syphilis therapy; (3) mass study of intensive syphilis therapy; (4) improved diagnosis, minimum dosage of sulfa drugs, and chemo-resistance of gonorrhea in females; (5) sulfonamide resistant gonorrhea in males; (6) the life cycle of the *Spirocheta pallida;* and (7) prophylactic agents.

Intensified and expanded civilian control activities and close cooperation among all agencies for civilian venereal disease control, together with the vigorous program of the armed services, undoubtedly accounted for the fact that no sharp increase in venereal disease had been reported among civilians up to June, 1944. A gratifying reduction of infection rates reported by the armed services also is attributable largely to these joint efforts.

Long wars accompanied by privation have always resulted in an increase in tuberculosis. During and after the last World War, all European nations, neutral and combatant, experienced a rise in tuberculosis mortality varying from 10 to 200 per cent. History is repeating itself in this war. In 1943, representatives of German-occupied countries reported that tuberculosis was raging with epidemic force in their nations, including France, Belgium and Greece. Even Great Britain, where living standards even in war were at a comparatively higher level, experienced a 13 per cent rise in tuberculosis mortality.

Crowding, fatigue, malnutrition, increased exposure, mass migrations of populations—all are factors which favor the spread of tuberculosis in wartime. Recognizing the potential threat, the Public Health Service sought a means to avert it. Prior to the outbreak of war in 1939, the Service became interested in the potentialities of the small-film x-ray as a public health method for mass case-finding. Intensive cooperative studies carried on for several years resulted in improvement of the technique to the point where its effectiveness could be clearly demonstrated.

In January, 1942, a Tuberculosis Control Section was established in the States Relations Division and began operation with funds allotted from Emergency Health and Sanitation appropriations. The Section carried out a program which included: (1) examination of workers in war industries and their families; examination of foreign workers brought to this country to work in war industry and agriculture; (2) consultation service to State health departments in the expansion of their control programs, with special emphasis on the development of follow-up procedures and record-keeping; and (3) cooperation with the Army, Navy and Selective Service in bringing men and women rejected for tuberculosis to the attention of their State health departments for follow-up and treatment.

In the two and a half years since its operation, the small-film technique has been improved so that a single unit can take and process, on the average, 500 films in an eight-hour day. With a double staff, the machine can work two shifts and complete 1,000 examinations in 24 hours. In 1943, a medical officer of the Service, Dr. Russell W. Morgan, perfected a phototimer for use with the fluorograph which doubles production and improves the quality of the pictures.

Budgetary limitations made it impossible for the Service to maintain more than 8 units at a time in the field; yet, despite these limitations, at the close of the fiscal year 1944, nearly three-quarters of a million persons—war workers and their families—had been examined.

The x-ray surveys disclosed that more than one in every 100 persons examined (1.3 per cent) showed evidence of reinfection tuberculosis. The encouraging significance of these findings has been the fact that 63 per cent of cases discovered in Public Health Service surveys were in the minimal stage. Thirty-one per cent of the cases were found to be moderately advanced and 7 per cent far advanced. (This is almost a complete reversal of past experience, when not more than 10 per cent of the patients receiving treatment for the first time were in the early stage of the disease.)

Up to June 30, 1944, mobile x-ray units of the Service had operated in thirteen States, the District of Columbia, Mexico and Jamaica. In addition, tuberculosis control officers of the Service operated State-and-city-owned units for State and local health departments requesting their services.

Migrant war workers presented a special problem. They were not always able to receive sanatorium care at public expense because they were not eligible under local residence laws. Many could not return to their original homes for care, because they had lost their residence there. State health departments, therefore, were greatly concerned with the problem of the non-resident war workers.

Impressed by the effectiveness of the program, the State and Territorial health officers of the nation, at their annual conference in March, 1944, unanimously recommended the expansion of the work of the Tuberculosis Section on a nation-wide basis, with emphasis on follow-up of newly discovered cases.

On April 17, 1944, identical bills (H. R. 4615 and S. 1851) were introduced by Mr. Bulwinkle of North Carolina in the House, and by Mr. Thomas of Utah in the Senate, to create a Tuberculosis Control Division in the Public Health Service. The Bulwinkle-Thomas Bill authorized the appropriation of $10,000,000 for the fiscal year 1945 and a sufficient sum for each year thereafter for research, grants-in-aid and other assistance to State health authorities, and interstate control of tuberculosis.

This legislation, sponsored by the National Tuberculosis Association and endorsed by the State and Territorial health officers, now makes possible a broader program which not only will serve to check the wartime threat of tuberculosis but should lead to the ultimate eradication of the disease in the United States.

Strategic and tactical considerations made it necessary to locate many of the larger training camps in the Southern States, where malaria is endemic. At the same time, troops from malarious areas were being transferred to non-malarious regions where malaria mosquitoes are plentiful. Furthermore, as war industry in the South was expanded, a vast army of workers and their families moved in. Thus malaria became a potential health hazard of the first rank, despite the fact that the prevalence of malaria in the United States at the beginning of the war was the lowest in history.

In April and May, 1941, engineering surveys made by the Public Health Service disclosed the need for controlling malaria and pest mosquitoes in 155 military, naval and industrial areas. In May, 1941, the Service initiated practical control measures in fifty critical areas in ten Southern States.

In February, 1942, the Office of Malaria Control in War Areas was established, with headquarters in Atlanta, Georgia, to organize and operate a control program. Control work outside military reservations was closely integrated with that carried on by the military authorities within the reservations. In industrial war areas, the projects were operated entirely by the Service in collaboration with the States. As of May 30, 1944, there were 1,600 projects in operation in twenty-two States, the District of Columbia and Puerto Rico. Approximately $1,400,000 was utilized for this work during the fiscal year 1942. During the fiscal years 1943 and 1944, nearly $6,500,000 and $8,000,000, respectively, were made available to the Public Health Service to continue operations and to extend control measures to new areas.

By April, 1944, the program had operated in 317 counties, providing protection for 1,200 war establishments and affording protection to several million persons. In 1943, the malaria rate among troops quartered in the United States was 0.3 per 1,000 per year, the lowest in the history of the United States Army, representing only a small fraction of the rate during the First World War.

At the request of the Surgeon General of the Army, the program was extended in 1943 to include 150 hospitals, prisoner-of-war camps and other military reservations receiving concentrations of troops and prisoners from malarious areas overseas. A number of mobile malaria-control units were organized by the Service, ready to move into any community where an outbreak of malaria occurred and to bring the situation swiftly under control. These units were utilized in the summer of 1944 to survey new threatened areas.

II

Prior to 1940, the Public Health Service was active in the development of means for the protection and improvement of the health of workers. It did so chiefly through field and laboratory investigations and by assisting State and local agencies in the organization and development of industrial hygiene services.

Even before the President declared a state of emergency, the Industrial Hygiene Division had made plans for converting its facilities and those of the States from peacetime to war effort. In October, 1940, the Subcommittee on Industrial Health and Medicine of the Health and Medical Committee (Federal Security Agency) requested the Industrial Hygiene Division of the Public Health Service to assume leadership in coordinating a nation-wide program in this field.

One of the first acts of the Public Health Service was to offer its industrial hygiene services to the Secretaries of War and the Navy, in anticipation of the enormous expansion of governmental industrial establishments (such as munitions factories, quartermaster depots, navy yards, etc.). A cooperative program was immediately developed by the War Department and the Industrial Hygiene Division, and put into action.

In February, 1941, a joint conference of Federal, State and local industrial hygienists was held with the Subcommittee on Industrial Health and Medicine.

A program was drafted which has been in effect since that date, with slight modifications. It called for a close working relationship between the Public Health Service, State and local industrial hygiene units, other official agencies, the medical profession, industry, labor and universities. The program had the following objectives:

1. The evaluation and control, in war industries, of the various health hazards resulting from exposure to dusts, fumes, gases, vapors and other materials and conditions.

2. The provision of advisory services to industry in connection with the construction of new plants and the renovation of old plants.

3. The promotion of physical examinations and medical services for the workers, in order that the benefits of preventive and curative medicine might be applied promptly to their individual health problems.

4. The control of communicable diseases among workers through programs developed in cooperation with local health departments.

The contribution of the Public Health Service to the program lay in four major activities: First, it recruited and trained several hundred persons for its own needs and for the States and industry.

Second, it gave direct assistance to the War and Navy Departments in the inspection of ordnance plants and other industrial military establishments, as well as in the conduct of research on special war problems. By June 30, 1944, the Division of Industrial Hygiene had made approximately 140 investigations in 90 government-owned industrial military establishments. In 1943, two liaison officers were assigned to the Office of the Chief of Ordnance, War Department, for the purpose of expediting the adoption of the recommendations resulting from these investigations.

Third, the Industrial Hygiene Division continued its assistance to the States in the development of additional services, so that in 1944 there were 47 units in 38 States employing approximately 360 personnel and spending nearly $1,300,000 for industrial hygiene activities. The Division loaned to the States scientific equipment and some 63 professional workers. During 1944, these various units devoted all their efforts to war industries and were able to inspect and render services to more than 11,000 plants employing 5,250,000 workers.

The fourth activity of the Division was in the field of laboratory research. More than 100 confidential reports were submitted to the armed services, covering special investigations relating to the physiologic evaluation of oxygen breathing apparatus, various types of combat clothing and related equipment, the toxicity and potential dangers of metals, explosives and solvents.

In June, 1942, the six war production leaders of the nation issued a joint statement appealing to the labor-management committees in war industries to reduce accidents and illness in the plants and in the communities. These committees were referred to the Public Health Service for advice. The Industrial Hygiene Division placed each committee requesting advice in direct contact with local industrial hygiene services and also furnished a detailed outline of an industrial hygiene program.

The War Production Board established a Section on Industrial Health and Safety, with which the Division cooperated actively. Investigations were carried on in the chromate industry and in other industries. In May, 1944, the Public Health Service and the War Production Board signed a formal agreement continuing these cooperative relationships. Similar agreements and studies were made with the War Manpower Commission.

Another cooperative relationship was with the United States Maritime Commission, involving investigations in the numerous shipyards operated for the Maritime Commission. In April, 1944, a research investigation of the health of shipyard workers was undertaken, with special reference to the effects of welding fume exposure.

Other cooperative relationships were maintained and active programs were carried on with the United States Department of Labor, the Army Industrial Hygiene Laboratory and the Provost Marshal General's Office.

In 1943, the Public Health Service joined with the National Society for the Prevention of Blindness in a cooperative program of eye conservation in industry. A specialist in ophthalmology was assigned to the task of developing this program. Work with the Industrial Hygiene Foundation was continued in conducting studies of sickness absenteeism, and with the American Standards Association in the development of codes for safe practices.

Other war activities of the Industrial Hygiene Division included a survey to determine the present practices of industrial nurses, and a survey of medical service facilities in plants.

Although nurses make up the largest single group of professional workers in the health field, a serious shortage of graduate nurses existed even before the war. Military and civilian authorities, therefore, anticipated that steps would have to be taken to avert critical shortages resulting from increased emergency demands.

At the request of the Nursing Council on National Defense, organized in 1940, the Public Health Service undertook to maintain an annual nation-wide census of registered nurses. The number of active nurses, as of April, 1943, was 170,599. Of this number, 77,704 were employed by institutions, 18,900 were in public health work, and 73,995 were employed as industrial nurses, private duty nurses, and in other occupations; 88,575 were inactive.

On July 12 and 13, 1941, the Subcommittee on Nursing of the Health and Medical Committee of the Federal Security Agency called a meeting with the Nursing Council and the National Committee on Red Cross Nursing Service. A master blueprint was drafted for mobilizing the country's nursing strength, and an intensified program of nurse recruitment was outlined. In July, 1941, Congress appropriated $1,200,000 for the establishment of refresher courses for inactive registered nurses, for postgraduate courses, and for increasing undergraduate enrollment. During the two-year period 1941–1943, a total of $5,300,000 was appropriated by Congress and made available through the Public Health Service to schools of nursing and other educational institutions for these purposes.

By 1942, schools of nursing had increased their student-nurse enrollment by 12,000. About 3,800 inactive nurses had been given refresher courses and some 4,800 graduate nurses had received postgraduate training.

However, military and civilian needs for nursing services had been mounting and, at the same time, the shortage of trained nurses had increased so rapidly as to outstrip the nurse education program. Schools of nursing and civilian hospitals found themselves in competition with the greatly expanded opportunities for employment of young women. Civilian hospital needs increased by 10 per cent in 1942 alone. War industries more than doubled their employment of nurses, and the Army and Navy, which had absorbed approximately 35,000 nurses, indicated that they would require 2,500 additional nurses each month during 1943.

In the fall of 1942, the nurse shortage had become so acute that hospital administrators and nursing leaders consulted with Federal agencies to see what could be done. In a series of conferences held by governmental agencies, the American Hospital Association and the National Nursing Council for War Service, the plan now implemented by the Bolton Act (Public Law 74, 78th Congress) was developed.

The Bolton Act, introduced by Mrs. Frances Payne Bolton, Congresswoman from Ohio, and sponsored by all interested groups and agencies, was passed on June 4, 1943, without a dissenting vote. The Act authorized the establishment of a United States Cadet Nurse Corps through the allotment of funds to participating schools of nursing; enlistment in the Corps provided tuition and fees, maintenance, outdoor uniforms, insignia and monthly stipends of at least $15 or $30 for each student nurse. The Act further provided that schools participating in the program shorten their training programs to 24 or 30 months. The period remaining before graduation was to be devoted to supervised practice either in the teaching hospital, a Federal hospital, or other civilian hospital or agency.

The administration of the program became the responsibility of the Public Health Service. The law also provided for the appointment of an advisory committee to be composed of at least five members, representing the nursing profession, hospitals and accredited nurse-training institutions. A Division of Nurse Education was established. Nurse recruitment was carried on through the National War Nursing Council and its State and local branches.

Congress appropriated a total of $55,200,000 for the fiscal year 1944 to implement the nurse education program. As of May 27,

1944, funds totaling $49,483,376.23 had been allotted to 1,064 nursing schools. Of the 94,761 students in these schools, 46,702 were first-year students. Forty-six schools had been allotted funds for the postgraduate training of 4,211 students.

The National Institute of Health was engaged in research directly relating to the war effort from 1939. By the close of the fiscal year 1941, 90 per cent of the Institute's resources—in scientific staff and facilities—had been channeled into confidential investigations for the Army, the Navy and the National Research Council. Many of the specific studies were initiated independently by the Institute; others were undertaken at the request of the armed services, which lacked research facilities comparable to those of the National Institute of Health. Scientists of the Institute served on committees and subcommittees of the National Research Council, on the special commission to develop the immunization program of the United States Army, on the United States of America Typhus Commission, and on other special bodies concerned with research problems.

A majority of the accomplishments of the National Institute of Health since 1940 were recorded in confidential reports to the Army and the Navy. As of June 30, 1944, 182 such reports had been made. Many other investigations which bear directly upon war problems, but which are not secret, have been reported in scientific journals and other literature of the subject.

The capacity of the Institute's staff to anticipate the need for investigation of new problems was an important factor in shaping the research program. This foresight was especially marked in the field of industrial toxicology; twenty years of experience in testing industrial substances had produced a keen awareness of potential dangers in new substances. For example, in 1941, the Institute became interested in the chemistry of the new high-octane gasolines which have been produced on a vast scale for military automotive equipment. Research upon potential hazards in the production, transportation and use of these gasolines was planned. Special funds for the project were not made available, but preliminary work was begun on July 1, 1943. On August 6, 1943, the Navy Department requested the Institute to undertake research along the same lines projected by the latter two years before. In another instance, planning and cooperation with the War Department made it possible for the National Institute of

Health to obtain complete information on the toxicology and potential hazards of PETN, a new explosive, before the munitions industry undertook mass production of the compound.

In 1941, the Rocky Mountain Laboratory of the Institute undertook to supply all the yellow fever vaccine required by the armed services. Methods of producing the vaccine were studied, with the result that certain potentially toxic substances in the vaccine were eliminated. A typhus fever vaccine developed by the Institute in 1939 was adopted by the armed services to protect military personnel, and has been produced by the Institute and by commercial biologic laboratories in enormous quantities.

The demand for biologic products of all types has risen sharply since 1940; this has placed a heavy burden on the Institute, which has the responsibility for the control of biologic products. The processing of blood plasma for the armed services, for example, required the investigation and supervision of laboratories engaged in processing enormous quantities of blood.

Since 1939, the Institute has made outstanding contributions to the knowledge of dysentery and its control among troops. Methods of diagnosis and treatment of the disease and sanitation of drinking water under various conditions have been studied.

In 1943, a study of burn shock and traumatic shock in experimental animals resulted in the discovery of the curative action of physiological salt solution administered by mouth.

Many studies in chemotherapy, especially in the effectiveness of the sulfa drugs and antibiotics, have been carried out at the Institute. For example, in 1944, the value of sulfadiazine in the treatment of bubonic plague was demonstrated.

Nutritional research relating to army rations, physical endurance, infections and poisoning has been productive.

In 1943, interest in tropical diseases prevalent in war theaters began to increase. As a result, independent and cooperative studies upon filariasis, schistosomiasis, onchorcerciasis, trypanosomiasis and leishmaniasis were organized by the Institute. Several years before the war, a unit in malaria research had been established, with special emphasis upon the synthesis of chemotherapeutic agents effective against the malaria plasmodium. The work of this unit expanded during the war, and the scientists in charge have been engaged in the coordination of cooperative studies in the same field.

Because the contributions of the National Institute of Health have been the result of confidential investigations, a complete history of the Institute's war research program cannot be told at this time.

The Public Health Service is responsible for the provision of medical and hospital care to the American Merchant Marine, the Coast Guard and certain other Federal beneficiaries. It was inevitable that as the war program gathered momentum, the medical and hospital services of the agency would increase.

Early in the Selective Service program, many localities were unprepared to meet the sudden demands for medical examinations. Therefore, certain of the Marine hospitals undertook to make special examinations of men referred to them by local Selective Service boards. Pending completion of Army hospital facilities, the Service was also called on to provide its excellent hospital facilities for Army personnel in certain areas. Army personnel were accorded the privilege of obtaining care in Marine hospitals. A situation without precedent arose when the Public Health Service was requested to furnish medical relief to detainees from certain foreign vessels seized by the United States.

As the numerical strength of the Coast Guard swelled from approximately 10,000 to 170,000 (exclusive of thousands of temporary reservists), medical and hospital services increased. Personnel of the Coast Guard were cared for at the Marine hospitals, at numerous stations, aboard vessels, and at hospitals under contract to the Public Health Service. In addition, a tremendous increase in medical personnel was required as the result of the new combat duties of the Coast Guard, which came to include land operations. The medical care of Coast Guard dependents also became a major undertaking.

The Public Health Service increased the number of medical and dental officers assigned to full-time duty with the Coast Guard from 46 in July, 1941, to 581 by May, 1944. These officers were assigned to naval transports, landing craft, cargo transports, destroyer escorts, patrol frigates, cruising cutters, and other necessary craft, as well as to shore duty. Since 1943, three Public Health Service officers have lost their lives while on duty with the Coast Guard.

After the beginning of the war, the volume of medical and hospital care required by Federal employees increased; many of these beneficiaries were workers in government arsenals and munitions plants. Yet, despite the increase in patients, no new hospitals were built, with the exception of one at Sheepshead Bay, New York, for United States Maritime Service trainees. The result has been overcrowding in the majority of the Marine hospitals. In the early part of 1944, the total capacity of the 25 Marine hospitals—6,630 beds—was severely taxed, with the patient load going as high as 6,364, or 96 per cent of the total capacity.

A neuropsychiatric service was developed at the United States Marine Hospital, Ellis Island, New York, staffed by competent psychiatrists and neurologists. Patients suffering from mental and neurologic conditions were received there from other Marine hospitals. A neuropsychiatric program also was made part of the training program at the United States Coast Guard Academy at New London, Connecticut. It included classification of cadets, special services, lectures and seminars, advisory service in disciplinary problems, and the development of new tests to fit the special needs of the Academy.

The Public Health Service also provided medical, dental and nursing care in a number of the alien detention camps of the Bureau of Immigration and Naturalization.

At the request of the War Shipping Administration, which was engaged in an extensive program of training officers and seamen, the Public Health Service supplied a complete medical service for that administration. In 1944, a total of 133 medical and dental officers—7 regular and 126 reserve—had been assigned to duty with the War Shipping Administration. For the first time in the history of the United States, a serious attempt was made to give merchant ships the services of hospital corpsmen. The United States Marine Hospital Corps School in Brooklyn, New York, was established, and there pharmacists' mates were given six months of intensive training and were then assigned to ocean-going vessels, where they were given charge of the ships' first aid, health and sanitation program.

The War Shipping Administration and the Public Health Service also carried out a joint program for the prevention and treatment of psychic effects of enemy attack on merchant seamen. These men were treated and rehabilitated in special nursing homes, and returned to their ships after convalescent care.

In 1941, the Public Health Service conducted a survey of health and sanitary conditions in Alaska and made recommendations with regard to health facilities and medical personnel. At the request of the Federal Works Agency, the Public Health Service on May 21, 1942, undertook the responsibility for the medical care of civilians engaged in the construction of the Alcan Highway, and for the supervision of sanitation on the project. The Public Health Service agreed to furnish the necessary medical, dental and sanitary officers; the Commissioner of the Public Roads Administration undertook to recruit all additional personnel, to build and equip hospitals, and to meet other non-professional needs. At the height of operations, there were nineteen regular and reserve officers of the Service on duty with the Alcan Highway.

The same kind of program was undertaken in connection with the construction of the Pan-American Highway, to which a group of medical and engineer officers were assigned in 1944.

On June 25, 1941, Dr. George Baehr of New York City, New York, was commissioned as a reserve officer of the Public Health Service with the rank of Medical Director, and was assigned to serve as Chief Medical Officer of the Office of Civilian Defense. Additional qualified physicians, chemists and engineers were recruited and commissioned by the Service for assignment to the Medical Division of the Office of Civilian Defense. A number of public health nurses and hospital administrators were also appointed to the staff. From June, 1941, to July, 1944, a total of 81 officers, 10 full-time and 29 part-time civil service employees were assigned by the Public Health Service to the Office of Civilian Defense. At the peak of operations, there were 64 officers and seven full-time employees of the Service on duty at the Civilian Defense agency. This staff planned and organized the Emergency Medical, Rescue, Sanitation, and Gas Protection services for the protection of the civilian population in the event of enemy attack.

The Public Health Service, as an operating agency, agreed to undertake the financing of the blood plasma program as well as the medical care and hospitalization of civilians injured by enemy action.

Congressional appropriations and grants from the President's funds, totaling $79,000, were made available to the Public Health Service for the expansion of civilian blood plasma reserves. Grants were made to 180 hospitals, which established plasma banks and developed reserves for emergency use totaling 77,700 units. In addition, 79,500 units of dried and frozen plasma were purchased and deposited where they would be available to the Emergency Medical Service.

The Federal Security Agency allotted to the Public Health Service $500,000 for the establishment of an Emergency Medical Section to cooperate with the Hospital Section of the Office of Civilian Defense in the care of civilians injured as a result of enemy action or civilian defense activities.

Some 2,272 physicians and dentists were commissioned in the Public Health Service inactive Reserve corps and organized in units of fifteen; and 1,700 nurses received consultant civil service appointments for duty at Office of Civilian Defense emergency base hospitals.

The Emergency Medical Section established a joint office with the Bureau of Old Age and Survivors' Insurance of the Social Security Board, which administered disability compensation and survivors' benefits for civilians injured or killed. More than 1,900 claims for medical service and hospitalization of injured civilian defense workers were considered by this office.

In spite of the fact that fewer vessels from foreign ports reached the United States in 1941, the work of all quarantine stations of the Public Health Service increased and was made more difficult. Among the factors which aggravated the problem of quarantine administration were: (1) the discontinuance by the International Office of Public Health in Paris of dissemination of information pertaining to the health status of ports in Europe, Asia, Africa and Australia; (2) the arrival of vessels from belligerent and non-belligerent countries without advance notice; (3) the diversion of American shipping to ports in Africa and the Far East from normal trade routes to Europe; and (4) the threat of bubonic plague due to the increasing number of rat-infested tramp cargo carriers in poor sanitary condition.

After Pearl Harbor, the problem of protecting the country from epidemics prevailing in foreign areas became even more complicated. Ships entered the country, coming from shores where epidemic typhus, plague, smallpox and other quickly spreading diseases were prevalent. At the same time, the acceleration of air traffic made it possible for passengers infected with quarantinable diseases to enter the country before symptoms actually developed. Furthermore, as conditions of war disrupted sanitary services in

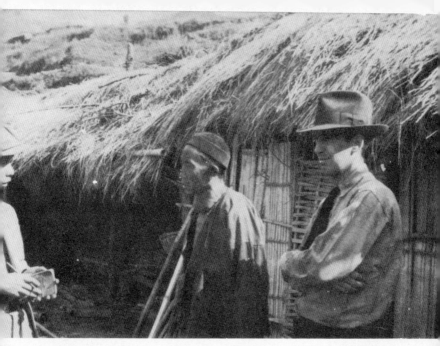

Jellison, of U. S. Public Health Service Commission, looks on as Chinese doctor health records from Chinese workman on Yunan Burma Highway. Note goitre, a prevalent condition in the area. (U. S. PUBLIC HEALTH SERVICE)

gation of old-type ships. Public Health Service men sealing hold of ship after cyanic acid soaked disks have been thrown into the lower holds to asphyxiate rodents. (U. S. PUBLIC HEALTH SERVICE)

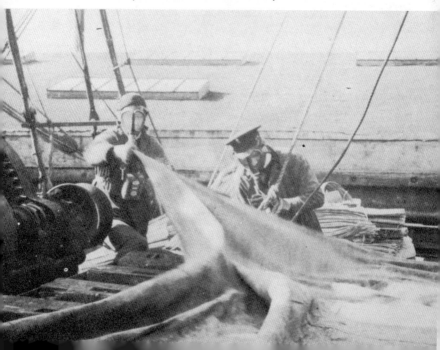

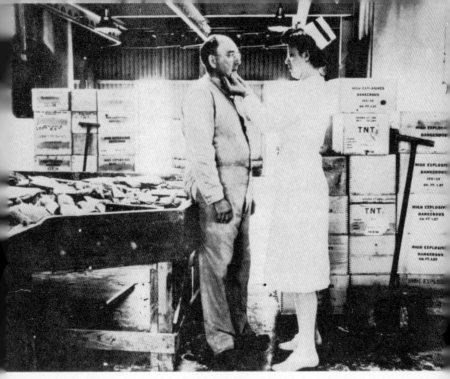

Plant nurse gives daily inspection to workers in hazardous jobs. Examination of TNT workers for poisoning includes observation of lips to note cyanosis.
(U. S. PUBLIC HEALTH SERVICE)

Preparation by doctor and staff for administration of five-day drip treatment for syphilis at a Rapid Treatment Center. (U. S. PUBLIC HEALTH SERVICE)

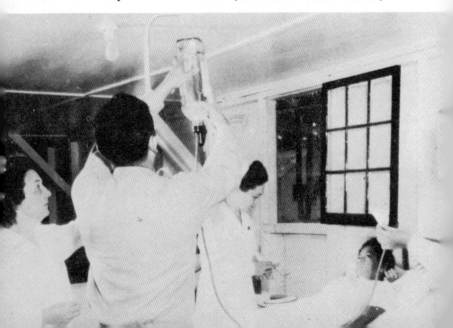

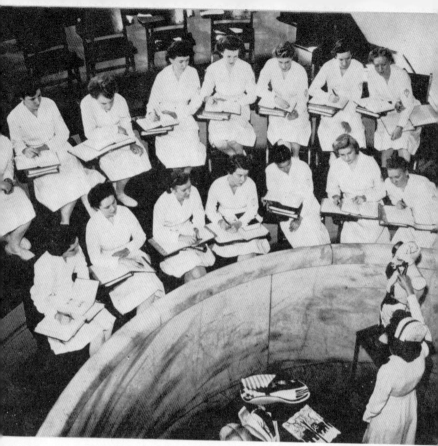

Student members of the U. S. Cadet Nurse Corps listen to anatomy lecture. These girls helped to meet urgent wartime need for nurses. (PHOTO BY HARRIS AND EWING)

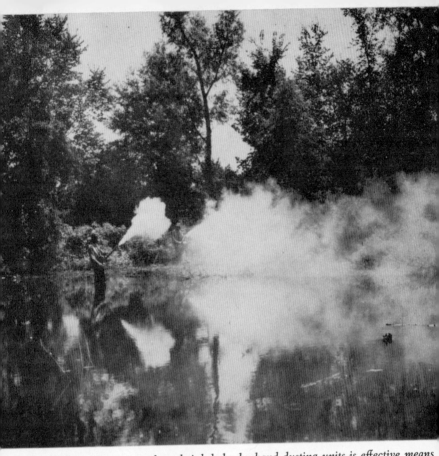

Laying poison dust on ponds and sink holes by hand dusting units is effective means of controlling breeding of mosquitoes in small areas. (U. S. PUBLIC HEALTH SERVICE)

distant areas, the vigilance of the Public Health Service had to be redoubled.

New procedures were developed to deal with the problem of air traffic, and the number of quarantine stations was increased, including a number of inland stations. In 1944, there were 21 major national quarantine stations and 163 minor stations. Air passengers were examined by medical officers for the presence of disease, and in certain instances, passengers were kept under surveillance during the incubation period of the suspected disease. All planes were disinsectized—before arrival by flight personnel, and on arrival by the foreign quarantine service—to guard against the transport of insect vectors of diseases.

As the United Nations anti-submarine warfare increased in intensity and was notably successful, fewer Allied merchant ships were sunk and more entered American ports. Quarantine service for incoming ships and prompt inspection of new ships before launching, in shipyards along the Gulf Coast and on the Pacific Coast, were important not only to the safety of the nation but to the maintenance of the United States Merchant Marine and transport of military personnel.

On August 2, 1943, by joint action of the Federal Security Administrator, the Secretary of War and the Secretary of the Navy, an Interdepartmental Quarantine Commission was established under the chairmanship of the Assistant Surgeon General of the Public Health Service in charge of foreign quarantine. The Commission was instructed to examine existing quarantine laws, regulations and enforcement procedures, and to recommend such changes or modifications as might be necessary to protect the United States and our military and naval personnel in other countries against the danger of the introduction of quarantinable and other exotic diseases. The Commission completed an extensive survey of health and sanitation conditions on several lines of communication and at foreign bases early in 1944. Recommendations were made, based upon a detailed report on air transport, conditions in foreign bases, and the impact upon civilian health of infected troops returning from abroad.

With the expansion of the war effort, officers of the Public Health Service were called on to serve in every theater of war, as well as on the home front. In addition to duty with the Coast Guard and the War Shipping Administration, officers were assigned to duty with the United States Typhus Commission.

At the outbreak of war, six medical officers of the Service were on quarantine duty in the Philippine Islands. At the request of General MacArthur, they were transferred to the Army to become part of the Medical Corps of the Army. Five of these doctors were later reported prisoners of war, and the sixth became medical aide to General MacArthur in Australia. The entire staff of the Public Health Service Medical Commission to China, assigned in 1941 in connection with the construction of the Burma-China Railroad, were reassigned to duty with the Army in India, under the command of General Stilwell, when the Japanese overran Burma.

At the request of General Eisenhower and Mr. Robert Murphy, five medical officers were assigned to supervise epidemic control and other health problems in North Africa, and a medical officer of the Service was assigned to the Office of Foreign Relief and Rehabilitation. The same officer was assigned to UNRRA, and other officers were detailed to assist in the recruitment of medical and sanitary personnel, and for direct relief work in foreign countries.

Cooperative work with the Pan-American Sanitary Bureau also increased in amount and complexity. A number of Public Health Service officers were assigned to duty in different parts of South and Central America. This work assumed increased military importance because of the presence of United States military forces in certain of these areas and elsewhere in the Americas.

In May, 1944, at the direct request of the Secretary of War, Dr. Warren F. Draper, Deputy Surgeon General of the Public Health Service, was assigned to serve as Director of the Public Health Section of Civil Affairs, on General Dwight D. Eisenhower's staff at Supreme Headquarters of the Allied Expeditionary Force in England.

After the establishment of the Procurement and Assignment Service for Physicians, Dentists and Veterinarians of the War Manpower Commission,* the facilities of the Public Health Service were made available to the Board of Directors of Procurement and Assignment. A medical officer of the Service acted as assistant director, and the chief of the Division of Public Health Methods served as chairman of the Advisory Committee.

* Originally in the Office of Defense Health and Welfare Services.

The Division of Public Health Methods analyzed all data on the number of physicians in the various States in relation to population served just prior to the war, and studied the effect upon medical services in States and counties of the withdrawal of men for the armed forces. Two physicians of the Division devoted part of their time to the Procurement and Assignment Service. One acted as chief of the Field Service Section and coordinator of statistics, the other developed standards in the procurement and assignment of nurses.

Studies of the weekly patient loads of private physicians were made in Maryland, Georgia and the District of Columbia. This was the first attempt to measure the amount of medical service physicians were giving and to determine the amount they could give. This knowledge was considered a prerequisite to the establishment of a rational program of withdrawal of physicians for the armed forces. The Division established the formula used by the Procurement and Assignment Service for the allocation of physicians to the Army and Navy by each State, and also conducted studies to establish quotas of nurses for military duty.

In 1942, a study was made of vacancies in health departments which disclosed that nearly 4,000 doctors, dentists, sanitary engineers and other health personnel were needed. In the same year, a study was made of the needs of medical schools for faculty personnel.

In 1943, a quota system was set up for the induction of interns on the basis of which arrangements were made with the Army and Navy for the deferment of commissioned interns to serve as residents in hospitals whose staffs had been seriously depleted.

Joint surveys were made by the Public Health Service and the Procurement and Assignment Service in certain areas where shortages of medical and dental personnel were believed to exist. In December, 1943, Congress authorized a special appropriation of $200,000 to the Public Health Service to be used during the fiscal year 1944 for the relocation of private practising physicians and dentists. The method by which the funds were administered was defined by the Act (Public Law 216, 78th Congress).

At the close of the fiscal year 1944, there had as yet been no widespread emergency to test the services available to the civilian population. However, the Public Health Service carefully scrutinized all developments with a view to dealing with emergencies.

The most romantic of all military activities in this war have been the far-flung operations of the Air Forces. Perhaps no other branch of the medical service has called for as much research, or for the development of as many technics, as has aviation medicine.

Major General David N. W. Grant, after receiving his doctor's degree from the University of Virginia in 1915, entered the Medical Corps of the United States Army in 1916. During World War I, he served in Panama and overseas with the Army of Occupation. When the Air Corps was developed in the Army, Dr. Grant was assigned to it in 1931, and he progressed from the position of post surgeon at Randolph Field, Texas, in 1936, to that of medical chief of the Air Corps in 1939 and became Air Surgeon in 1941.

Many experts believe that evacuation of the wounded by air accounts in large measure for the marvelous record that has been made in this war in saving the lives of the wounded. The flight surgeon, as General Grant points out, is a combination family physician, psychologist and father confessor. He lives with the pilots and the members of the crew. Flight Surgeons are hand-picked; to them must go much of the credit for the manner in which our fliers "kept 'em flying."

CHAPTER XII

THE MEDICAL MISSION IN THE ARMY AIR FORCES

By
MAJOR GENERAL DAVID N. W. GRANT
The Air Surgeon

I

IF ANY ONE quality may be said to characterize the work of a Flight Surgeon and his medical associates in the Army Air Forces, it is the urge to participate. Fundamentally, the Flight Surgeon's participation is that of a medical officer assigned to provide the professional services of a physician to military personnel who fly or who make up the system supporting the flier.

The inseparable relationship of the flier and his airplane requires, however, that the Flight Surgeon extend his interest to the technology of flight. The Flight Surgeon must team with the engineer in the mutual adaptation of man and machine, and with the tactician in the relation of the human organism to combat. It was the technical and tactical application of his medical knowledge that inspired the aphorism, "To do his job, the Flight Surgeon has to have his nose in everybody's business."

Whether the motivation was his sense of duty, the infectious nature of enthusiasm for flying, the team spirit of the AAF, the desire to share the risk, the spirit of the inquiring mind, or simply an itch for action, the typical officer in the AAF medical services could be expected not only to accept but to seek the opportunity for adventurous missions.

An Aviation Psychologist, for instance, left his desk in Washington and toured four overseas Air Forces to see how pilots, bombardiers and navigators selected through aptitude tests developed under his supervision were measuring up in combat.

He wound up flying missions in a B-17 heavy bomber, an A-20 attack bomber and a P-40 pursuit plane.

An Aviation Physiologist in the next office headed for a mountain peak to spend two months at altitudes up to 20,000 feet and temperatures down to 20 degrees below zero, wearing an oxygen mask and arctic clothing for aero medical research purposes.

In the China-Burma-India theater, a Flight Surgeon, flying on a jungle rescue mission, saw below a crashed transport airplane and the panel code signal, "Need first-aid supplies." Of his own volition, he made a parachute jump to provide medical assistance, and was closely followed by two medical aides, a sergeant and a corporal.

Another AAF medical officer parachuted to a station within the arctic circle to perform an emergency appendectomy on the camp cook, and then took over the latter's duties while he recovered.

A Flight Surgeon, who had made several jumps with paratroopers at the Fort Benning, Georgia, Parachute School, made a jump into the ocean with two other volunteers to prove that a flier can safely release himself in the water from the regulation parachute.

In England, an AAF psychiatrist quit hospital duty to fly a series of heavy bombardment missions so that he could determine how the introverts and the extroverts, the emotional and the phlegmatic, reacted under fire.

A Flight Surgeon flew over Tokyo on the famous Doolittle raid and, after his B-25 made a forced landing in the China Sea, provided medical care for injured crew members in the long days of escape through the Chinese underground.

In the Solomon Islands, a Flight Surgeon, air-evacuating military patients, was severely injured in a mountain crash, but in the 36 hours before help arrived, gave them first aid, supervised their overland evacuation to a native village, and set up a dressing station.

In the same South Pacific area, a Flight Nurse rushed to warn a crew member in danger of being crushed by a 1,600-pound airplane engine during the ditching of the transport plane on which she was attending patients. The engine struck her, but despite serious back and leg injuries, she placed rations and medical equipment on the life raft before the plane sank in the water.

In Albania, thirteen Flight Nurses and fifteen Staff Sergeants from an AAF Air Evacuation Squadron in Italy survived a forced landing after their transport plane became lost in bad weather. They spent 60 strenuous days eluding the Germans with the aid of guerrillas before they were safely evacuated.

A Flight Surgeon, testing a bail-out oxygen bottle for high-altitude jumps, made a parachute descent from an altitude of 40,200 feet (nearly eight miles up), setting an American record.

Another Flight Surgeon, observing that some young pilots in transition training were afraid to fly the B-26 "Marauder," learned to pilot this medium bomber. He then volunteered as co-pilot for any pilot who would like to have a physician at his side on his first flight.

To prove that it was safe, an Aviation Physiologist underwent explosive decompression in a low-pressure chamber, subjecting himself to an atmospheric pressure reduction equivalent to being projected instantaneously from 10,000 to 35,000 feet altitude. A large number of Flight Surgeons followed suit.

These are only a few representative episodes in the everyday practice of military aviation medicine from the equator to the poles, and from sea level to the stratosphere. The more heroic resulted in appropriate decorations—the Distinguished Service Medal, the Silver Star, the Purple Heart, the Distinguished Flying Cross, the Legion of Merit and the Air Medal. Some missions, where good luck failed to support great courage, ended in death for Flight Surgeons, Flight Nurses and enlisted men. Living and working with men for whom heroism was as commonplace as a burst of flak, the people in the AAF medical services proved they belonged to that select company.

This proof was, of course, a prerequisite to the success of a Flight Surgeon, whose mission was first the maintenance of the physical and mental fitness of the flier, and secondly to provide medical care for AAF ground personnel. The job of the Flight Surgeon, as far as the ground personnel were concerned, was pretty much like that of any other medical officer in the Army. In dispensary and hospital service, he saw the diseases and injuries common to military life, and on his post he had the same problems of sanitation, hygiene, supply and administration that confronted any Army doctor.

In the care of the flier, however, military medicine must pin-point on a target with special characteristics. This is the field of aviation medicine. Aviation medicine borrows from most of the major branches of the medical sciences as well as the basic sciences. Yet it assumes a sum and substance which identify it as a definite field of specialization, owing to the inescapable fact that man in flight is a different animal from that earth-bound creature with whom other medical specialists are accustomed to deal.

One good look at the environment of the combat flier will explain the difference. Take, for instance, the operation of a B-17 Flying Fortress. A glance at the pilot's cabin will convince you that the flight of a 30-ton B-17 is actually a complex engineering operation demanding a coordination of manual and mental skills which put the driving of a five-ton truck or even a streamlined locomotive in the kiddy-car class of human learning. The compartment is lined—front, sides, ceiling and part of the floor—with controls, switches, levers, dials and gauges. I once counted 130.

The efficient operation of all these gadgets would be difficult in the swivel-chair comfort of an air-conditioned office. *But*—cut the size of that office to a five-foot cube, engulf it in the roar of four 1,200-horsepower engines, increase your height above ground to four or five miles, reduce the atmospheric pressure by one-half to two-thirds, lower the outside temperature to 40 or 50 degrees below zero. Then, to meet these interesting conditions, get into bulky flying clothes with suit, gloves and boots all heated through an electric cable, strap on your parachute harness, put on a "Mae West" life preserver vest, put on a flying helmet with earphones and another wire attachment, cover your face with an oxygen mask containing a microphone, making sure that the oxygen supply hose is connected and the microphone wire is plugged in, add a heavy flak helmet and about 23 pounds of body armor.

You are now ready to go to work, not alone, not on a single problem, but as a member of a team of ten men working on a multitude of problems. With them you will solve, while flying from one pin point on the map to another perhaps 600 miles away, the higher mathematical relationships of engine revolutions, manifold and fuel pressure, aerodynamics, fuel consumption, oxygen supply, barometric pressure, altitude, air speed, ground speed, wind drift, compass heading, position, and plane altitude. You and your crew will do all this whether you can see the ground or are flying through an overcast, and you will do it not as a single unit but in relation to your position in a formation of several dozen other bombers.

Of course, there may be occasional individual interruptions in flight operations due to an earache from pressure changes, a joint pain from aeroembolism, a cramp from intestinal gas expansion, a little dizziness or nausea from airsickness, a frostbitten hand, a general numbness from cold, or the subtle, deadly comatosity of anoxia.

Now consider the impact of these *unearthly* forces on your central nervous system. Flight destroys the sense of security and well-being which man, as the result of thousands of years of evolutionary adaptation, derives from "keeping his feet on the ground." The spirit of adventure and the thrill of flying are so strong that they quickly overpower the natural anxiety induced by projection into a strange environment. Yet, while man learns to like the idea of flying and develops a sense of mastery in the air, he remains either consciously or subconsciously afraid of his new habitat and, when he gets into trouble in the air, becomes acutely aware of his fear of falling. This is the psychological picture in *peaceful* flight.

Interject the greater fears of combat—the enemy fighter plane closing in with guns blazing, the setting of a steady course through a seemingly impenetrable wall of flak, the sickening bump when a shell tears a hole through wing or fuselage, the sight of other planes in the formation going out of control and at times exploding in mid-air, the danger of gasoline catching fire and engulfing the plane in flame, the sitting-on-a-keg-of-dynamite feeling of carrying a bomb load, the ordeal of dead or seriously wounded crew mates on board, the danger of asphyxiation or freezing if the oxygen or electrical system is shot out, the hazard of having to bail out and clear a spinning plane with one's parachute, the possibility of a crash landing or a ditching at sea.

In this bizarre situation of intense concentration amid intense distraction, the fear of death becomes very real.

The maintenance of the health and efficiency of the flier in the face of these stresses and strains is the task of military aviation medicine. It is not easy. The aeronautical engineer has carried the mechanical performance of aircraft far beyond the physiological limits of the human body; technological warfare has imposed an abnormal load on the psychological motivations of the human spirit.

The problem is to take a man whose body is adapted to function in a ground environment and whose mind is conditioned to seek peace and security and fit him for the life of a flying, fighting animal. Since we cannot build the flier to specifications or wait for evolution to turn him into a superman, our only alternative is to select and train the individuals best fitted physically and mentally for this duty, and then provide them with devices and methods for protection against their limitations. Because the ideal or the perfect is fundamentally incompatible with aerial war, success is measured in terms of working compromises.

In the four years beginning with 1939, the AAF Training Command graduated approximately 150,000 pilots, bombardiers and navigators. The physical standards for the selection of these men, emphasizing not only general physical fitness but also normal function in vision, hearing, equilibrium and psychological behavior, were developed between World Wars I and II in the well-known "six-four" examination for flying. The educational requirement of two years of college existing at the time the present war began was inadequate, however, to meet the needs of an air force which was to undergo a 3,500 per cent expansion in the next two years. It became the responsibility of the Air Surgeon to develop scientific tests for the selection of aviation cadets and their classification for pilot, navigator and bombardier training on the basis of aptitude. This became a function of Aviation Psychologists.

Selection began with the age restriction of 18 to 26, which limited the source of aviation cadets to a physically active population group. Self-selection was a second important factor, inasmuch as the candidate had to volunteer for flying training. Definitive selection started with a three-hour pencil-and-paper test known as the Aviation Cadet Qualifying Examination. This examination, which was substituted for the college requirement in January, 1942, involved about 150 multiple-choice questions which were sifted from 2,600 items to provide a measure of native alertness, understanding of mechanical principles, interest in aviation, and aptitude for learning to fly. From the viewpoint of education, the proportion of candidates qualifying ranged from about one-third for those who had not finished high school to more than three-quarters for those who had spent some time in college. Among those who did qualify, however, the amount of education had no effect on the probability of success in pilot training. Nearly one million candidates took the Aviation Cadet Qualifying Examination in the first two years of its use.

Those who passed this written examination were given a final type of physical examination for commissioned officer service. Roughly, 50 per cent survived these preliminary screening devices to reach an AAF Medical and Psychological Examining Unit. The Unit administered the "six-four" physical examination and a battery of twenty psychological tests. The latter were developed by Aviation Psychologists to provide a reliable prediction of the individual's aptitude for flying success and to classify his special aptitudes as pilot, navigator and bombardier. These tests, each designed from the requirements for a specific flight operation, were introduced in the spring of 1942 and subsequently subjected to continuous evaluation and periodic refinement during a two-year experience with nearly half a million candidates.

Fourteen pencil-and-paper tests were given in the course of one day. Six apparatus tests took another half day. The paper tests included such subjects as the reading of dials and tables, understanding of mechanical instruments and principles, reading comprehension, mathematics and spatial orientation. This last subject, the interpretation of aerial photographs and the location of the points pictured on topographical maps, was one in which navigators and bombardiers needed eagle-eye proficiency. The apparatus tests, to a great extent developed at the AAF School of Aviation Medicine, were important in determining individual capacity for learning the psychomotor coordination required for superior piloting. The machines measured finger dexterity, ability to divide attention between two different hand operations, speed of mind-and-muscle reaction to light signals, coordination of hands in mechanical operations, coordination of eyes, hands and feet in a complex stick-and-rudder operation, and coordination of the sense of equilibrium with rudder movements. This last, the rudder control test, was accomplished by sitting in a cockpit which tipped continually and unpredictably, but could be righted by manipulations of the rudder with the feet.

All the scoring and timing in the twenty tests was done by electricity, so the human factor in judging the candidate was eliminated. Each candidate received three scores on a nine-point scale, one for his aptitude as pilot, and the others for his aptitude as navigator and bombardier. The highest qualifying score in relation to personal preference determined the individual's classification. About 60 per cent were disqualified on the basis of their psychological test scores and the results of the "six-four" examination, which meant that fewer than 20 out of every 100 original candidates became aviation cadets.

The severity of this selection system was a continual source of disappointment to the many boys who were eager to fly but unable to make the grade. Statistical analysis of the aptitude scores in relation to the cadet's success in flying training, however, proved beyond a doubt that the system conserved time, money and manpower. It was found that the pilot candidate scoring highest (9) had a 96 per cent chance of passing primary training against a 22 per cent chance for the one scoring lowest (1). The score was found to have a relationship not only to "wash-outs" in primary training, but also to the risk of crashing, to success in training for tactical operations, to the percentage of hits in fixed gunnery, and to superiority in actual combat.

In a follow-up study of both bomber and fighter pilots in the European Theater, it was determined that pilots who had had high psychological classification scores at the outset tended to be rated by their squadron commanders as more successful in combat. Likewise, those with the minimum acceptable scores appeared to be more frequently "missing in action" than those with the highest aptitude rating. The combat results were equally impressive for navigators, but owing to the influence of many variables beyond the individual's control, were somewhat less predictive of success among bombardiers.

On the whole, the Aviation Psychology Program achieved an outstanding record. Starting without military or aviation experience, its members developed the most comprehensive mass psychological testing program in history, and selected the raw ma-

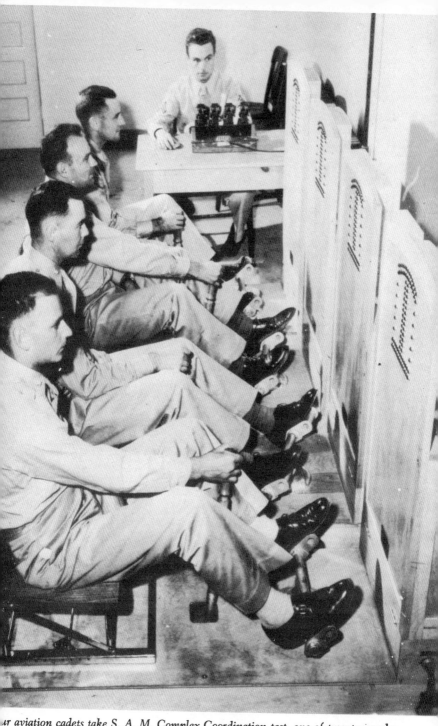

ur aviation cadets take S. A. M. Complex Coordination test, one of twenty psycho-
ical tests for flying aptitude. This test measures speed and skill with which individual
can make a series of complex reactions. (ARMY AIR FORCES PHOTO)

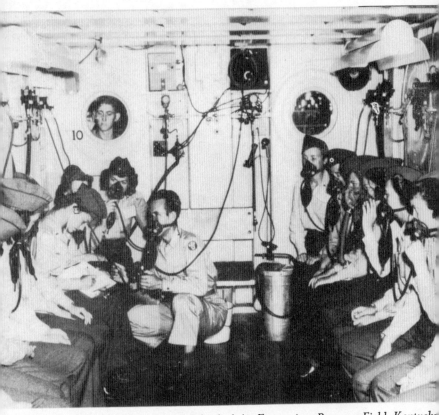

Army nurses in training at AAF School of Air Evacuation, Bowman Field, Kentucky, for duty as flight nurses get indoctrination in low-pressure chamber as part of the altitude training program. (ARMY AIR FORCES PHOTO)

terial for a combat flying force which compared favorably with any in the world.

Having done everything practicable to pick the best-qualified man, the AAF's next task was not simply the training of the aviation cadet in the technic and tactics of aircraft operation. It was also his training in the physiological effects of flight and how he could protect himself against the forces of barometric pressure, temperature, centrifugal force and gravity. Any one of these forces is sufficient to kill a flier if he makes any serious mistake or loses control in the operation of a technological maze of instruments and apparatus.

Two important activities were established by the AAF medical services for the aero medical protection of the flier. One was the Altitude Training Program, which indoctrinated aircrew personnel in the physiological effects of flight and the use of oxygen equipment. Simulated flights to a pressure altitude of 38,000 feet were made in 65 low-pressure chambers operated in the zone of the interior and theaters of operation by Aviation Physiologists. Altitude chamber "flights" by aircrew members totaled more than 275,000 in 1943.

The second activity was that of the Personal Equipment Officer, an Air Corps position in the tactical unit originated by Flight Surgeons but later a function of operations. It was the duty of the Personal Equipment Officer to maintain all personal and emergency equipment of the aircrew and instruct the fliers in its proper use. This equipment included oxygen masks, regulators and cylinders; oxygen "walk-around" and "bail-out" bottles; electrically heated flying suits, boots and gloves; first-aid kits; fire extinguishers; body armor; life rafts and "Mae West" life preserver vests; parachutes; sun and dark adapter goggles; emergency rations, and special equipment for survival in the arctic, desert, tropics and sea. Experimentation in the aero medical aspects of all these items extended wherever the AAF flew, but was centered in the Aero Medical Laboratory, AAF Matériel Command, Wright Field, Ohio, and the Research Laboratory, AAF School of Aviation Medicine, Randolph Field, Texas, the latter being under AAF Headquarters command. While both laboratories conducted physiological research programs, the Aero Medical Laboratory's main interest was in the development and standardization of aero medical matériel, whereas the School of Aviation Medicine emphasized its application in the care of the flier.

While such equipment as gloves, fire extinguishers and parachutes was primarily someone else's business, the Flight Surgeon's interest in preventing frostbite, burns and death or injury gave him, as a part of the "flying family," a direct interest in the development of adequate equipment and its propr use.

No better example could be cited than that of the invention of the "flak suit" by Brigadier General Malcolm C. Grow, a Flight Surgeon and founder of the Aero Medical Laboratory. As Surgeon of the Eighth Air Force in England, General Grow observed that 79 per cent of wounds among heavy bomber crews returning from missions over Europe were from low-velocity fragments of cannon shells, and that 85 per cent of the fatal wounds occurred in head, neck and trunk regions which could be protected by armor. He investigated the various types of body armor of medieval England and, with the collaboration of a British swordmaker, developed a quick-release vest, apron and helmet of shingled steel. The flier's fear of flak from antiaircraft guns, something against which he cannot fight back, made the body armor immediately popular. Study of a series of cases in which flak-suited fliers were hit by enemy missiles of all types showed that 69 per cent were uninjured and an additional 21 per cent only slightly wounded.

From a cartoon-illustrated book entitled "Your Body in Flight," a popular training aid prepared by the Aero Medical Laboratory, the flier undergoing altitude indoctrination learned that the foremost effect of atmospheric pressure reduction is anoxia. It had been established that fortification of the partial pressure of oxygen in the lungs was required in all daylight missions above 10,000 feet. At night, the oxygen mask was needed from the ground up, owing to the impairment of vision by even the slightest amount of oxygen want.

The development of AAF oxygen equipment was the responsibility of the Aero Medical Laboratory, where Flight Surgeons, Physiologists and aeronautical engineers worked in collaboration to make equipment as nearly foolproof as possible in the prevention of anoxia accidents. The Laboratory had a B-17, the "Nemesis of Aeroembolism," for the flight testing of equipment at high altitude. A demand type of oxygen system was developed and installed in AAF aircraft. The demand regulator did away with the risk of human error latent in the necessary manual adjustment of the older continuous flow system with every marked change in barometric pressure. The demand system automatically supplied all the oxygen the body required up to an altitude of 38,000 to 40,000 feet. Since the oxygen flowed through the demand system only upon inspiration, the waste of oxygen involved in continuous flow was eliminated. The mask underwent consecutive modifications to reduce dilution of the inspired oxygen by air leakage, and to minimize the danger of icing.

Other problems resulting from changes in barometric pressure are aero-otitis media, aero-sinusitis, aeroembolism and intestinal gas expansion. The creation of a negative pressure in the Eustachian tube or sinus during descents from high altitude may prove troublesome if the flier is unable to keep these passages clear. The problem is considerable in climates conducive to head colds, and congestion and inflammation of the upper respiratory passages are common causes for grounding a flier.

Aeroembolism, commonly known as the bends or decompression sickness, is the formation of gas bubbles, mainly nitrogen, in the joints and fatty tissues during ascents to high altitude. It may result in crippling pain. It is not an important problem in flights below 30,000 feet, however, and only a small percentage of flying personnel is susceptible to the bends above that altitude in actual flight. The gas normally present in the gastro-intestinal tract triples in volume in ascent from sea level to 27,000 feet, and in individuals with a sensitive gut, may produce severe cramping. Most individuals are able to pass the expanding gas without difficulty, but those who are susceptible to distress present the Flight Surgeon with the problem of guarding the flier's diet against certain gas-forming foods.

The altitude chamber was of great value to the Flight Surgeon in diagnosing ailments associated with low barometric pressure and in distinguishing between organic and psychological causation. Fliers whose chamber experiences demonstrated that they were unfitted for the physiological stress of high altitude were removed from flying status or assigned to types of aircraft which customarily fly at low altitudes.

Low temperature is second only to low pressure as a physiological hazard in high-altitude flight. Anoxia is far swifter than sub-zero cold but no less deadly. High-altitude frostbite, principally of the hands, constituted a leading cause of battle casualties in heavy bomber operations over Europe, where temperatures of 40 to 50 degrees below zero are "normal" between 25,000 and 30,000 feet altitude. Waist, tail and ball turret gunners in the more exposed portions of the bomber suffered most, since they did not have the benefit of the cabin heating system. A few minutes' exposure of the hand, such as in clearing a machine gun of a jam, is sufficient to produce frostbite, and two or three frozen fingers will incapacitate a gunner as effectively, and sometimes as permanently, as the loss of a whole arm.

The problem of general body warmth was solved by improved types of electrically heated flying suits, gloves and boots which eliminated the excessive bulk and restriction of movement inherent in insulated clothing adequate for prolonged exposure at these low temperatures. The heat requirements of various portions of the body were scientifically determined and incorporated in the later types of electrical clothing. Frostbite of the hand was reduced by teaching the gunner that with practice he could field-strip his gun as fast with his gloves on as off.

Centrifugal force—which keeps the water in the bucket when you swing it over your head—may cause the pilot to black out at the end of a steep dive or sharp turn, when the direction of the airplane is suddenly changed. Blacking out is a visual phenomenon due to an interruption of the blood supply to the brain. Unconsciousness may occur if the force is continued. The problem is of tactical importance only in certain types of pursuit maneuvers and dive-bombing.

Several research attempts were made to combat the effect of centrifugal force on the blood column, and one preventive device received extensive testing. The object was to restrict the volume of blood moving through the body in the direction of the centrifugal force. This the pilot could do to some extent himself through muscular tension created by "yelling like hell."

In another direction, the AAF medical services established methods for testing and improving the flier's night vision. The correct use of the eyes at night was of importance in night fighter and bomber operations.

Whereas the *cones* in the central portion of the retina are the principal organs for distinguishing color and detail in daylight, night vision is largely a function of the *rods* in the outer area of the retina. These rods detect the movement of an object and picture it in different shades of gray. The rods are 1,000 times as sensitive in dim light as the cones. For most efficient function at night, however, the flier must adapt his eyes to darkness by protecting them from light for thirty minutes prior to use—a protection which must be continued during the period of night operations. This was accomplished without the necessity of remaining in darkness by the use of dark adapter goggles containing red lenses. Furthermore, the flier had to learn the off-center method of gazing at objects at night to bring his rod vision into full use and to avoid the night blind spot presented by the center of the retina in gazing directly at the object. The flying candidate's night vision was tested in connection with the "six-four" physical examination for flying.

Important research in night vision was carried on at the School of Aviation Medicine, which developed a portable night vision tester for training use. Night vision indoctrination, including simulated firing at targets under moonlight and starlight conditions, was especially valuable in aerial gunnery training.

A history of swing, train, sea or other types of motion sickness was sought in the physical examination for flying, and the aviation cadet was continually observed during training for susceptibility to airsickness. Actual flight constituted the best index. Study conducted at the School of Aviation Medicine, based on the use of a swing test and on reports of the relationship between airsickness and individual fear of flying, disclosed that the syndrome is a composite of two factors: motion and emotion.

Airsickness primarily due to motion has important differences from the preponderantly emotional type. In the former, which occurs only during rough weather or acrobatics, nausea is relieved by vomiting, symptoms disappear upon landing, and an immunity is acquired. The emotional type may occur before or after take-off and produce nausea not relieved by vomiting, sickness during smooth flight, headache, and symptoms after landing.

Sixty-five per cent of navigation cadets and 30 per cent of pilot cadets experienced airsickness early in training, but only about 10 per cent of all navigation cadets, and 1 to 3 per cent of pilot cadets, were eliminated because of airsickness. The symptoms of those eliminated fell predominantly in the emotional category and were linked with fear of heights or of flying, and other factors impinging upon emotional stability. Conditions commonly associated with airsickness, such as current diet, aircraft odors, temperature, vibration and the sight of others being sick, were discounted as having any stimulus in airsickness other than lowering the threshold at which disturbances of the sense of equilibrium might produce symptoms.

The Flight Surgeon is on the flying line when the aircrew takes off and when it returns, but during flight, which may continue for several hours in the course of a bombing mission, emergency medical treatment depends upon the knowledge of the crew members. For this reason, aircrew instruction in the use of aeronautic first-aid kits was emphasized. The treatment of shock, control of hemorrhage and pain, the prevention of infection, and the technic of resuscitation were common practices during bombing missions, and many fliers' lives were saved by their fellow airmen. In at least one instance, a life was saved by a flier's administration of blood plasma during flight.

II

When all efforts of the Flight Surgeon, the Aviation Physiologist and the Aviation Psychologist to select and train fliers for high-altitude life are exhausted, they still have a human being and not an aerial automaton on their hands. The air the flier breathes can be fortified and his body can be insulated, but there is no simple device for fortifying or insulating his central nervous system against the impact of fear and fatigue in combat flying. Each man has his flying efficiency curve, and even the best will reach a point in that curve where he will break down himself or crack up his plane.

The breakdown common to combat fliers is called operational fatigue. This syndrome, which does not differ fundamentally from the nervous breakdown of an overworked desk worker with a tyrannical boss or a nagging wife, is not ordinary tiredness. It is, rather, an illness made of emotional and fatigue symptoms, generally manifesting itself in a state of anxiety. The typical symptoms may be any number of the following: a tired appearance, irritability, depression and moroseness, insomnia and nightmares, mental confusion or inability to concentrate, free floating anxiety or phobias, overactivity of the sympathetic nervous system, startle reactions, tremors, loss of appetite, weight loss, sweating, palpitation and other psychosomatic symptoms. The syndrome does not appear suddenly among combat airmen but is usually the result of a chain of distressing, harrowing, fatiguing, conflicting and terrifying events, any one of which could be tolerated but which together impose a stream forcing even the emotionally "tough" airman to squeeze out in some direction and develop symptoms of anxiety.

Because it may occur in individuals who are basically stable but simply have passed their tolerance point for repeated stress, operational fatigue differs from a true neurosis, or psychoneurosis, which usually denotes the presence of symptoms basically dependent on unconscious conflict arising early in childhood. Although there is a close similarity between the clinical manifestations of operational fatigue and psychoneurosis, the differences in their origin merit the use of distinctive terms.

Fear and inability to obtain adequate expression of the fear instinct through motor release form the core of the psychological conflict. This last factor is reflected in the greater incidence of operational fatigue among bomber crewmen than among fighter pilots. Even the bomber pilot has little chance to act in response to flee-or-fight impulses; every man stays at his station and every bomber holds its position. The fighter pilot has more freedom of action in his maneuvers.

At times when the air casualties have been high, the hope of survival has presented a high emotional hurdle. The flier knows he has little chance for survival. To this knowledge the "average man" became reconciled early in his combat tour and carried on without developing a marked anxiety about it. His sense of duty and discipline was strong. All his colleagues were doing the same thing, and the social pressure of the group dictated that he continue to fight as a member of a team. Reconciliation on such a fatalistic basis does not mean that the flier forgets his fears. "Being afraid" is a topic that combat flying personnel often talked about and freely admitted.

About the only persons who deny fear of combat are those who repress anxiety, develop psychosomatic symptoms, and eventually have to be removed from flying status. Such individuals usually state that they have little or no fear and want to return to combat "as soon as I am well." This is a variation of a common situation observed by the Flight Surgeon: The average flier will conscientiously attempt to keep on combat status even though he has marked operational fatigue, and some manage to complete their operational tour despite definite symptoms. It's a matter of loyalty to their crew or squadron mates. Admission of their symptoms among their fellows carries no implication of being "weak" or "yellow." The individual is simply described as being "flak-happy" or having the "Focke-Wulf jitters."

While most fliers experienced some symptoms of operational fatigue in the course of a combat tour, only a very small percentage became cases for medical disposition. Psychiatric studies of airmen in the major theaters of war supported the conclusion expressed by one psychiatrist: "The outstanding fact was not the few men who 'broke,' but that the great majority of flying personnel tolerated these extreme stresses and dangers in a 'normal' manner and without becoming psychiatric casualties. This is a tribute to the stamina and courage of the American airman."

The incidence of psychological failures in combat flying due to true psychoneurosis, or a fear reaction, was much smaller than for operational fatigue. Psychosis was a rarity and so was malingering.

At least 70 per cent of operational fatigue cases can be returned to full flying duty. Unlike ordinary physical fatigue but similar to a neurosis, operational fatigue will not respond to rest treatment alone. The symptoms are self-perpetuating and repetitive even though the individual is removed from all flying duties. The syndrome has been successfully treated with narcosynthesis, or narcosis, which aids in breaking the vicious circle. This, of course, requires hospitalization. Following such therapy, the regimen is a week or ten days of psychotherapy, physical reconditioning, good food and rest.

When military conditions permitted replacement, the Flight Surgeon could prevent the development of operational fatigue by recommending grounding and rest when the flier showed incipient signs and symptoms of this syndrome. To do this effectively, the Flight Surgeon had to combine the talents of a country doctor and a clinical psychiatrist in a role unique in military medicine. He had to live, eat, sleep, fly, play and work with the men in his squadron or group. This intimate association was the only way he could observe his patients early enough to prevent a complete break in their efficiency.

Adequate rest and recreation were most important in prevention. An outstanding measure in this direction was the establishment of rest camps where the fatigued flier could be sent at any time during his combat tour for a few days or a week of loafing, athletics and amusement far from the flying field and in a non-military atmosphere which would aid him in "getting back to normalcy."

A medical measure found to be of considerable value in aborting operational fatigue in individuals who had just undergone exceptionally harrowing experiences was heavy sedation for a period of 12 to 24 hours.

The adoption, in so far as military necessity permitted, of a definite number of missions or hours, after which the flier was relieved from tactical flying duty, was an important preventive measure. The setting of a goal, which was recommended to the commands by Flight Surgeons, helped the flier to "see it through," inasmuch as even the toughest were motivated by the desire to "get the hell out."

Any contribution to morale, ranging from an acceptable explanation of why we were fighting down to the Flight Surgeon's occasional prescription of a drink of whisky following combat, aided in the prevention of operational fatigue. It was a help to brief an aircrew on why they were attacking a certain target, and after the mission, to review what had been accomplished.

Nothing contributed more to morale, and hence to mental health, however, than good leadership within the tactical unit. A follow-up survey of flier selection methods disclosed widely divergent performance records in two groups operating the same type of airplane on identical missions from adjacent fields in the same theater of operations. The differences, which involved not only bombing accuracy and aborted missions but also the incidence of anxiety neurosis cases, were attributed to the quality of leadership provided by the group commanders and group surgeons. This judgment was confirmed by the records when the second group was given a strong commander and a strong Flight Surgeon.

Observations in the AAF, as well as in the Army Ground Forces, showed that a strong leader imparted strength to the weaker members of his outfit to an extent where even the psychologically unstable might perform well, and even heroically, under fire.

The previously mentioned AAF psychiatrist who flew a series of heavy bombing missions had an opportunity to observe this equalization of diverse personalities under combat stress. On one mission, the B-17's controls were damaged, forcing it out of formation before reaching the target, but thanks to the skill and strength of the pilot, the plane continued and made an effective bomb run. After turning home, the lone bomber was under a 45-minute attack by about 100 German fighters, and most of the crew were wounded, three severely. More damage was done to the control, oxygen, hydraulic and electrical systems of the Fortress. A small fire broke out in the bomb bay, and the tail appeared to be ready to break off. There were holes in both wings and two of the propellers. The crew expected that the plane would have to be ditched in the sea, crash-landed, or abandoned by parachute.

For the psychiatrist, the scene had been set for a comparison of the reactions of a number of personality types. These ranged from the easy-going, stable unaggressiveness of the pilot, a highly intelligent introvert, through various degrees of introversion and extroversion, sensitivity and toughness, aggressiveness and shyness, irritability and indifference, to the definite manic-depressive tendencies of the temperamental co-pilot. Despite these wide variations, the psychiatrist was surprised to find that all the crew members, even those who were severely wounded, reacted alike in the face of extreme danger. Each carried out his assigned duties and obeyed orders. Far from exhibiting panic, confusion, faulty judgment or self-seeking, all were quiet, quick, decisive, dependable, loyal, efficient, careful and even cheerful. And all got back alive.

This psychiatrist and others subsequently made a study of a group of fliers who had successfully completed their combat tours. They classified 48 per cent of them as having a family predisposition to emotional instability, and 57 per cent as having a personal predisposition to emotional unadaptability. Yet all "wore well," despite the fact that most had experienced some symptoms of operational fatigue.

Such observations are a reflection of the prophylactic power of good leadership. The function of the Flight Surgeon as a teammate of the Commanding Officer makes him a prime factor in the leadership-morale equation and its relation to the psychiatric casualty rate.

All this responsibility of the Flight Surgeon for the care of the flier adds up to the fact that the effective performance of his duties required a man of exceptional talent and tact. Consequently, a premium was placed on the attainment of the designation of Flight Surgeon. The candidate had to be a medical officer with some experience in the AAF medical services. He had to be recommended and accepted for appointment to the postgraduate training course at the AAF School of Aviation Medicine, the primary function of which was to train Flight Surgeons. At the school, the candidate was instructed in the physiology of flight, the theory of flight, the employment of aviation in the AAF, air transportation of the sick and wounded, methods for the selection and care of the flier, neuropsychiatry, tropical medicine and other subjects, all given in a nine-week course designed to test him for alertness and stability as well as for his medical and military ability.

Following graduation, the candidate could apply for designation as an Aviation Medical Examiner. His subsequent acceptance as Flight Surgeon was dependent on the fulfillment of certain requirements. He had to pass the physical examination for flying.

Unless assigned overseas, the A.M.E., before applying for his wings, had to serve a year in the AAF medical services, with full service credit, however, for overseas service prior to attendance at the School of Aviation Medicine. If he was not assigned overseas, the A.M.E. had to have put in a minimum of 50 hours' flying time in military aircraft. Lastly, his Senior Flight Surgeon was required to state that he had demonstrated the requisite professional and military qualifications, personality and character. The designation of Flight Surgeon was made by the Air Surgeon, acting for the Commanding General, AAF.

The number of Flight Surgeons on duty at the time of Pearl Harbor was approximately 400. By 1944, the School of Aviation Medicine had trained in the vicinity of 4,000 Aviation Medical Examiners, approximately half of whom had attained the Flight Surgeon's designation.

In the early phase of expansion, preference for training at the School of Aviation Medicine was given to young doctors best adapted for the rugged, vigorous life of a surgeon in a tactical unit. As procurement objectives permitted, the policy of giving all AAF medical officers an opportunity to become Flight Surgeons was adopted, in recognition of the fact that postgraduate training in aviation medicine gave the AAF hospital staff physician a better understanding of the flier cases coming to his attention. Likewise, a better patient-physician relationship could be maintained if the flier found that a Flight Surgeon was providing his care in the hospital as well as on the flying line.

As a result of a procurement program which increased the AAF medical officer total from 800 to nearly 10,000 in the two years following Pearl Harbor, the medical roster stood at approximately 8,300 early in 1944, following a series of transfers to the Army Service Forces. Many of those 8,300 were recognized specialists in civilian practice who later occupied key positions on the staffs of the more than 230 AAF regional and station hospitals and seven convalescent centers in the Continental United States. The mission of these medical installations was to provide, during training and following return from combat, the highest quality of medical care for the airmen and the more numerous ground personnel who supported them. The hospital system was organized to effect the maximum utilization of medical manpower, with emphasis on regional distribution of hospital services for definitive surgical and medical treatment. The qualified specialists were organized into regional consultation service available to lower echelon medical units. The consultation service was intended to carry the patient to the consultant, or the consultant to the patient, by air whenever appropriate.

A point was made of qualitative selection and proper placement of the hospital medical officer, with the result that more than 98 per cent of AAF medical specialists were assigned in their own fields of work. Approximately 60 AAF hospitals were approved for resident training by the Council on Medical Education and Hospitals of the American Medical Association.

All AAF hospitals operate a Convalescent Training Program, which probably has been the most popular achievement of the AAF medical services. The idea of utilizing the otherwise lost time of military hospital convalescence in physical reconditioning and useful military training was given its original application in the AAF by Lieutenant Colonel Howard A. Rusk, who describes this major development in military medical service in a separate chapter. Following the program's introduction throughout the AAF in December, 1942, the principles of the Convalescent Training Program were adopted by the Surgeon General for application in Army Service Forces hospitals. Stemming from pre-combat convalescent training was the program carried on for physical and psychological rehabilitation of sick or wounded personnel returning from combat. Seven AAF Convalescent Centers were established to accomplish the objective of retraining the handicapped soldier for military service, or if this was not possible, for a self-respecting, self-supporting role in civilian life. Because the handicapped veteran of combat had valuable training and experience which could be utilized in various ground duties, the loss of a leg or an arm was no longer regarded as cause for a medical discharge from military service.

The medical officer is by no means the only class of personnel of importance in the AAF. Including all medical services—hospital, training, research, tactical and administrative—the AAF had approximately 22,000 Medical Department officers on duty early in 1944. In addition to medical officers, this total included 6,000 nurses, 3,800 dentists, 3,000 medical administrative officers, 360 veterinarians, 200 sanitary officers, 180 hospital dietitians, 135 aviation physiologists, 130 aviation psychologists and 40 physical therapy aides. In addition, Medical Department enlisted men amounted to approximately 70,000, bringing the total of AAF medical services personnel to nearly 100,000.

Reflecting the *esprit de corps* and the team concept of the AAF, the medical services commanded by the Commanding General, AAF, and directed by the Air Surgeon operated on the morale-building principle that the Army Air Forces would take care of their own personnel within the limits of their organic function as a component force of the United States Army. One important exception to this principle was where general hospital service was provided by the Army Service Forces, particularly overseas. Another, in the opposite direction, was air evacuation service, in which AAF medical personnel provided care in flight for casualties of all branches of the American and Allied armed forces. The swift, comfortable transportation of casualties from forward areas to base hospitals equipped for definitive medical care placed air evacuation in a group with blood plasma, sulfa drugs and penicillin as one of the four greatest life-saving measures of modern military medicine.

Air evacuation of non-effective was equally important from a tactical standpoint. The success of a campaign was often linked to an army's ability to perform the essential function of prompt removal of the sick and wounded from the field of battle. The introduction of mass air evacuation in World War II came as an answer to a problem which has traditionally perplexed the military commander. The evacuation of casualties is likely to reach its greatest volume at a time when surface routes to the rear are vitally needed for the forward movement of reserve troops and ordnance. The high-speed mobility of modern warfare, increasing the possible distance of a striking force from its base and decreasing the practicability of maintaining hospital units in the forward area, merely served to magnify the difficulties inherent in this historical problem of logistics.

Flight Surgeons of the old Army Air Corps clearly recognized the air as an open road for evacuation of casualties and advocated the feasibility of this method prior to World War II. It fell to the German Luftwaffe to provide, during the Spanish Civil War and the invasion of Poland, the first air demonstrations of mass evacuation of the sick and wounded over great distances.

Air evacuation achieved American acceptance as the result of absolute military necessity. Airplanes proved to be the only available means for casualty evacuation in the building of the Alcan Highway to Alaska and in the Allied retreats from Java, Burma and China. The need for air evacuation was even more pressing in August, 1942, in our first offensives against the Japanese—the Allies' Papuan campaign in New Guinea and the Navy-Marine landing in Gaudalcanal. These attacks occasioned the first large-scale evacuation operations by American aircraft, the AAF supplying the aircraft and personnel in Papua and joining facilities with the Navy and Marines in the Solomon Islands. In Papua, the problem was one of traversing a 9,000-foot mountain range; in the Solomon Islands, it was one of a 1,000-mile flight over water at a time when sea transportation was inadequate and unsafe.

The demand for AAF air evacuation continued in the British Eighth Army's elastic campaign against Rommel's Afrika Korps through Libya early in 1943, and in the Allies' Tunisian, Sicilian and Italian campaigns in 1943. Tunisia was typical: medical units in the battle zones had to be held to a minimum and land routes to the rear were poor. Ground evacuation from the Tebessa area to general hospitals in the Constantine areas, 230 miles distant, was confined to one narrow-gauge railway and one good motor road. Motor ambulances, of which there was a shortage, took 12 to 15 hours and a hospital train 20 to 22 hours to cover this distance.

In contrast, air evacuation from advanced flying fields required about one hour, and it was only about one or one and a half hours more to the hospitals in Algiers and Oran.

The importance of air evacuation of casualties was reflected in the total of approximately 173,000 sick and wounded patients of United States and Allied forces who were evacuated by American military aircraft throughout the world in 1943. Of this total, which includes both battle and non-battle casualties, more than 161,000 were evacuated in theaters of operations, nearly all aboard AAF Troop Carrier airplanes. Nearly 9,000 patients were carried between theaters of operations or into the United States along the global routes of the Air Transport Command. Some 3,000 were transported by the AAF within the United States.

These totals speak for themselves as a measure of the degree to which air evacuation was accepted as the most efficient method of evacuating non-effectives of air, ground and service forces. But their significance cannot be appreciated without an understanding of the basic factors upon which the success of air evacuation depends: (1) availability of large transport aircraft adapted for carrying litters; (2) the medical risk to the patient; (3) the provision of medical personnel trained, equipped and organized for flying duty.

In the first place, the shortage of military aircraft was so acute early in the war that it was obvious that no aircraft could be used as a single-purpose air ambulance. But hundreds of troop and cargo carriers were returning to their bases empty from their flights into forward areas. They were assigned the secondary mission of air evacuation. Each airplane, of which the C-47 (DC-3) was the most common type, was equipped with removable metal litter racks, which could be installed to provide space for eighteen litter patients following removal of the cargo. Replacement of the metal litter supports with a lighter, more compact and more rapidly installed webbing-strap litter support was begun in March, 1944. This latter type, developed at Wright Field, permits the loading of twenty-four litter patients in six to eight minutes.

In addition, each plane was equipped with an airplane ambulance chest containing ample medicines and instruments for the care of patients in flight. Blood plasma, oxygen, morphine, heat, control of hemorrhage, and relief of gas distention were among the treatments which could be given aboard the plane. Since the troop and cargo carrier is engaged primarily in a military mission, it cannot carry a red cross or operate under the Geneva Convention, as is the custom for motor ambulances and hospital ships. This did not prove a deterrent to the practical success of air evacuation, which was carried on only in areas over which the Allies had air supremacy or air parity.

Air evacuation in troop and cargo transport airplanes has solved the logistical problem of casualty evacuation without any addition of vehicular equipment to Medical Corps units, and has contributed considerably to the tactical success of the major land offensives involving American forces. Furthermore, it has reduced the need for hospitalization in forward areas.

The medical risk to the patient, the second factor in the success of air evacuation, is epitomized in the number of deaths occurring during more than 173,000 patient flights in 1943. The total was 11. The rate was .006 per cent, or six per 100,000 patient trips. It has been possible to evacuate safely at low to moderate altitudes nearly all types of casualties with the exception of those in a state of shock, in which case transportation by any method is contraindicated. Chest, head and abdominal wound cases have been transported comfortably in considerable numbers.

The selection of patients for air evacuation is a matter for

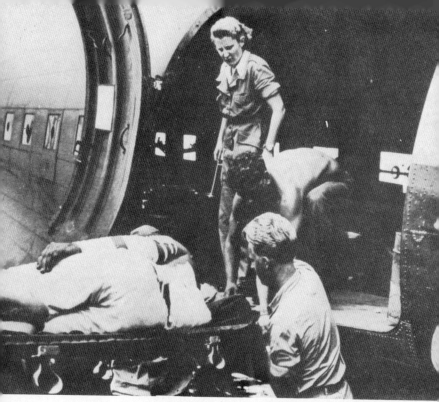

Air evacuation nurse watches as soldier wounded in Bougainville fighting is unloaded from plane for treatment at base hospital on Guadalcanal.
(OFFICIAL U. S. ARMY SIGNAL CORPS PHOTO)

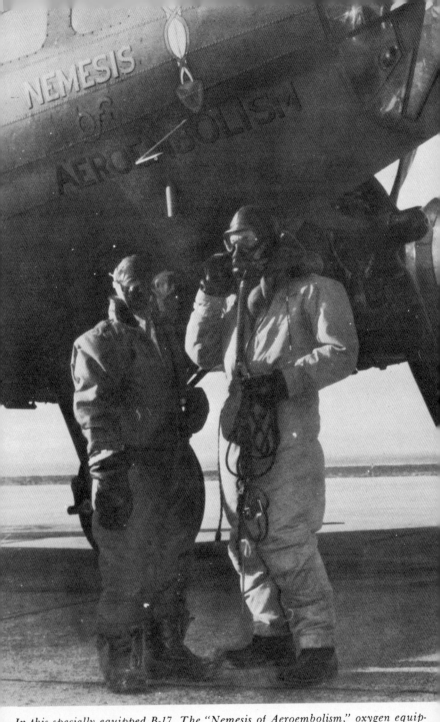

In this specially equipped B-17, The "Nemesis of Aeroembolism," oxygen equipment and flying clothing were flight-tested at high altitudes by the Aero Medical Laboratory, Wright Field, Ohio. (ARMY AIR FORCES PHOTO)

individual medical judgment. The risk has proved to be only moderate even for patients who are seriously ill, if they are carefully attended and given oxygen or other treatment whenever indicated. In any event, the risk is far outweighed by the advantages of removing the casualty with little loss of time from the stress and strain of the combat zone to a general hospital where definitive medical care is available in an atmosphere of peace and quiet. On the basis of AAF experience, it can be concluded that air evacuation is the method of choice for the quick, safe and comfortable transportation of virtually all types of sick and wounded patients.

The final factor in the success of air evacuation is the efficiency of the people who run it. These are the Flight Surgeons, Flight Nurses and enlisted men who make up the squadrons engaged in air evacuation service. The medical personnel of the first "air ambulance battalion" were activated at Fort Benning, Georgia, in May, 1942, and in October, 1942, were moved to Bowman Field, Kentucky, to become the training nucleus of the basic air evacuation squadron established at that time. This training activity was taken over by the AAF School of Air Evacuation at Bowman Field in June, 1943. Five hundred Flight Nurses were trained and 20 air evacuation squadrons activated throughout 1943.

While plans and training were pushed to fruition, Flight Surgeons in theaters of operations were directed to improvise air evacuation service from available medical personnel in tactical units. This they did with great success, drawing mainly on the Troop Carrier and Air Transport units, which also furnished the planes. During 1943, regulation air evacuation squadrons went into service in all major theaters of operations, and by the end of the year, the 802nd Squadron was cited by General Eisenhower for having evacuated 50,000 patients with only one fatality.

In addition to ground personnel, each air evacuation squadron included five Flight Surgeons, 25 Flight Nurses and 24 Staff Sergeants trained as surgical technicians. Ordinarily, a team of one Flight Nurse and one Staff Sergeant would fly with each airplane carrying patients, although a Flight Surgeon was in attendance on planes carrying patients in critical condition. The Flight Surgeon's main responsibility was to select the patients for air evacuation and keep the system operating efficiently. He supervised the loading and unloading of patients at the airdrome. He coordinated the complex system under which casualties were moved from evacuation hospitals or holding stations in the forward areas to the flying field at the time that planes arrived, and at the end of the flight were moved from the air base to the nearest general hospital. He had to know how many patients awaited evacuation and how many airplanes would be available. He was also responsible for the stocking of the airplane with medical supplies and the exchange of such equipment as blankets and litters between rear and forward areas.

Many members of these air evacuation squadrons were decorated or cited for distinguished service, and a few gave their lives in the line of duty.

One may dwell upon one activity or another of the AAF medical services only at the expense of other projects of major scope. The setting of requirements for aero medical supplies to be used in air operations over jungle swamps, arctic snows, desert sands and the seven seas was itself a major task involving painstaking devotion to detail. The procurement, training, organization and placement of qualified personnel and the maintenance of facilities were tasks made unending by the fact that war is fluid and the needs constantly changing. Venereal disease, a perennial military problem, required intensive and never-relaxing effort, but fortunately responded to conscientious effort: the AAF reduced its venereal disease rate 25 per cent in 1943 and cut the time lost from duty because of venereal infection by one-third.

Because of the thousands of man-days lost owing to rheumatic fever, streptococcic infections and respiratory disease, a preventive and control program was established at forty large air bases; this included a system for air-evacuating convalescents from areas of high incidence to climates where they would do well.

In response to the need for wider dissemination of current information on military aviation medicine, both in the theaters of operation and in the zone of the interior, a monthly journal called *The Air Surgeon's Bulletin* was established. The planning of a history of aviation medicine in the AAF is another important function. Because so much has been learned, and learned so quickly, this history will form an invaluable prospectus for the day the Flight Surgeon puts away his uniform and becomes the industrial surgeon of the skyways. At the same time, it will provide a permanent military record of what was done in Army aviation medicine and by whom—a monument, in effect, to the efforts of the Flight Surgeon and his associates to support the fliers who rained death and destruction upon our enemies.

The strains and stresses of this war have given us a higher percentage of men who have cracked up and who have had to be brought back to efficiency than in any previous war.

Not long ago, the American Design Award of $1,000, with a citation, was presented to Lieutenant Colonel (now Colonel) Howard A. Rusk, chief of the Convalescent Branch in the Office of the Air Surgeon, for his program of convalescent reconditioning now in effect throughout the country. Through this program, wounded men and those broken down by the strain of combat have been prepared both mentally and physically for recovery so that they were able to return to combat or to re-enter productive civilian life.

Colonel Rusk initiated a novel program for convalescent soldiers while at Jefferson Barracks in Missouri, teaching them, by means of lectures, moving pictures and other technics, subjects that would be useful to them regardless of the careers which they were capable of following when they left the hospital. The program included such interesting topics as camouflage, radio, model airplane building, the classics, mathematics and chemical warfare. Thus, men convalescing for a long time were able to make use of their time and not simply lie staring at the ceiling, wondering about the next step in their careers. A constructive concept emerged from a war of destruction. This story of rehabilitation Dr. Rusk himself tells in the chapter that follows.

CHAPTER XIII

CONVALESCENCE AND REHABILITATION

By
COLONEL HOWARD A. RUSK
Chief of the Convalescent Training Division, Army Air Forces

I

DURING AND FOLLOWING the last war, great strides were taken in the rehabilitation of the seriously disabled, but the normal convalescent patient was left to convalesce in the normal, undisturbed routine fashion. When war came again, unprecedented numbers of men were called into military service and with millions of men being assembled for training, it was only natural that thousands of them should become hospitalized with the usual civilian sicknesses and injuries, aggravated by the arduous activities of military life and by some sicknesses and injuries peculiar to military life. The period of convalescence in all these cases was longer than that in civilian life. In the Army, a soldier is either "on full duty" or "sick in hospital." There is no in-between period, as in civilian life, where the doctor can send his patient home with instructions to "stay at home and take it easy for a few days."

In this training phase of the war, great emphasis was placed on devoting every possible hour to the physical conditioning and technical training necessary to turn rookies into efficient fighting men. Time was precious and had to be utilized to its maximum extent. Yet, in Army hospitals thousands of men spent millions of hours convalescing in the traditional routine manner. They amused themselves in the traditional manner, worked the traditional jigsaw puzzles, read the traditional comic books, and were finally returned to duty, often in worse general physical condition than when they entered the hospital.

The remedying of this paradox began in December, 1942, when

the Air Surgeon initiated the Army Air Forces Convalescent Training Program in all Army Air Forces hospitals. The program had as its objectives: to get a man into physical condition to meet the rigorous demands of full duty in the shortest possible time, to utilize hitherto wasted time with a planned program of military and general education, and to provide a reorientation from the routine of hospitalized life to that of full duty.

This last objective, to provide a reorientation from the routine of hospitalized life to that of full duty, although secondary to the principal aims of the program, was still important, because there is a large variance between the two routines. When a man entered the hospital, it was easy for him to adjust himself to the much less strenuous hospital life, but going back to full duty was very different. In the hospital a man had time to think about affairs at home, discipline and routine, and other phases of Army life which might be distasteful to him. The program was definitely planned with some measure of military discipline, and was designed to keep the soldier extremely busy, and to assist him in bridging the gap so as to make him not only physically but psychologically ready for full duty.

Obviously the first objective, to get a man into physical condition to meet the rigorous demands of full duty in the shortest possible time, was of paramount importance. In this phase, the standard technics of physical therapy were utilized, but the program's approach to and use of carefully graded physical exercise, both in the immediate postoperative and in the later ambulatory stages of convalescence, were especially interesting.

Patients were divided into four groups on the basis of physical condition. The Class IV group consisted of those in immediate postoperative stages and those just over the acute stages of illness; Class III consisted of those semi-ambulatory patients who could take light conditioning exercises and individual corrective exercises for specific disabilities; Class II were those who could take general conditioning exercises graded downward in terms of strenuousness and length of performance; and Class I consisted of men taking strenuous, full-duty exercises. Small bed tags of red, yellow, blue and green were used in an ascending scale to designate the patient's class. Often the ambulatory patient's convalescent suit had a similar tag.

Patients coming into the program were classified by the Ward

Officers and placed in their proper groups. Progression was on an ascending scale, and was made solely on the basis of the patient's needs and abilities as prescribed by the medical officer. No specific amount of time was to be spent in any group, nor were all cases started in Group IV. For example, a man with laryngitis might be placed initially in Group II and progress rapidly to Group I, or an orthopedic case might spend a relatively long time in Group III as compared with his rapid progression through Groups II and I. All initial classifications and all progressions were made by the medical officer and were based entirely on the individual progress of the patient. Convalescent training was on a prescription basis, and men were placed on the program by prescription in the same manner that drugs and diet are prescribed.

II

Experience showed that, to attain maximum results, carefully graduated mild exercises had to begin at the earliest possible moment following injury, or as soon as the patient became free from fever. These exercises were given to the patient by a trained physical therapist upon prescription of the medical officer. A systematic record of the types of exercises, length of performance, original restrictions and increases in range of motions in joints, strength and patient cooperation was kept. Exercises within the group classification were graduated in the usual sequence of (1) forced passive, (2) free passive, (3) passive plus "thinking the movement," (4) active assistive, (5) active plus forced passive, (6) active, (7) active plus light resistance, (8) active against gravity, (9) active plus resistance against gravity, (10) concentric, (11) eccentric and (12) weight-bearing.

The groundwork for enthusiastic cooperation on the part of the patient was laid during the Group IV period. By a close informal "soldier-doctor-physical therapist" relationship, the soldier was taught what he was doing and why he was doing it. He was encouraged to take an objective view of his disability or sickness, and shown not only the value of exercise but also the disastrous conditions that might result from lack of exercise.

Group III was composed of ambulatory patients, some of whom had been transferred to special convalescent wards. The exercise classes were held in the ward itself, in the hospital or post gymnasium, in barracks converted to this specific use, or outdoors.

The physical instructor was given the diagnosis and prescription for exercise by the medical officer and the records of the patient's activities while in Group IV. A set of individual corrective exercises was designed for each patient and approved by the medical officer. Such exercises were given to the patients individually or in small classes if similar disabilities permitted homogeneous groupings. Deep breathing and mild conditioning exercises were given in addition to the correctives prescribed. Again, systematic records were kept of the types of exercises, length of performance, increase in range of motion in joints, strength and patient cooperation.

Group II exercises were given after the patient's disability and general physical condition had improved to such an extent that he could perform general conditioning exercises graded down in terms of strenuousness and length of performance. The instructor watched closely for shortness of breath as an indication of overexertion, but at the same time gave his men a work-out commensurate with their physical condition. Again emphasis was placed on letting the patients know what they were doing and why they were doing it. In this group, applied psychology and super-salesmanship were chiefly relied upon by the good physical instructor.

When the patient moved up to Group I, his exercises became the vigorous and strenuous calisthenics of the full-duty soldier. He did "burpees," "squat-benders," "sit-ups" and "trunk-twisters." He participated in guerrilla exercises, grass drills, combatives and relays. He often took hikes of five, seven or ten miles for "graduation." He was no longer a patient, but a soldier, physically prepared for the arduous demands of full duty.

In many Army Air Forces hospitals, all men were given the standard Army Air Forces Physical Fitness tests on the day of discharge, consisting of chin-ups, push-ups and running against time. Several hospitals reported that these men discharged from the hospital indicated an over-all physical condition as much as 4 or 5 per cent better than the average for non-hospitalized men at the same field or base.

Correlated with the reconditioning exercises was a widespread, carefully planned program of adaptive sports. In all instances possible, recreational therapy and adaptive sports were used as the means to the end of physical fitness. Such activity was introduced

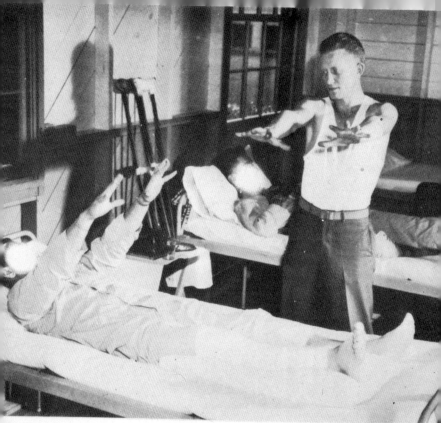

dividual bed exercises are given as soon as possible following trauma. Randolph Field, Texas. (AIR FORCES PHOTO)

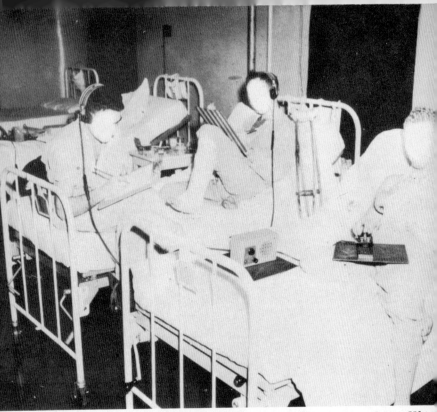

If the man can't come to the class, the class is brought to the man. Fort George Wrig Washington. (AIR FORCES PHOTO)

at the earliest possible moment. For a contracture of the palmar surface of the hand and fingers following a gunshot wound, patients played croquignole, did card tricks, typed, or studied piano. Semaphore flags, lariats and diabolos supplanted tedious arm exercises. The use of recreational therapy and adaptive sports was limited only by the ingenuity of the patients and the staff. After both knew what goal was wanted in terms of muscles and movement, they set to work with results that were both interesting and successful.

Full programs of inter-ward competition were carried on in many hospitals, with leagues in basketball, volleyball, softball, horseshoe pitching, shuffleboard and kindred sports. Through the careful use of adaptive sports, even the men in casts received the same exhilaration that comes to all men from planned competitive team play. The inter-ward athletic program was patterned after the intramural programs used in schools, and even though confined within certain physical limitations, the play of the men was hard and the competitive spirit high.

An example of the functional aspect of physical conditioning can be found in the swimming classes. Along with recreational swimming and learning the fundamentals of swimming, men were taught the technic of using barrack bags and trousers to keep afloat, how to abandon ship, swimming through burning oil and surf, methods of combating sharks and barracuda, and safety in swimming. The common denominator of swimming, like all activities on the program, was its functional value.

Every effort was made to correlate the physical activities of the soldier with the educational training he was receiving by utilizing this military training as "military-occupational therapy." Patients in Groups I and II took part in close-order drill, school of the soldier, manual of arms, and firing positions in marksmanship. The technic of knot-tying and camouflage net construction supplanted the traditional weaving and beadwork. Patients regained finger dexterity by assembling and disassembling carburetors, field-stripping machine guns and carbines, and repairing and reconstructing radio equipment. Work experiences in camouflage construction, digging foxholes and slit trenches, and building sand tables and tactical boards combined the standard procedures of occupational therapy and practical military training. With activi-

ties of this type, which are purposeful rather than merely diver-
sionary, the goals of physical reconditioning and military efficiency
were attained together.

Like the physical training phase, the educational activities were
built around the needs and abilities of the individual soldiers on
the program. They were correlated with the general type of
training activities being carried on at the base or field which the
hospital served. If the station hospital serviced a basic training
center, the educational activities of the Convalescent Training
Program were built around basic military training. If, for example, the hospital was located at an advanced two-engine flying
school, lectures were given on inspection, taxiing, trimming, stalls,
landings and formation flying with this type of aircraft. Trained
educators with military experience were used as instructors, but
every effort was made to utilize qualified patients as instructors.
The program had at its disposal all the Army Air Forces training
aids, publications and equipment used in regular Army Air Forces
training and combat units, and much of this material was adapted
to specific use within the hospitals.

It was not an uncommon sight in Army Air Forces hospitals to
find carburetors, tachometers, altimeters and radio equipment on
bedside tables instead of the usual jigsaw puzzles. In some wards,
cutaway sections of aircraft engines and hydraulic systems were
mounted on rollers and moved to the bedsides of embryonic
mechanics. Classes, lectures, demonstrations and training films on
such subjects as detection of booby traps, camouflage, medical aid,
marksmanship and map reading were brought into the wards to
the patients.

When the patient became ambulatory, he was enrolled in a
regularly scheduled series of classes, some of which were required
while others were elective. His instruction paralleled as closely
as possible the instruction or training he would be receiving if
he were not hospitalized, and often upon discharge he was able
to resume his training at the same level that he would have reached
had he not been hospitalized. Because the classes were small and
informal and the soldier was not greatly fatigued and therefore
was receptive to learning, he often learned more while in the
hospital than if he had been in regular training.

This was particularly true in hospitals where special classes were
formed for men educationally retarded. With these groups the

material was adapted to their ability level, and the slow learner had an opportunity to learn slowly. In small classes under instructors who were specialists, military problems which seemed complex became simple. Men were taught to sign their names and serial numbers, and the stigma of being branded an illiterate, at least once a month when signing the paybook, was gone.

Particular emphasis was placed in all hospitals on army orientation and current news. Most wards had bulletin boards where, through clippings, maps and pictures, the men traced the activities in the theaters of combat. Such newsboards were assigned to an interested patient as a special project, and it was his duty to gather and display the materials. Using films, guest speakers and particularly discussion technics, the men studied the backgrounds of the present conflict and learned why they were fighting and some of the problems to be expected in the postwar world. Again, small groups made it possible for each man to enter the directed discussion and to participate actively. Through military, governmental and civilian agencies, a wealth of posters, charts, maps and pamphlet materials was available for use.

Hospital libraries have long been noted for their abundance of fiction, particularly mystery stories. Under the Convalescent Training Program, they were equipped with technical manuals, field manuals, training aids, history, biography, political and military science, technical books and other pertinent non-fiction. Some hospitals reported a 100 per cent increase in withdrawals of these technical books since the inception of the program. In some hospitals, bed patients were required to participate in a supervised reading program where work-type reading exercises and tests were used both for checking the retention of the material read and to speed up reading rates.

Men were also encouraged to enroll in Armed Forces Institute Courses where, for a small sum, special self-teaching correspondence courses were available in subjects of all types, both military and general. Courses could be taken for the knowledge alone or for high school or college credit. Staff members assisted the patients with enrollment, supervised preparation of the lessons, and obtained needed reference materials from post or nearby civilian libraries. Many of the Armed Forces Institute texts were used as textbooks for group classes in subjects ranging from shorthand to auto-mechanics.

Although most of the training was along military lines, opportunities were usually present for hobby-type activities, many of which had definite military value. Craft shops, woodworking shops and complete photographic darkroom facilities were often available within the hospital. Art groups and classes made posters, training aids and signs for general hospital use. Photography classes took, developed and printed pictures for the Public Relations Office and for use in local hospital newspapers. In many hospitals, mimeographed, photo-offset or printed convalescent newspapers were written and edited by the patients with a minimum of supervision, and in some hospitals all the printing was done in the Convalescent Training Program print shop.

All patients were required to do fatigue duties according to their physical condition. Even though a man was a hospital patient, he was still a soldier, and the men performed their own "military housekeeping" tasks and other light duties around the hospital and grounds. Whenever possible, an attempt was made to correlate this detail work with training. If a man was enrolled in a course in Military Administration, he might perform clerical duties and typing. His woodworking shop course might embrace carpentry in small construction work or utility repair. Every effort was made to make all training and all activities as highly functional as possible. Over two hundred victory gardens in AAF hospitals were used to combine the effects of heliotherapy, light exercises and productive enterprise. In addition to working in the gardens, many hospitals had varied agricultural projects, such as reforestation and the raising of chickens. Field trips of an educational nature were taken to observe and study other activities on the base or field, industrial plants, civic activities, historic spots and nearby airfields.

The personnel for the program was carefully chosen from specialists who had the necessary understanding and patience to deal with hospitalized men. Patients qualified as instructors were utilized wherever possible. In some hospitals, as much as 80 per cent of the teaching was done by the patient-instructors. Nurses, doctors, officers and enlisted personnel taught classes, as well as guest instructors from post organizations, local community groups and nearby schools. The Red Cross coordinated its recreational and craft activities with the program, and often the bulk of the individual academic instruction in the wards was given by the Gray Ladies of that organization.

The entire program, whether in the physical training, educational or recreational phase, was built on the specific needs and abilities of the patients. The soldier was treated as an individual rather than a mere name and serial number, and treatment and activities were based on the total person, his needs, abilities, problems and personality, for the maximum benefits could be obtained by treating the individual rather than his disability. A great deal of careful work was done in building up a close patient-doctor relationship. The soldier gained confidence in the medical officer and had the same friendly cooperative attitude he had in civilian life toward his family doctor.

In hospitals utilized for treatments of a specialized nature, convalescent training programs were established to deal specifically with these patients. For example, a number of special centers were established for treatment of rheumatic fever patients. In these centers, where it was known that the patient would be under treatment for a period of six months, long-range programs of both group and individual instruction were planned in keeping with the slower physical progression of the patients.

The same procedure was followed in neuropsychiatric sections, where particular use was made of adaptive therapeutic sports and occupational therapy. Emphasis was placed in such programs on physical activities both simple and complex, depending upon the levels of regression. The more alert types were carefully inducted and motivated to play games they had learned as boys, while the more regressed types were reactivated upon the reflex level through elementary exercises such as bowling, horseshoes, shuffleboard and pitch and catch. One hospital reported that before inauguration of the convalescent program, 44 per cent of the patients had required sedatives at night, while under a planned program of physical and mental activities, only 3 per cent required sedatives. Increased patient cooperation in the wards was also noted after the inception of the program.

III

The Convalescent Training Program went into effect in Army Air Forces hospitals in December, 1942. During the first eighteen months, more than thirty million man-hours of physical and educational training were given. The teaching rate in 1944 exceeded three million man-hours per month. *The results of this convalescent training program were to reduce hospital readmissions by sending men back to duty in better physical condition, to shorten the period of convalescence in certain of the acute infectious and contagious diseases, and to eliminate in the majority of cases the necessity for sick leave. The results of the convalescent educational training were to increase the soldier's military knowledge, to increase his general knowledge, to practise preventive neuropsychiatry by establishing a series of "patient-doctor" talks designed to assist the soldier in orienting himself to his new environment, and to assist the soldier being discharged on Certificate of Discharge for Disability.*

Numerous research projects were carried out in connection with the AAF Convalescent Training Program. In a study by Van Ravenswaay, Erickson and others, published in the January, 1944, issue of the *Journal of the American Medical Association* (Vol. 124, pp. 1–6), of 645 controlled cases of atypical pneumonia, running two parallel groups, the group permitted to follow normal convalescence in the routine manner averaged forty-five days of hospitalization with a 30 per cent recurrence rate. The second group was kept in bed until the sedimentation rate reached 10 mm. in half an hour, and then put in a Convalescent Training Program, beginning exercises for half an hour the first day and increasing progressively until the twelfth day, when the patient was participating in a full six-hour day of physical training, mass games and various types of supervised recreation. At the end of thirty-one days, this second group was returned to duty with a 3 per cent recurrence rate—forty-five days' average hospitalization, unsupervised; thirty-one days with graduated conditioning. This was a 30 per cent recurrence rate as compared with a 3 per cent recurrence rate.

The period of convalescence in certain other acute and infectious diseases was reduced in many instances from 30 to 40 per cent. One hospital reported a reduction from eighteen to eleven days in patients with measles and a drop of thirty-three to twenty-three days' hospitalization for patients with scarlet fever. Spot checks in various hospitals indicated that hospital readmissions were reduced in some cases as much as 25 per cent.

A tangible but immeasurable result of the program was the increased morale of the men hospitalized. Formerly, men were bored by the enforced inactivity of hospitalization, but the new program kept them interested and busy. The soldier no longer had time to brood over personal problems or imaginary complaints. He knew that his training was continuing and that he would be able to resume his place with his organization when he returned.

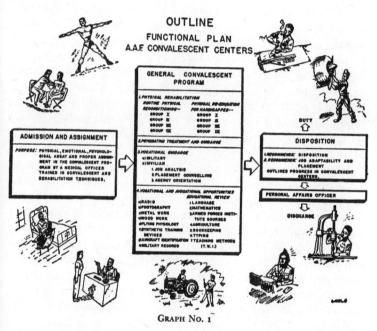

GRAPH NO. 1

Practical clinical experience gave the medical officer a yardstick whereby a patient's vitality loss and gain could be accurately evaluated. (See Graph No. 1.)

It is upon the experiences of the Convalescent Training Program that the Army Air Forces based their system for rehabilitation of Army Air Forces casualties returning from overseas. The popular concept of the word "rehabilitation" is not exact as far as the Army Air Forces program is concerned. The aim of the program was not to give straight, formal job training, but rather to provide each returning soldier with an individualized reorientation to military or civilian life by short exploratory work experiences while he was still a patient. Such a program not only improved morale, but started the soldier working and thinking in his broad field of interest and allowed him to prepare himself for a reassignment in the Army Air Forces, or if that was impossible, assisted him in his integration to civilian life. The progress made in the training program became an integral part of his clinical record which followed him to the Veterans Administration or other similar agencies.

The Army Air Forces program was primarily intended to retrain soldiers for return to military duty, and secondarily, to do vocational, aptitude and functional testing in order to give a man returning to civilian life or discharged to the Veterans Administration adequate guidance on the vocational possibilities open to him in terms of his disability or handicap. Those soldiers returning to military duty were given physical reconditioning which enabled them to return to their new duties in excellent shape. Refresher courses were given so that these men would be brought up to date with the latest technics in the field.

For example, with his combat experience a soldier might make a valuable instructor, so he was trained in the principles, practices and methods of teaching, and thus was enabled to impart his knowledge so that it would be most effective. A man who had made his way through the booby trap fields of the Germans at Salerno and Cassino could provide vivid lessons on what to do and what not to do at the front; and a pilot who had been shot down and had drifted for days on a rubber life raft in the Southwest Pacific could make the cold type in the booklet on survival realistic. On the entire program, patients with specific skills contributed altogether about 75 per cent of the teaching done, and as teachers they themselves learned as much as they taught.

Every skill and effort was centered on the task of reconditioning as many men as possible for military service with the following sequence of possibilities: (1) return to original Army Air Forces assignment; (2) return to Army Air Forces in a new assignment; (3) return to assignment within the Army; (4) return to civilian life as a self-sufficient individual, both socially and economically; (5) discharge to the Veterans Administration for further medical care and training.

For men being discharged from the service, there was an intensive program of physical reconditioning and other training de-

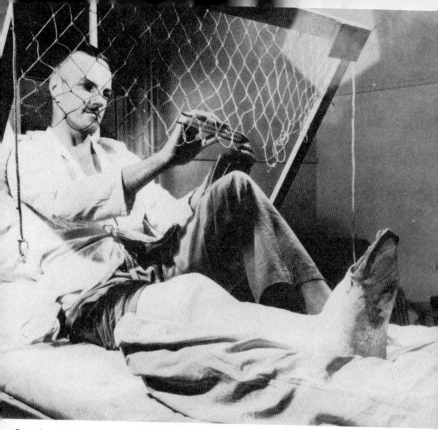

Occupational therapy has definite military value. Jefferson Barracks, Missouri.
(AIR FORCES PHOTO)

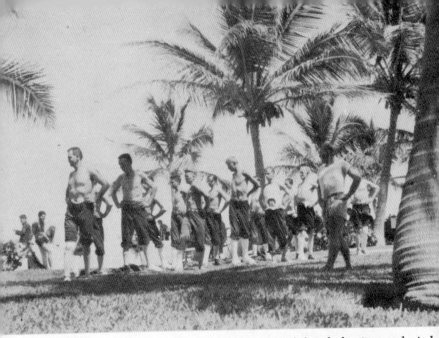

Casts don't stop AAF men from keeping the rest of their bodies in top physical condition. Miami Beach, Florida. (AIR FORCES PHOTO)

Before being returned to duty, patients often take ten-mile hikes. Camp Bable Missouri. (AIR FORCES PHOTO)

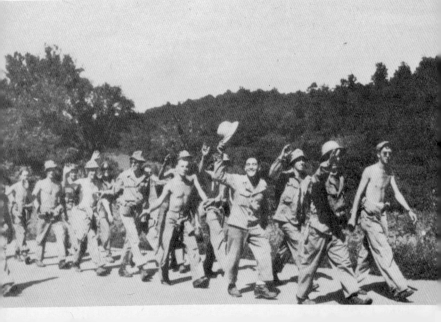

signed to restore them to active participation in their communities. They received transitional vocational guidance and job orientation. Through a series of short, broad work experiences and functional testing, they learned what they *could do* in relation to what they were *able to do;* i.e., their physical abilities were correlated with the job opportunities in the fields of their interests. They were taught their rights and privileges as veterans, and were aided in so far as humanly possible to return to their daily lives as self-respecting, self-sustaining, dignified citizens with a definite community contribution to make.

Through interviews with counselors and psychological social workers, the disabled were taught that every man is in this world to produce and that only through production of something of value can a man gain self-respect. No punches were pulled as the men were told that though their production might be limited because of disability, or it might be necessary to divert their productive efforts to some new channel commensurate with their disabilities, there was no place in American society for a drone and there was no need for an Army Air Forces veteran to become a drone.

Short work experiences were provided in a host of vocational fields. Men had a chance to learn not only of the job opportunities, but of their own aptitudes and interests in such fields as photography, commercial subjects, auto-mechanics, aircraft mechanics, printing, sheet metal work, woodworking, machine shop practice and a score of similar fields. Then, by analyzing the interests and aptitudes shown, the current vocational opportunities, and the physical limitations of the soldiers, the vocational counselor was able to give each man being returned to civilian life an objective vocational profile. Or, if a man was going to the Veterans Administration, he knew what type of training being offered by their huge vocational program was best suited for him.

Again, a definite attempt was made to make these short work experiences productive, not only from the standpoint of knowledge and insight gained for vocational guidance, but also in the production of concrete and tangible products of value.

At several of these large convalescent hospitals, animal husbandry and modern agricultural methods were taught in the classroom along with real experience in the shops, fields, gardens and barns of the hospital, producing foodstuffs which were used in the hospital kitchen. At one hospital, the remains of a jeep which had been relegated to the salvage pile were converted into a usable vehicle which gave its renovators more than eight thousand miles of service.

Again, in both the physical and educational instruction, the emphasis was placed on functional activities. In some centers, there was a room which contained a reproduction of a city street crossing, complete with traffic lights and curbs. Here men, after they learned to walk with either crutches or artificial legs, learned to cross the street within the necessary number of seconds before the light changed. Men relearned to climb stairs, open doors, and the hundreds of other activities of daily living which had become forced conscious actions because of their disabilities.

For the men who were going back to the Army Air Forces, in either original or new assignments, military instruction was provided. If a man's physical abilities required that he be placed in a new duty assignment, it was the convalescent hospital's task to start his broad training in the field of his prospective assignment.

In 1944, there were seven Army Air Forces convalescent hospitals, situated at strategic points throughout the continental United States, for servicing overseas returnees. Physicians, educators, physical therapists, psychologists and psychiatrists who had already demonstrated their abilities on the Convalescent Training Program were used to staff these convalescent hospitals. But again, wherever feasible, men returning from overseas combat who were qualified for these specialized assignments were utilized in the convalescent hospitals. Many of these men were given intensive special postgraduate courses at the famous Institute for the Crippled and Disabled in New York City, where they received instruction in the most practical use of artificial limbs and prosthesis, functional re-education, trade training for the disabled, technics for vocational placement of the physically handicapped, physical therapy as applied to casualties, and other courses designed to make the soldier who will have to relearn many ways of life self-sustaining.

By 1944, there were several thousand patients at the seven convalescent hospitals located at Coral Gables, Florida; Albuquerque, New Mexico; Pawling, New York; Denver, Colorado; Nashville, Tennessee; St. Petersburg, Florida, and Fort George Wright, Washington. This load, it was expected, would increase materially as the casualty lists grew, but it appeared from experience that the majority of these men could be returned to military duty in some capacity. In 1944, more than 80 per cent of all the returnees were able to go back to duty as active members of the Army Air Forces.

That men returning from combat were interested primarily in being discharged from the service is the misconception of many laymen. It is true that when men first came back to the United States, their morale was low, owing to the mental and physical stress they had endured. Time and a carefully planned program of activity were necessary for their return to normal. The task of the Convalescent Training Program was to reawaken within them the qualities of spirit which they originally took into combat. This could not be done through appeals to patriotism, but only through a well-rounded program of carefully supervised activities, both physical and educational. When this was accomplished, nearly every wounded man was anxious to get back to duty, either in his original assignment or in some new assignment, where his experiences and skills could be utilized.

The program was charged with getting every patient possible back to duty. Because of their training, skills and experiences, they were valuable men. If they had to be discharged, the very close liaison between the Air Forces and the aircraft industry was utilized to make available these highly trained men who could make a definite contribution to that industry. Similar close liaison was maintained with the Veterans Administration and other agencies, both governmental and civilian.

The Army Air Forces Convalescent Training Program has been big, both in the number of men involved and in the results attained. The effect of what has been learned on future military and civilian medical practice in convalescent care may be pronounced, but with more than thirty million man-hours of experience with thousands of patients having hundreds of disabilities and illnesses, certain fundamentals manifested themselves so repeatedly that they can now be classed as the prime requisites of good convalescent care. They are:

1. Treatment must be started at the earliest possible moment following trauma or illness.
2. Treatment must be for the whole individual rather than his disability.

3. Treatment and training must keep the patient *purposefully* occupied every day during the entire period of convalescence.
4. Treatment and activities, both physical and educational, must be functional.

Based on these four principles, any convalescent program, whether military or civilian, for one individual or for large groups, can produce results.

The fundamental philosophy of the Army Air Forces Convalescent Training Program, simply stated, is: "The debt of disability shall be paid in the currency of opportunity."

THE VETERANS ADMINISTRATION

Most of the veterans of World War I are today scattered in many occupations in civilian life. Many, however, are permanently invalided in veterans hospitals. The veterans of World War II, already far exceeding in numbers those of World War I, are likely to ask of the nation even more in the way of medical and hospital service than has previously been made available.

The Medical Director of nearly one hundred veterans hospitals and head of all the medical activities for America's war veterans is Dr. Charles Marion Griffith, a native of Jasper, Tennessee, who served as a captain in the Medical Corps overseas with the 109th Infantry during World War I and with the United States Public Health Service before taking up his duties with the Veterans Bureau. He rose to his position as Medical Director in 1930 from a post as chief of a veterans hospital.

What medicine has to offer to the veterans is elucidated in Dr. Griffith's article on the Veterans Administration.

CHAPTER XIV

THE VETERANS ADMINISTRATION

By
CHARLES M. GRIFFITH, M.D.
Medical Director, Veterans Administration

I

BENEFITS GRANTED BY Congress to ex-members of the armed forces of our country are dispensed through the Veterans Administration. That agency, which is an independent establishment created in 1930 by an Executive Order, and not a bureau of any Federal department, is the largest of its kind in the world. Moreover, its workload is enlarging steadily and can be expected to be at least trebled in a few years, when its potential beneficiaries will approximate sixteen million men and women.

The activities of the Veterans Administration are of unprecedented variety and volume. Its claimants and beneficiaries consist of living soldiers, sailors and Marines who served in former wars (the Civil, Indian, Spanish-American, Philippine Insurrection, Boxer Rebellion and First World War) and in World War II, and surviving dependents of deceased veterans. It also administers benefits authorized for ex-members of the peacetime regular establishment and their dependents.

Besides furnishing hospital and out-patient treatment, and awards of disability compensation, disability pension, service pension, and pension to dependents, the Veterans Administration makes payments to retired emergency and other officers of World War I; furnishes domiciliary care, vocational rehabilitation, and guardianship supervision; administers government life insurance granted to members and ex-members of the armed forces; and guarantees to commercial insurance companies the premiums on insurance policies carried by persons in active military or naval service, under the provisions of the Soldiers and Sailors Civil Relief Act of October, 1940.

In the central office at the national capital, and in 115 field stations scattered over the continental United States and in two insular possessions (Hawaii and Puerto Rico), a force of nearly 50,000 employees is engaged in a mounting effort to keep current the administration of those various benefits. During the fiscal year 1943, 223,963 beneficiaries were provided hospitalization and 800,000 treatments were rendered out-patients, while there was an even larger total of physical examinations. Net disbursements from appropriations and trust funds of the Veterans Administration for the fiscal year 1943 ran to $643,406,394, while its budget estimate for the fiscal year 1944 was $1,259,310,500.

This large and expanding organization is the product of an evolutionary process which began with the amendment of October 6, 1917 (six months after our entrance into World War I), to the War Risk Insurance Act.*

Prior to the date of that amendment, the national policy was to pay pensions to persons separated from the armed forces. At first, those pensions were awarded to the disabled only, but later they were granted as well for military or naval service in itself. But, except for such medical service as was incidental to domiciliary care in the National Home for Disabled Volunteer Soldiers (created just after the Civil War), no specific provision was made for treatment benefits.

The Act of October 6, 1917—the announced purpose of which was to put an end to the "pension system"—was a well-balanced, comprehensive body of legislation which reflected modern concepts of the legitimate obligations of the nation to its defenders. Monetary payments, for disability incurred or aggravated in armed service, based largely upon the practices of State employees compensation laws, and called "disability compensation" instead of "pensions"; payments to dependents for death of veterans due to service-connected disease or injury; allotments and allowances to

* The War Risk Insurance Act of September 2, 1914, established a Bureau of War Risk Insurance in the Treasury Department, to administer provisions for the insurance, by the United States, of American vessels and their cargoes against the risks of war. An amendment of June 12, 1917, authorized insurance of the officers and crews of such vessels against loss of life or personal injury by the risks of war, and compensation (at the same rate as the earnings of the individual) during detention following capture by the enemy.

the families of men in active service; and government insurance in amounts from $1,000 to $10,000 covering death and total permanent disability, were features of that novel and enlightened program of benefits. Subsequently, in June, 1918, another Act was approved which authorized vocational rehabilitation of disabled persons discharged from the armed forces.

The administration of this legislation became vested, however, in three independent organizations. The Bureau of War Risk Insurance, then a part of the Treasury Department, was responsible for disability evaluations and awards of monetary benefits. The United States Public Health Service, which at that time was also a bureau of the Treasury Department, conducted physical examinations of claimants upon which those monetary awards were based, and provided hospital and out-patient treatment for beneficiaries of the War Risk Insurance Bureau. And the Rehabilitation Division of the Federal Board for Vocational Education took over the vocational training of disabled ex-members of the military and naval forces. This divided jurisdiction caused many complaints of confusion and delay in the dispensing of benefits, and the growing dissatisfaction resulted, on August 9, 1921, in the act creating the United States Veterans Bureau. In that newly established agency were amalgamated the functions and powers which had pertained to those three separate agencies.

The success of that first merger pointed to the desirability of the absorption into a unitary agency of two other Federal organizations which were concerned with the administration of related benefits. The first of those organizations, the Bureau of Pensions, was administering pensions to persons who had served in the Civil War, Indian Wars, the Spanish-American War, Philippine Insurrection and Boxer Rebellion, and to their dependents. The second, the National Home for Disabled Volunteer Soldiers, was providing, through the several branches over the country, domiciliary care for ex-members of the armed forces. But it was not until July, 1930, that legislation came whereby those two agencies were consolidated with the United States Veterans Bureau to form the present Veterans Administration. As the head of this new organization, with the title of Administrator of Veterans Affairs, Brigadier General Frank T. Hines, who had been the Director of the United States Veterans Bureau, was appointed.

The men and women separated from active service in World War II are returning to a home country that is much better prepared to meet their needs than was the case at the close of World War I. The mass demobilization of the spring of 1919 was unexpected, and the then rather small organization of the War Risk Insurance was inundated by a flood of claims for disability benefits. Much more serious, however, was the inadequacy of facilities for medical treatment, particularly hospitals. The United States Public Health Service strove energetically to meet the heavy demands for hospitalization—by use of all available beds in its Marine Hospitals, negotiation of contracts with State and private hospitals, occupancy of the temporary hospital buildings in abandoned Army cantonments, and utilization of beds in National Soldiers' Homes. But it was inevitable that anything like standardized methods of diagnosis and therapy could not be realized in such heterogeneous facilities, nor could direction and supervision be at all sufficiently exercised.

It was because of this situation that Congress decided upon a policy of erecting modern, fireproof hospitals for disabled beneficiaries of the First World War, and since the first act of March 3, 1919, authorizing such construction, that policy has continued. In twenty-four years, a total of $218,703,912 had been made available for alteration and expansion of existing facilities, and for construction of new hospitals, out-patient units and domiciliary accommodations.

In 1937, the President approved a program of construction of hospitals and domiciliary homes, recommended by the Federal Board of Hospitalization, which proposed the attainment, over a period of ten years, of a goal of 100,000 beds. That number of beds, it was estimated, would suffice to meet the future peak requirements of what was then the total of potentially entitled beneficiaries, viz., survivors of former wars and persons discharged for disability from peacetime enlistments in the regular establishment. But the immense expansion of the armed forces which, beginning in 1940 with the calling into Federal service of the National Guard, continued later in that year with the induction of registrants under the Selective Training and Service Act, and culminated in December, 1941, with the declaration of war against the Axis Powers and their satellite nations, demanded a drastic revision of the 1937 program. Accordingly, on April 2, 1942, the President approved a recommendation of the Federal Board of Hospitalization that the Administrator of Veterans Affairs be empowered to accelerate all remaining projects comprehended by the previous ten-year construction program, and the carrying out of that authorization was begun at once. By March, 1944, the Veterans Administration had made available 87,000 beds for hospital treatment and domiciliary care in the 94 field stations operated under its direct and exclusive jurisdiction. It is expected that by the end of 1945 this total will reach 94,134 and, a year later, close to 104,000 beds. A further increment of 100,000 beds has been planned to come from the taking over of Army and Navy hospitals upon termination of the war. But the final objective is 300,000 beds, to be acquired over a period of twenty to thirty years after demobilization of the forces. The peak of requests for hospital treatment or domiciliary care is anticipated in 1975, when it is estimated a total of 298,400 beneficiaries will require such treatment and care. Of that total, 207,000 will be persons who served in World War II, and 91,400 will be survivors of other wars.

It is not generally understood that Veterans Administration plans for construction of new hospitals or enlargement of existing hospitals are based upon that provision of the laws which grants hospitalization or domiciliary care not only for injuries or diseases incurred or aggravated in former armed service ("service-connected"), but also for any illness or injury that the veteran of a war may develop at any time in his life. Preference in available beds is given the applicant who needs hospital treatment for a condition attributable to military or naval service, and all that is required of such an applicant is exhibition of an honorable discharge. But hospitalization can also be furnished without cost, under very liberal conditions, to the applicant who needs it for a disease or injury in no way related to former armed service. He does not have to meet any requirement as to length of service; one day will suffice. Nor is an honorable discharge insisted upon; all that is required is that he shall not have been dishonorably discharged. He is required to make affidavit that he is unable to defray the expense of the hospitalization or of the transportation to and from the hospital. This benefit was conferred by Congress upon veterans of World War I by the act of June 7, 1924, or some five and a half years after the armistice of November 11, 1918; and since that time, more than 80 per cent of all admissions to hospitals of the Veterans Administration have been for conditions not related to former military or naval service. During the fiscal year 1943, more than 92 per cent of all such admissions were of that character.

Men and women (including members of the Women's Army Corps, Women's Reserve of the Navy and Marine Corps, and Women's Reserve of the Coast Guard) of the armed forces in World War II received an earlier grant of this valuable benefit. It was authorized for them in the act of March 17, 1943, and it may be expected that in years to come they will avail themselves of it to much the same extent as did their fathers.

II

The present 94 hospitals operated by the Veterans Administration were designed primarily for three clinical types of patients—tuberculous, neuropsychiatric and general medical or surgical—but emergent illness or injury of any kind can be treated at any of them. Twenty-nine of these hospitals are for neuropsychiatric beneficiaries, who make up about three-fifths of the entire hospital population, and who largely influence all plans for hospital expansion and new construction. All hospitals are staffed by full-time physicians, whose services are supplemented by attending specialists and consultants of the neighboring communities. Approved by the American College of Surgeons, these "facilities" as they are termed, are equipped with every modern diagnostic and treatment device. Physical therapy in all its modalities is available, and there are few, if any, other hospitals of the country in which occupational therapy has been so highly developed. For psychotic patients, particularly, a wide variety of outdoor and indoor (shop) projects are available. Group therapy, including bibliotherapy, occupational therapy, physical exercises and recreational activities, is under the coordinated direction of a trained physician, the "reconstruction officer."

Special facilities include three diagnostic centers (in Washington, D.C., San Francisco, and Hines, Illinois, a suburb of Chicago); nine chest surgery centers, for such major collapse therapy procedures as cannot be done in tuberculosis hospitals; six tumor clinics, one of which, at Hines, Illinois, is among the largest and best equipped in the world; four centers for major neurosurgery; five for finer plastic surgery; six hospitals for the study and treatment of tropical diseases; and an allergy clinic in the facility at Pittsburgh, where allergens are prepared for supplying other field stations.

Out-patient treatment is furnishable at more than one hundred field stations, but only to applicants requiring it for diseases or injuries attributable to armed service. When the condition of such a beneficiary forbids travel to an out-patient unit, attendance by a physician of his community can be authorized.

The Veterans Administration has an allocation of beds in a number of hospitals of other Federal medical organizations (Army, Navy, Public Health Service, Federal Security Agency), and carries a large number of contracts with State and private hospitals. Such contract hospitals can be utilized only for emergent service-connected illness of male beneficiaries; but women beneficiaries can obtain treatment in them for any condition, regardless of its relation to armed service, when facilities under direct jurisdiction of the Veterans Administration are not readily available.

Physicians and dentists of the Veterans Administration within the required age limits and physical requirements of the Medical Corps of the Army have been given commissions by the Surgeon General, War Department, with assignments to the service of the Veterans Administration. And the Veterans Administration, as a war agency, has been accorded priority in the procurement of other classes of personnel.

Besides the physical and mental reconditioning which disabled ex-members of the armed forces in this war are supplied through the hospitals and out-patient resources just described, the Veterans Administration provides vocational rehabilitation under authority of an act, Public No. 16, 78th Congress, approved March 24, 1943. To be entitled to such rehabilitation, an applicant must have been in active military or naval service after December 6, 1941, and during World War II; have been honorably discharged from active service; have a disability, mental or physical, incurred or aggravated by such service, for which pension is payable under laws administered by the Veterans Administration; and be in need of vocational rehabilitation to overcome the handicap of such disability.

Training will be arranged in accredited colleges, universities and educational institutions, and in well-established business enterprises to effect "training on the job." No course of instruction may exceed four years, and no training may be initiated later than six years after the termination of the war. The full cost of the instruction and of necessary books, tools, instruments and other supplies will be borne by the Veterans Administration, which will also furnish any medical treatment required to prevent interruption of the training. Further, maintenance and support during the training and for two months after the trained beneficiary has been placed in employment will be furnished through increase of pension payments.

A single person will receive a pension of $80, and a married person $90 monthly; while $5 monthly will be granted for each dependent child, and in addition, $10 monthly for each dependent parent. Payments by employers during "training on the job" are also permissible; but when such payments, added to the increased pension, exceed what the employer is paying a qualified employee in the job for which the veteran is being trained, a decrease in the increased pension will be made to correspond with the excess payment received. Medical staff members designated as medical consultants, and in some cases, ward physicians, will counsel as to an applicant's physical or mental fitness for any vocational training, and as to choice of objectives for those who are judged ready to begin training.

Ex-members of the forces who have a disability determined by the Veterans Administration as not incurred or aggravated in military or naval service ("not service-connected") can be supplied training, like employable handicapped civilians in general, through State vocational rehabilitation officers, in conjunction with the Federal Security Agency.

A generous pension is granted by the Veterans Administration for disability that was incurred or aggravated in line of duty in active armed service. Determination whether a disability is so attributable, and percentage evaluation of its degree, are responsibilities of rating boards, whose members (consisting of medical, legal and occupational specialists) consider detailed reports of the physical examination of the claimant and the records of the branch of the armed service from which he was discharged.

The percentage of disability assigned is based upon the average degree of impairment in earning capacity which would result from the injury in a civil occupation similar to that of the claimant at the time of his enlistment. And the law expressly provides that there shall be no reduction in the rate of payment because of the beneficiary's success in overcoming the handicap of his injury. It matters not what income accrues to him from a salary or business; no attempt is made to commute the pension awarded him against such other income. Increase or decrease in his pension is to be made, however, commensurately with increase or decrease of his disability, as shown by periodic physical examination. Permanent conditions, particularly amputations, ankyloses, deteriorating psychoses, etc., are assigned permament disability ratings, and re-examinations are not required in such cases.

Disability pension payments ordinarily range from $10 to $100 monthly, in multiples of 10, dependent upon the relative degree of disability as determined from a schedule of ratings. A beneficiary with a total disability, entitling him to a pension of $100 monthly, can be paid $50 additional for aid and attendance, if shown to be in need thereof. But besides the ratings assignable under the schedule of disability ratings, the law provides awards for certain specific conditions, and those are granted in addition to the payment under the schedular evaluation. Thus, a claimant who loses an eye, leg or arm receives $35 monthly for such injury, but besides, is paid the percentage rating for the disability, which may range from 40 to 90 per cent ($40 to $90). The level of the amputation of an extremity determines the disability evaluation. Loss of a leg at the knee joint entitles a claimant to a schedular evaluation of 60 per cent ($60), but in addition, he receives a statutory award of $35 monthly, so that his monthly payments for life would be $95. Other special statutory awards are made for loss, or loss of use, of a part or parts, and as high as $250 monthly can be paid for certain combinations of such injuries.

In general, the evaluations of disability prescribed in the disability rating schedule of the Veterans Administration are higher than those provided by employees' compensation commissions of the States. Important, too, is the principle that income from employment, regardless of its amount, shall not affect the evaluation of disability and the monetary benefit awarded by the Administration. And as stated in the foregoing, the grant of one benefit—vocational training—does not entail surrender of another—the disability payments the trainee is receiving. On the contrary, his pension payments can be increased to cover his maintenance and support (and that of his dependents) while he is being vocationally rehabilitated.

On the death of an ex-member of the armed forces from a service-connected condition, a pension becomes payable by the Veterans Administration to his widow and minor children. Indeed, a child may continue to receive the prescribed payment until he or she reaches the age of 21, if such child is completing education at an approved school or college. Parents, too, are pensionable if shown to have been dependent upon the dead veteran. A widow and child or children are held automatically entitled to a pension, and do not have to prove dependence or need of the payment. No limitation as to private income attaches to the grant made them. Death pension rates are: for a widow, $50; a widow and one child, $65, with $13 for each other child; no widow, but one child, $25; no widow, but two children, $38 equally divided, and $10 for each additional child, the total to be equally divided; a dependent parent, $45; and dependent parents, $25 each. The total monthly pension to dependents may not exceed $100 for a widow and children.

III

While a pension is a government gratuity, insurance is a contract. The insured must have applied for it, and must pay premiums to vest it and continue it in effect. He may request that the premiums be deducted monthly from his service pay. Should the insured be continuously disabled for six months or more from a condition which began after the date of application for insurance, while the insurance was in force under premium payments, and prior to the insured's sixtieth birthday, premiums may be waived upon application while total disability continues.

During the first 120 days of his military or naval service, the applicant is insured without precedent physical examination;

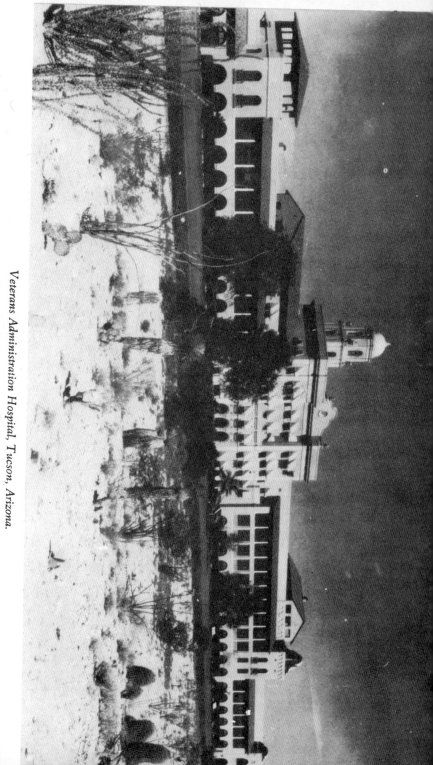

Veterans Administration Hospital, Tucson, Arizona.

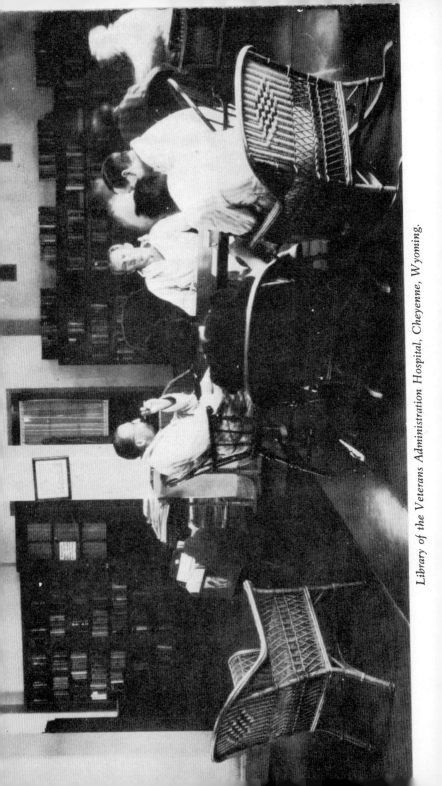

Library of the Veterans Administration Hospital, Cheyenne, Wyoming.

thereafter, and while he is in active service, he must submit satisfactory evidence that he is in good health. The premium rates vary according to the insured's age. They are comparatively low, because the government pays all administrative costs, besides assuming the extra hazards of military or naval service.

Issued as a five-year term policy, the insurance, after one year, may be converted into an ordinary life or 20-payment or 30-payment policy without physical examination. The applicant may take out a policy of from $1,000 to $10,000 in multiples of $500. Payments upon death of the insured to his beneficiary or beneficiaries (confined to wife, children, parents, brothers or sisters) are made in the form of annuities, the amount being based upon the age of the recipient at the time of death of the insured.

At the end of April, 1944, 14,880,000 applications for National Service Life Insurance had been filed by members of the armed forces in the present war, representing the stupendous total of more than 110½ billions of insurance. Besides, 580,379 policies of United States Government life insurance, representing $2,500,004,491 of insurance, have been kept in effect by veterans of the First World War and by those members and former members of the armed forces who were granted this insurance after entrance into active service, after the termination of the First World War and prior to October 8, 1940, the date of enactment of the National Service Life Insurance Act.

As of April 30, 1944, the beneficiaries of deceased veterans of World War II, awards of National Service life insurance to the face amount of $400,163,700 have been made; and to totally and permanently disabled veterans and beneficiaries of deceased veterans of World War I (including totally and permanently disabled veterans and beneficiaries of deceased veterans who had served in the armed forces after the termination of World War I and prior to October 8, 1940), war risk insurance benefits totaling $2,200,083,422 have been paid, and in addition, United States Government life insurance awards to the face amount of $418,640,251 have been made. The immensity of this insurance function alone conveys some realization of the scope of the activities of the Veterans Administration.

Members of the armed forces who held insurance with commercial companies need have no fear of their policies lapsing while in active service. Under the provisions of the Soldiers' and Sailors' Civil Relief Act of October, 1940, the Veterans Administration will guarantee payment of their premiums pending their return to civil life. That legislation, moreover, affords protection, during the period of active service and for six months after, against suits for collection of debts, fulfillment of contracts, repossession of property, collection of certain taxes, sale of property for delinquency in taxes, and eviction of their families for non-payment of rent. Legal counsel in the assurance of these rights is furnishable without fee by State chairmen of the American Bar Association, the Legal Aid Society, or local boards of the Selective Service System.

The Veterans Administration maintains supervision, in cooperation with the State courts, over payments of any benefits made to guardians on account of minor or insane beneficiaries, to insure proper application of such benefits. In the absence of appointment of a guardian, the Veterans Administration is authorized by law to release payments to the wife of a mentally incompetent veteran, to the chief officer of the hospital in which such veteran is being maintained, and to legal custodians for minors.

The Veterans Administration maintains twelve facilities in various sections of the continental United States at which domiciliary care is provided for men and women ex-members of the forces who are suffering from disability which incapacitates them from earning a living for a prospective period of time. At the end of April, 1944, there were 9,500 persons (termed "members") residing in these domiciliary homes. This is lower than the average domiciled population, and the reduction in the number of these beneficiaries is due to the exceptionally favorable opportunities for industrial employment, even of disabled persons, which exist at present.

It would appear that the principal interest of the general public and of the men in the service is that employment opportunities await the returning soldier, sailor and Marine. The responsibility for procuring positions for persons separated from the armed forces has not been directly placed upon the Veterans Administration, except in so far as "training on the job" is involved, though the Veterans Administration has cooperated with the other Federal agencies more directly concerned, viz., the United States

Employment Service and the Selective Service System, in this duty.

However, the creation, in February, 1943, by Executive Order, of the Retraining and Re-employment Administration, in effecting the Baruch-Hancock reconversion recommendations, insures coordination of all associated government agencies in the re-employment of ex-members of the armed forces and persons who had been engaged in war work. The direction of the Retraining and Re-employment Administration is entrusted to Brigadier General Frank T. Hines, the present Administrator of Veterans Affairs, who will be assisted in his great task by an advisory board composed of representatives of the Department of Labor, the Federal Security Agency, the War Manpower Commission, the Selective Service System, the United States Civil Service Commission, the War Production Board, the Departments of War and of the Navy, and the Veterans Administration. Leaders of labor and industry in the States and local communities will be consulted.

The Selective Training and Service Act of September 16, 1940, defines the right of reinstatement in their prewar employment of returning service men and women, provided that application therefor is made by them within forty days after discharge from military or naval service, and that they are qualified at that time for the duties of the occupations. It was stipulated that the employer must restore the applicant to the position he had held, or to one of "like seniority, status and pay, unless the employer's circumstances have so changed as to make it impossible or unreasonable to do so." Similar protection was afforded to returning employees of the Federal and local governments who had gone into military or naval service. Should the applicants fail to procure the reinstatement they sought, the law provides that United States attorneys shall represent them in the district courts, and the courts are directed to expedite hearings in such proceedings.

Executive Orders promulgated over the past two decades provide liberal preferences for persons who had served in the armed forces, in respect to examination and rating, appointment to and retention in the Federal Civil Service. They are given 5 points in addition to an earned rating upon examination, and need earn a rating of only 65, which, with the granted 5 points, places their names on the register of eligibles. Disabled veterans, their widows, and the wives of those who, because of service-connected disability are themselves not qualified, are granted 10 points in examinations and need earn a rating of only 60. That rating not only makes such examinees eligible for appointment, but, more important, their names are placed above all others on the register of eligibles.

Except as to positions exempted by regulations of the United States Civil Service Commission, persons entitled to veterans' preference may be examined without regard to age, and physical requirements for the position may be waived for a disabled applicant. The name of a preference eligible on a register cannot be passed over by an appointing official unless a reason is supplied. An employee entitled to military preference cannot be discharged or dropped from the Federal civil service, or reduced in rank or salary when a reduction in force is being made, if his record be good or his efficiency rating be equal to that of any competing employee in a like type of work.

S. 1617, a bill introduced on January 11, 1944, to "provide Federal government aid for the readjustment in civilian life by returning World War II veterans," contains, among a variety of other proposed benefits (academic education, extension of hospital facilities, vocational training, loans to finance purchase, construction or repair of homes, farms or business properties), provisions for a special employment service and unemployment payments. The measure, upon its unanimous passage by the Senate, authorized payments of from $15 to $25 a week, for a maximum of one year, to unemployed ex-members of the armed forces.

The immediate financial need of persons who, upon discharge from the armed forces, do not procure early employment, will be considerably relieved by the mustering-out pay authorized by Congress, as follows: $100 to those who had less than 60 days' service; $200 to those who had service of 60 days or more, not foreign; and $300 to those who had foreign service of 60 or more days. Ranks above captaincy are not eligible for this benefit.

It would appear that the program of the Federal Government for the civil readjustment of returning ex-members of the armed forces is comprehensive and generous. The disabled man or woman is assured not only skillful medical reconditioning, but for disability attributable to military or naval service, other rehabilitation benefits, such as vocational training to overcome occupational handicap and liberal monetary awards. Well-planned coordinated efforts on a large scale will be made to procure employment, both for the disabled and the non-disabled, as promptly as possible after they are separated from the armed forces.

In 1944, Americans contributed more than five million pints of blood in the blood donor centers of the American Red Cross. The National Director of the Blood Donor Service has been Dr. G. Canby Robinson, widely known as a medical investigator and a medical educator, who in 1941 accepted the responsibility for the special service associated with the development of blood plasma, listed by many leaders in medicine as among the first three contributions of medicine in the present generation.

Dr. Robinson, who was graduated from Johns Hopkins University School of Medicine in 1903, has been at various times associated in positions of leadership with Vanderbilt University Medical School, Johns Hopkins University School of Medicine, Cornell University Medical College, Peiping (China) Union Medical College, and also with many of the leading medical societies of America. He has made investigations on the use of digitalis and studies dealing with the circulation of the blood, medical education and the social aspects of medicine. From the Chinese government he received a Medal of Honored Merit for long service as chairman of the Baltimore chapter of the American Bureau for Medical Aid to China. His portrait was presented to Vanderbilt University when he resigned as dean of the School of Medicine to accept a position with Johns Hopkins.

In no other activity of the war have as many individuals contributed personally as have been concerned with the Red Cross Blood Donor Service. Here is its history and a record of its contribution.

CHAPTER XV

WARTIME MEDICAL ACTIVITIES OF THE AMERICAN RED CROSS

By

G. CANBY ROBINSON, M.D., LL.D., Sc.D.

National Director of the Red Cross Blood Donor Service

I

TWENTY-FOUR DAYS AFTER the attack on Pearl Harbor, the Red Cross mercy ship *Mactan,* evacuating wounded men from Manila to Australia at the request of General Douglas MacArthur, plowed its way through the South Pacific. Aboard, Red Cross doctors and nurses cared for the wounded. There were no reporters present to chronicle the story. There was simply a job to be done, and the Red Cross was there.

Months later, enclosed in a letter to Red Cross national headquarters from one of the passengers, a crude snapshot provided the first pictorial proof of the value of a Red Cross project which, by 1944 was considered the most dramatic civilian undertaking of the war. In a crowded wardroom aboard the *Mactan,* a doctor was giving a blood plasma transfusion to a seriously wounded man.

Literally hundreds of pictures have since been released showing plasma saving lives in combat. At Guadalcanal and Tarawa, in North Africa and in Italy, in England and in France, plasma processed from the blood of volunteer donors enrolled by the Red Cross helped to save the lives of thousands of wounded men.

"Stories of plasma are legion at the front," wrote Turner Catledge in the *New York Times.* "It is giving the surgeons a chance to get at and save men who otherwise would die from the shock of wounds. All up and down the mountains in Italy one runs into empty plasma bottles and cartons showing where wounded men were given a new lease on life or at least a new hope because people at home gave blood through the Red Cross."

On the other side of the world another reporter, Lewis B. Sebring, Jr., of the *New York Herald Tribune*, wrote a vivid account of a hill on Cape Gloucester where so much plasma was used that the Marines called it "Plasma Ridge."

"Marines ordered to take the hill," he wrote, "had been ambushed. by snipers and machine-gun nests. Wounded men were pinned to hastily dug foxholes. Then the Navy Medical Corpsmen crawled forward on their bellies, carefully shielding precious bottles of plasma. Everywhere you looked you could see men in foxholes getting plasma. Plasma is the great savior of the war. I never realized how much it means to our wounded men until I heard about it at Cape Gloucester."

Such stories, vividly portrayed by the press and radio, were fully authenticated by medical reports from our doctors at war. According to the Surgeons General of the Army and Navy, blood plasma was the foremost lifesaver of the war. Speaking over a radio network five days after the invasion of France, Major General Norman T. Kirk, the Surgeon General of the Army, said that 97 out of every 100 wounded men were being saved, a record attributable in large part to the use of plasma.

Captain French R. Moore of the Navy, Division Surgeon of the Fifth Marine Corps, which spearheaded the Tarawa occupation, reported that of the 2,519 wounded on Tarawa, only 2.7 per cent were lost. "We gave an average of a thousand plasma transfusions a day," he reported. "At least half of the seriously wounded men owe their lives to plasma."

Another report, made by Captain Saul Hochheiser of the Army Medical Corps at the Fort Hancock, New Jersey, station hospital, declared that plasma from the blood of 320 donors was used to save the lives of thirty-five badly burned survivors of the U.S.S. *Turner*, which exploded in New York harbor—an average of nearly ten pints each. One sailor, burned on 65 per cent of his body, required twenty-four units of plasma. Another required twenty units. Basing its figures upon reports from the combat zones, the Army Surgeon General's Office estimated that the average casualty requiring plasma received 1,200 cc., the amount procured from four pints of blood.

These reports are typical of hundreds received. Yet the Blood

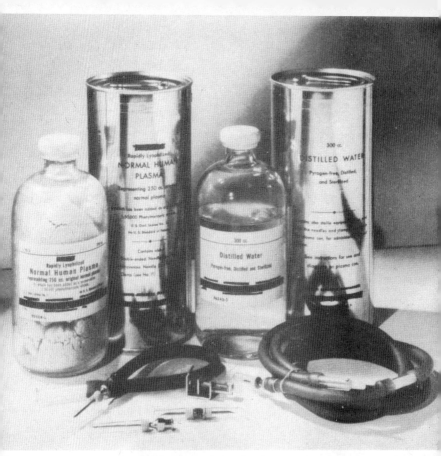

Contents of a blood plasma carton. (AMERICAN RED CROSS)

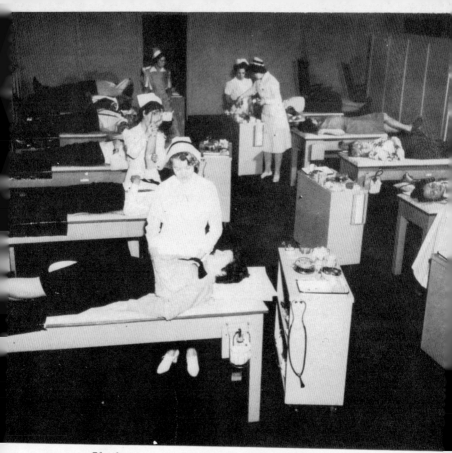

Bleeding room in a fixed center where donations are made.
(RED CROSS PHOTO BY WALLER)

Donor Service was only one of many Red Cross activities through which the people of America kept faith with the men overseas. Any summary of Red Cross medical or medical-social wartime activities must include also the surgical dressings prepared in Red Cross workrooms by the women of America, the recruitment of nurses for the Army and Navy, the work of Red Cross recreation and social workers in Army and Navy hospitals, and numerous other activities. And while it is sometimes difficult to separate the medical or medical-social from other Red Cross wartime activities, the underlying principle of service to the armed forces runs throughout all reports.

The place of the American Red Cross in the medical picture of the war goes back to a Congressional Act of 1905. Under the Congressional charter then issued, the principal functions of the Red Cross in time of war were "to furnish volunteer aid to the sick and wounded of armies, . . . to perform all the duties devolved upon a national society which has acceded to [the Treaty of Geneva], . . . to act in matters of voluntary relief and in accord with the military and naval authorities as a medium of communication between the people of the United States of America and their Army and Navy." The Red Cross was also charged "to continue and carry on a system of national and international relief in times of peace and to apply the same in mitigating the sufferings caused by pestilence, famine, fire, floods and other great national calamities, and to devise and carry on measures for preventing the same." It is thus a quasi-governmental organization, although its funds are dependent upon voluntary contributions from the public.

The Treaty of Geneva, upon which the Red Cross is founded, was inspired by a Swiss layman named Henri Dumont who, in 1859, haunted by the cries of the wounded during the battle of Solferino, issued a stirring appeal for the alleviation of the suffering and pain of men wounded in battle. This led to the Treaty of Geneva, which was ratified by the United States in 1882, and the founding of the International Red Cross. It was largely through the efforts of Clara Barton, the founder of the American Red Cross, that the treaty was ratified by this country.

Beginning in a small way, the American Red Cross grew until, in 1944, the organization was made up of 3,755 chapters and 6,000 branches which covered almost every community in the nation. Time after time, with the support of the public, the Red Cross banner of mercy was raised in this country and abroad. When war came again in 1941, with American forces engaged all over the world, Red Cross activities expanded manyfold. Never in its history was the Red Cross called upon to perform so many tasks.

Outstanding among these activities, because of its great emotional appeal as well as its value in saving lives, was the Red Cross Blood Donor Service. This service owes its origin to the soldiers who died unnecessarily on the battlefields of France during the First World War. It was observed then by medical officers that many men were lost as a result of traumatic shock who could have been saved had blood transfusions been available.

Much effort was expended during the First World War, both at the front and in the laboratories at home, to find methods for the treatment of traumatic shock, a condition often responding favorably to blood transfusions. The problems of having donors available, of typing and cross-matching the blood of donors and recipients, of preserving blood so that it could be used for transfusions, could not be solved to supply the great number of blood transfusions that were needed on the field of battle. Nor was a satisfactory and efficient blood substitute discovered that was satisfactory for the treatment of traumatic shock.

Traumatic shock is a condition that has received extensive study in recent years, largely stimulated by the medical experiences and futile efforts of the last war. Traumatic shock has been described briefly by Professor Carl J. Wiggers as "a combination of symptoms resulting from depression of many functions of the body, but in which reduction of the effective circulating volume and blood pressure are of basic importance, and in which impairment of the circulation steadily progresses until it eventuates in a state of irreversible circulatory failure. Reduction in the volume of blood returned to the heart is the keystone of all modern conceptions of shock."

Treatment for traumatic shock must be given as promptly as possible after its manifestations appear in order to restore the blood volume before irreversible circulatory failure occurs. Blood transfusion not only restores the volume of the blood, but the liquid portion of the blood, the plasma, has the property of drawing fluid from body tissues back into the circulation.

The value of blood plasma in the treatment of shock was reported by Captain Gordon R. Ward, a British medical officer, toward the close of the last war. He pointed out that the liquid portion of human blood after the cells had been removed was effective for this purpose. With the cells removed, blood typing was no longer necessary, so that the plasma from the blood of any person could be administered indiscriminately to anyone requiring a transfusion. The prolonged storage of plasma also did not present the difficulties that are encountered in the preservation of whole blood. This observation was therefore of much significance as a practical means of solving some of the problems in the treatment of shock that had been encountered during the last war.

During the years following the war, through the work of a number of investigators, methods were devised for the preservation of plasma for years by reducing it to a dried state. With these basic facts established, the Division of Medical Sciences of the National Research Council undertook, at the request of the Surgeons General of the Army and Navy, to develop technical methods by which dried human blood plasma could be made available for the treatment of traumatic shock under conditions of modern warfare. The studies of its Subcommittee on Blood Substitutes, supplemented by those of the Army and Navy, resulted in the development of methods of preparing dried plasma on a large scale and in devising means by which the plasma could be safely transported and simply and quickly administered wherever it might be needed.

In the original package for the distribution of plasma, there were two tin cans, one containing a bottle of dried plasma derived from one pint of blood and the other a bottle of sterile distilled water. Within these cans were also put the rubber tubing, needles and other small apparatus used to introduce the water into the bottle of plasma and to administer it to the patient. The plasma goes quickly into solution when the water is added. These packages were dated and the plasma could be administered for at least five years from the time of its production.

Experience in the treatment of shock under battle conditions indicated the desirability of making two changes in the use of the blood derivatives. One was to double the amount of plasma in each package and the other was to reduce the size of the package. To meet the first of these conditions, most of the packages later contained the plasma from two pints of blood. To meet the second condition, methods for the production of serum albumin were devised. This blood derivative contains most of the substances of the plasma that draw fluid from the body tissues back into the circulation, and when a solution of serum albumin is injected into the vein of a patient in shock, it has much the same beneficial effects of plasma. The serum albumin derived from three and a half pints of blood is dissolved in 100 cc. of physiological salt solution, and three vials of this size are contained in a carton somewhat smaller than an original package of plasma. This reduction in the bulk of the package was desirable for certain types of military and naval operations.

The production of serum albumin had an added advantage in that certain by-products were obtained that had medical uses valuable for the Army and Navy. They were also expected, when produced in excess of the needs of the armed forces, to be of value to the civilian population as a preventive of measles, as a means of controlling hemorrhage in surgical practice, and for other purposes not yet fully determined.

Dried blood plasma and serum albumin are the two substances that were recommended by the National Research Council to the Surgeons General of the Army and Navy for the treatment of shock where transfusions were indicated. The extensive laboratory investigations and technical studies that were required to develop these substances have been described elsewhere.

The production of plasma and serum albumin presented two major problems to the Army and Navy. One was how to obtain the large volumes of human blood needed, and the other was how to organize the mass production of these substances. These problems were under consideration in the early part of 1941, when it was decided that the American Red Cross should be requested to act as the agency to procure the blood, and that commercial firms with experience in the production of medical biological substances, such as sera and antitoxins, should be depended upon to process the blood into dried plasma and later into serum albumin.

The project was inaugurated on a small scale in February, 1941, when a pilot blood donor center was organized in the Presbyterian Hospital, New York, the donors being recruited and enrolled by the New York Chapter of the Red Cross. The blood was shipped from New York to the one laboratory then equipped for the processing of dried plasma at Glenolden, Pennsylvania, near Philadelphia. The project at that time had as its objective the production of 15,000 units of plasma. The technical operations were carried on under the direction of the Blood Substitutes Committee of the National Research Council in collaboration with representatives of the medical services of the Army and Navy, and of the National Institute of Health of the United States Public Health Service.

During this period, many of the basic problems for the conduct of the service were worked out, such as the safest and most efficient method of procuring blood from a large number of donors, methods of refrigerating and transporting the blood, necessary tests and procedures to assure a reliable, safe and uniform product from the laboratory, and the best method of packaging plasma so that it could be safely transported and be ready for immediate use. Steps were taken also to organize other blood donor centers, and in May, 1941, centers were opened by the Red Cross in Philadelphia and Baltimore, to be followed soon after by centers in Buffalo and Rochester.

During this period of trial and investigation, operational plans were also formulated that resulted in formal requests of the Surgeons General of the Army and Navy to the American Red Cross and to the Division of Medical Sciences of the National Research Council to organize a cooperative project for collecting human blood plasma for the medical departments of the Army and Navy.

The Red Cross was requested to establish and maintain facilities in a number of cities for procuring blood from volunteer donors, to recruit and enroll the donors, and to arrange for the rapid transportation of the drawn blood to laboratories selected by the Army and Navy to process the blood.

The Division of Medical Sciences of the National Research Council was requested to assume general supervision of the professional services involved in the collection and storage of blood plasma, and to provide competent professional personnel, both for a national supervising group and for the local collecting agencies.

On the basis of these requests, an agreement was signed on

May 12, 1941, by the Chairmen of the American Red Cross and of the Division of Medical Sciences of the National Research Council to undertake the joint project with a division of responsibility along the lines of those requested, the administrative responsibility being assumed jointly through individuals designated for the purpose. A plan of operation was made part of this agreement, defining more specifically the joint responsibilities and those assumed by each organization separately.

It may be stated briefly that the joint responsibilities covered determination of policies and principles of operation, determination of budgets for technical operation, designation of cities in which the collection of blood was to be made, and the control of scientific publications. The National Research Council agreed to appoint an advisory committee to supervise the technical phases of the project, to select the personnel in each community to carry out the technical phases of the project, and to determine the type of equipment to be used.

The American Red Cross, through its national organization and chapters, agreed to conduct the enrollment of volunteer donors in communities where blood donor centers were developed, to provide the equipment for collecting the blood, and to arrange for its shipment to processing laboratories. The Red Cross further agreed to provide nationally necessary funds for support of the technical operations, while the respective Red Cross chapters were to meet the expense of enrolling volunteer blood donors.

It was stated as part of the agreement that the Army and Navy would cooperate with the Red Cross and the National Research Council in this project, and would acquire the prepared plasma from the processing laboratories, reimbursing them for their services at a rate agreed upon.

This joint agreement may be regarded as the charter of the Red Cross Blood Donor Service. In order to carry out its provisions, a National Director of the Blood Donor Service was appointed by the Red Cross, on the recommendation of the National Research Council, and a national staff was developed to carry out, on the one hand, the technical direction of the service and, on the other hand, to direct and stimulate the methods of recruiting and enrolling donors in the blood donor centers as they were developed. By this method, the responsibilities of the Red Cross and of the National Research Council were centered in one staff, with a National Director, representing and reporting to both organizations.

Doctors well qualified in the field of blood transfusions were appointed by the National Research Council to serve as technical supervisors in each city selected for the development of a blood donor center by the local chapter of the Red Cross. These supervisors, who served on a voluntary basis, rendered a service of conspicuous value in organizing the technical facilities and staffs under the general direction of the technical director of the national staff, and took an important part in the development and conduct of the service.

From the small beginning described above, the Red Cross Blood Donor Service was extended to larger cities in all parts of this country. The rapidity of its expansion, which was made systematically in line with the increasing Army and Navy needs as the war progressed, is indicated by the fact that while less than 50,000 pints of blood were procured in 1941, 1,325,000 were procured in 1942 and 4,280,000 pints in 1943. To attain the military requirements of 1944, 5,000,000 additional pints of blood had to be obtained, which meant a weekly quota of 100,000 pints.

To meet these requirements, Red Cross chapters in thirty-five of the larger cities had established blood donor centers by the end of 1943. By this time, sixteen processing laboratories had been organized in twelve plants, nine processing plasma and seven processing serum albumin, both operations being carried on in four of the plants. All these laboratories were licensed by the National Institute of Health of the United States Public Health Service to process the blood. The licenses were issued on the basis of a carefully controlled technic, which included not only the prescribed methods of procuring the blood and its protection from contamination, but also definite specifications which had to be fulfilled before the finished product was acceptable by the Army or Navy. Constant testing was required.

Each blood donor center was attached to a particular laboratory, to which it sent the freshly drawn blood every day. Some laboratories received all their blood from a single center, while one received it from as many as seven.

The project developed into an assembly-line mass-production operation which required the setting of weekly quotas for each center in order to correlate closely the production of blood with the processing capacity of each laboratory. This laboratory capacity was determined by its equipment and personnel, which were in turn determined in relation to the size of its contract with the Army or Navy and the rate of production required to meet the terms of its contract. The contracts for dried plasma were made by the Surgeon General's Office of the Army, and the contracts for serum albumin by the Bureau of Medicine and Surgery of the Navy. The needs of the Army and Navy for the two products were met by an agreement between services governing their distribution after delivery by the laboratories. Blood was also processed into liquid plasma in Denver and Washington by the Army and Navy. It was distributed to military hospitals in this country.

The following table indicates the production schedule of the Blood Donor Service in operation during 1944:

Weekly Production Assignments of Laboratories and Blood Donor Centers

LABORATORY A—18,500
Plasma, 16,000; Albumin, 2,500
New York 9,000
Brooklyn 4,000
Rochester 1,500
Schenectady 1,500
Buffalo 2,500

LABORATORY B—17,500
Plasma, 14,500; Albumin, 3,000
St. Louis 3,500
Indianapolis 2,000
Cincinnati 2,500
Atlanta 1,750
Louisville 2,000
Columbus 2,750
Milwaukee 3,000

LABORATORY C—12,500
Plasma, 10,500; Albumin, 2,000
Boston 5,500
Philadelphia 5,500
Harrisburg 1,500

LABORATORY D—7,500 Plasma
Pittsburgh 4,000
Washington 3,500

LABORATORY E—5,000 Albumin
Baltimore 2,500
Hartford 2,500

LABORATORY F—4,000 Plasma
Cleveland 4,000

LABORATORY G—5,000 Plasma
Detroit 5,000

LABORATORY H—14,000
Plasma, 11,500; Albumin, 2,500
Los Angeles 5,500
San Francisco 4,250
Oakland 1,750
Portland 2,500

LABORATORY I—5,500 Plasma
Los Angeles 3,500
San Diego 2,000

LABORATORY J—6,750 Plasma
Kansas City 2,750
Minneapolis 2,250
St. Paul 1,750

LABORATORY K—5,000 Albumin
Chicago 5,000

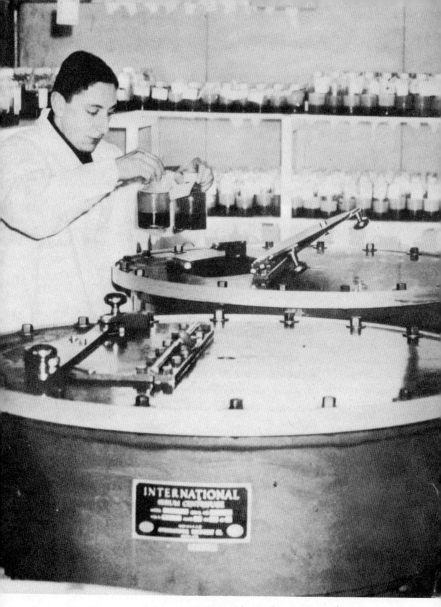

Blood is removed from centrifuge. Plasma has risen to the top.
(AMERICAN RED CROSS PHOTO)

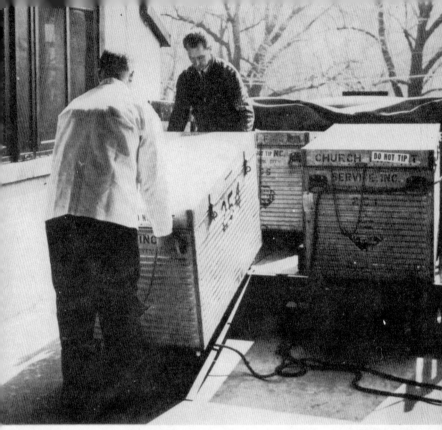

Blood is shipped in refrigerated Church containers. (RED CROSS PHOTO BY JOHNSON)

LABORATORY L—7,000 Albumin
   New Orleans 2,000
   Dallas 2,000
   San Antonio 1,500
   Fort Worth 1,500

ARMY AND NAVY LABORATORIES—
2,250
   Denver 1,750
   Washington 500

TOTAL PLASMA 81,250
TOTAL ALBUMIN 27,000
TOTAL LIQUID 2,250
                    ——————
                    110,500

The organization of the Blood Donor Service consisted primarily in establishing a series of blood donor centers by selected Red Cross chapters in accordance with the national plans of organization and operation. These plans were presented mainly in two manuals, one entitled "The Organization and Operation of the American Red Cross Blood Donor Service," and the other called "Methods and Technique Used in Red Cross Blood Donor Centers." The first manual described the functions and relationships of all who participated in the Service, set forth certain general policies, and explained the financial operations to be followed. It also contained the essential portions of the agreement between the Red Cross and the National Research Council, so that their respective responsibilities might be generally understood.

The so-called technical manual described in detail the duties of the technical personnel and how all procedures were to be carried out in each blood donor center. The manual stated that "the prime objective of the American Red Cross Blood Donor Service is to provide human blood in sufficient quantities for the preparation of dried plasma and serum albumin for the armed forces. In the assembly-line type of production necessary to fulfill such an objective, the first consideration has been and is the care and protection of the donor; the second is the prevention of spoilage of blood obtained. All methods and techniques have been developed with these considerations in mind."

The development of a blood donor center was, like the Service as a whole, a joint undertaking between the Red Cross and the National Research Council. The Red Cross chapter was represented by its Blood Donor Service Committee, the chairman of which played an important part, and by the Center Director, a full-time employee of the chapter. The National Research Council was represented by the Technical Supervisor, who was a well-qualified doctor of the community, appointed by the Subcommittee on Blood Substitutes of the National Research Council.

In cooperation with the national organization, the local group rented or borrowed a suitable building and equipped it for the required functions. The blood donor centers contained reception rooms and office space for recruiting and enrolling donors, recording their histories, and making simple examinations, and, as the center of operations, the large room in which the blood was withdrawn. The center also contained rest rooms for donors, a canteen for their refreshment, and space for the care of their outer clothes and for presenting them with emblems and certificates. They were furnished so as to provide a friendly and attractive atmosphere.

The technical operations also required ample refrigeration for the blood, facilities for the preparation of blood for shipping, sterilizing equipment, and accessories such as storeroom, staff dressing rooms and offices. Each blood donor center was developed according to the weekly production that it was expected to meet, which naturally varied with the size of the community in which it was situated.

An important development by which about half the total number of blood donations were obtained was the mobile unit organization. Each center operated from one to four mobile units. These were ton-and-a-half vanette motors, equipped with cots, refrigerators, sterile bleeding equipment and all the supplies needed for blood procurement. Each mobile unit was accompanied by a technical team consisting of a doctor, five or six nurses, a technical secretary and a blood custodian.

The mobile units visited Red Cross chapters within a radius of about seventy-five miles of the blood donor center. They operated on a definite schedule which was arranged weeks or even months in advance. Each cooperating chapter set up its own organization for the recruiting and enrolling of donors, and arranged all local details for the visit of the mobile unit, which might last for a day or a week. A special assistant attached to each center visited the chapters to organize them for the service and was responsible for coordinating the cooperating chapters with the blood donor center. By this means, about 900 Red Cross chapters participated in the Blood Donor Service. The mobile unit was also used for visits to industrial plants within the jurisdiction of the center-chapter.

Each mobile unit collected on an average about 150 bleedings per day. The blood was either brought back to the center in portable refrigerators for shipment to the laboratory or shipped by Railway Express in large refrigerated Church containers directly to the processing laboratory. The 35 centers operated 63 mobile units. The success of this phase of the Blood Donor Service required thorough organization, in which many people participated.

II

The organization and operation of a blood donor center included the activities dealing with the public as a whole and those dealing with the individual voluntary donor and with the blood that he contributed. Although this was a natural division, these activities were closely integrated and required the exercise of teamwork and understanding by all the many volunteer and paid workers who participated in the conduct of a center. The Red Cross chapter was primarily responsible for the public relations of the service and supported from its chapter funds the expense of recruiting donors, the operations required for their enrollment, the furnishing and serving of refreshments, and the general administration of the center.

The activities that had to do with individual donors and with the blood that they contributed included the technical operations of the center, and were under the control of the technical supervisor, who engaged the technical staff and was responsible for the maintenance not only of professional standards, but also of the supplies and equipment required for the proper performance of the technical operations. The expense of the technical operations was borne by the funds of the National Red Cross. Although originally the National Red Cross bore the expense of the bleeding equipment and the cost of transporting the blood to the laboratories, as the magnitude of the operations increased, the Army and Navy agreed that these costs should be met by government funds. All costs of processing the blood were also borne by the government.

The first consideration in the operation of a blood donor center was the procurement of a sufficient number of voluntary donors to meet the weekly quota of the center. The people of the community had to be aroused to the urgency of the cause; they had to be reassured that donating a pint of blood was a relatively harmless and painless operation. Further, they had to be brought to feel both a personal and communal responsibility for the success of their blood donor center, and organized and regulated so that donors came to the center in a steady, even flow. They had to be encouraged by all means to make definite appointments and to keep them religiously, so that for days ahead the center could be assured that its prescribed number of donations would be obtained.

The problem of recruiting was solved by local efforts, backed up, stimulated and instructed by the national staff. The usual methods of newspaper support and radio talks and announcements were used extensively, and very generous cooperation was given by the press and radio. The giving of blood to save the lives of our fighting men had, of course, the strongest sort of public appeal, and the whole nation in many ways expressed its desire to urge this project onward. The national organization distributed posters and leaflets of information, publicity kits, photographs, movies and other promotional material for the use of the centers and of the cooperating chapters. Plans of recruiting in motion picture theaters were worked out with motion picture organizations on a national scale, and plans for the organization of group donations from industrial and business firms were promoted.

Much enthusiasm and ingenuity were shown by the centers in organizing speakers and in appealing to all sorts of religious, social, labor, business and civic groups. A large amount of the recruiting was done by the donors themselves, who were proud of their donation and ready to urge others to follow.

Nation-wide publicity came from magazine articles, national hook-up radio programs, motion pictures, and especially from the news stories from the battle fronts which extolled plasma as a means of saving the lives of our soldiers and sailors. Although this type of publicity was of great value to the Blood Donor Service, it also caused frustration by creating an emotional urge in many people to donate their blood, who lived in parts of the country where there were no centers, or who were below or above the age limits of 18 to 60 years. It also produced in many communities the feeling that they had been left out of a great opportunity to serve and were being discriminated against. This situation required frequent explanations that the existing centers were those most favorably placed geographically in relation to the processing laboratories, and that these centers had the facilities for procuring all the blood needed to meet military requirements.

The enrollment of donors who applied for appointments in person, by telephone, by filling out forms and by mail required a carefully planned operation, as appointments had to be given on the basis of so many donors every fifteen minutes, and every effort was made to suit the convenience of donors and to expedite their donations. The importance of not breaking an appointment was constantly emphasized.

Volunteer Red Cross workers performed many essential functions in the centers; they received the donors, assisted in filling out their registration cards, conducted the canteen for their refreshment, and presented the donors with their blood donor certificates and emblems. These emblems, much prized by many donors, indicated the number of donations made. A bronze emblem was given after the first donation, a silver emblem after the third, and when eight donations, the total number allowed in a twelve-month period, had been made, a small red ribbon was placed behind the silver emblem. This denoted that the donor had given a gallon of blood and was a member of "The Gallon Club." White and blue ribbons were added when donors had given sixteen and twenty-four pints of blood, respectively.

Other members of special Red Cross volunteer services served as motor corps drivers, and those who were qualified as nurses' aides took part in some of the technical operations. It was estimated that more than 15,000 Red Cross volunteers participated in the Blood Donor Service.

The Center Director represented both the local chapter and the national organization. He was the administrator of the center and was responsible to the chapter in seeing that the national program was carried out as prescribed. The Center Director had a relation to the Technical Supervisor and his staff similar to the relation of a hospital superintendent to the professional staff of the hospital.

The technical staff and facilities of the center were organized and directed by the Technical Supervisor, under the general direction of the Technical Director of the national staff, and according to the methods prescribed by the Committee of the National Research Council and approved by the National Institute of Health of the United States Public Health Service. The technical staff of a blood donor center was organized as teams consisting of a doctor, five or more registered nurses, a technical secretary and one or more blood custodians. Each team procured from 750 to 1,200 bleedings a week, and with an over-all weekly production of 100,000 bleedings, approximately 125 doctors and nearly 1,000 nurses were required to meet the needs of all the centers. The teams in the centers worked under conditions that allowed them to procure considerably more blood per week than those operating with the mobile units.

In the early days of the Service, technical supervisors were able to man the centers with doctors from their own communities, who in most instances devoted their full time to the blood donor centers. This method of operation became more and more difficult as the production of the centers rose and the call on civilian doctors for the armed forces increased, so that it became impossible to conduct the centers without the aid of medical officers from the Army and Navy. From a small beginning, a plan was finally adopted by which sixty medical officers were assigned to the Blood Donor Service by the Army and forty by the Navy to supplement the doctors employed by the Red Cross. All these officers were on limited service because of physical disabilities which were present when they were commissioned, or which were the result of injury or illness while on active service at the battle fronts. A small number of women physicians and physically disqualified or over-age medical men were retained, and a few doctors in essential teaching positions completed the required number of doctors.

A careful survey was made of all nurses in the Blood Donor Service in collaboration with the Red Cross Nurses Recruiting Service and the Office of Procurement and Assignment of the War Manpower Commission. All nurses eligible for military service were released except for a few head nurses of long standing in some of the centers, who were considered in essential war-work positions.

The doctors in the centers or on the mobile units supervised the technic of venepunctures generally performed by the nurses, who after training in the procedure, became very skillful. The doctors passed on all donors where there was any question as to their physical fitness or other matters needing a professional opinion. They cared for all donors who might react unfavorably following the withdrawal of blood, or who fainted, and conferred with donors whose blood might be reported by the laboratory as unsatisfactory on the basis of a serological examination for syphilis performed on every donation.

Donors were accepted only when judged to be qualified to give a whole pint of blood without harm. Donor requirements were specifically stated and rigidly adhered to. All donors were required to sign a form releasing the Red Cross and those connected with the procurement of blood from responsibility for the effects of the blood donation. They had to be under sixty years of age or over eighteen, and unmarried minors had to have a release signed by a parent. Limits of blood pressure and temperature and especially of the hemoglobin contents of the blood were prescribed. A series of questions was asked by a graduate nurse and the answers recorded. All questionable cases were referred to the physician in charge. Donor requirements are discussed in the first three publications listed in the references.

An important point in the protection of the donor was to make sure that blood was not withdrawn from a person with anemia. Much attention and study were given to this point by the technical director and by various technical supervisors in the course of the service. An accurate method of estimating the hemoglobin content of the blood was used so that all those who fell below a critical level were rejected. Because of this control, and because of its impracticability when dealing with such a very large number of people who were not under medical supervision, no directions as to diet or the use of drugs were allowed in the centers.

After a person was accepted as a donor, he or she (men and women donated in about equal numbers) was conducted into the donating room and reclined on a high couch. The vein at the elbow was exposed, the skin about it sterilized with iodine and alcohol, and a small injection of novocaine made over the vein, which was made prominent by a tourniquet above the elbow. A hollow needle attached to a rubber tube leading to the bleeding bottle was inserted into the vein. The bleeding bottle contained 50 cc. of a sodium citrate solution which prevented the blood from clotting. In four to ten minutes, a pint of blood was collected, the needle withdrawn and a small sterile dressing attached over the site of puncture. Donors were required to rest for ten minutes on the couch, and were then invited into the canteen, where volunteer Red Cross workers served light refreshments. Donors were then presented with a blood donor emblem if they did not already have one, and their donations were recorded on a certificate given to them. Nearly all donors returned to their usual occupations or activities immediately after completing the routine of donating.

Although varying considerably from day to day, approximately 10 per cent of donors had some reaction following the withdrawal of blood. A thorough study of the complications of blood donations was made when about 7,000,000 donations had been procured. The result of this study, which is the seventh publication in the references, indicates that serious complications were so rare in relation to the great number of donations that we feel justified in speaking of the procedure as harmless.

At the completion of a donation, the bottle of blood was placed immediately in a refrigerator, and at the end of the day, it was shipped in refrigerated containers from each center to its particular laboratory within twenty-four hours of the time it was procured. Most of the blood was transported by Railway Express, and in order that it might be carried without damage, it was packed into large insulated chests (known as Church containers) holding 80 bottles of blood and weighing, when filled, nearly 400 pounds. The transportation of blood on fixed schedules and on designated trains, sometimes as much as 500 miles, was a problem which the transportation company and the railroads solved by exceptional service and cooperation. By the terms of the specifications under which the blood was processed, the plasma had to be brought to the frozen state within seventy-two hours after it was withdrawn, so there was no time to be lost.

As soon as the blood reached the laboratory, the bottles were removed from the chest. That which was used for dried plasma was placed in large centrifuges, and rotated at a speed of about 2,200 revolutions per minute for about forty minutes. This treatment throws all the red and white blood cells to the bottom of the bottle, and the clear plasma at the top is drawn off.

The plasma of about 50 bottles of blood was "pooled" by mixing it in a large container, and after samples were taken to test its sterility, the plasma was measured off into the bottles in which it was frozen and dried.

The freezing of plasma was accomplished rapidly by rotating the bottles in a solution brought to about 70° below freezing by a mixture of dry ice. This process was known as shell freezing because the plasma was frozen about the sides of the bottle with an open space in the center which facilitated the drying.

The drying of plasma was begun when it was in the frozen state, and practically all the water was withdrawn by means of vacuum pumps and a gradual rise of temperature, bringing the plasma, after a number of hours, to a light brown powder. The dried plasma was then sealed under sterile conditions, and was ready for packaging, with its accompanying bottle of sterile water and the equipment for its use in the treatment of traumatic shock.

The blood used for the production of serum albumin was treated differently, the red blood cells being separated from the plasma by a machine similar to a cream separator, and somewhat complicated chemical processes known as plasma fractionation were employed for the production of serum albumin and other substances of medical value to the armed forces.

After the dried plasma and serum albumin were finally placed in cartons in which they were transported to the far corners of the globe wherever our fighting men had been sent, a label bearing a small red cross was attached to each carton, saying that the plasma or serum albumin in the package had been processed from blood obtained from volunteer donors enrolled by the American Red Cross. Photographs from the battle fronts showed these cartons being carried forward on the back of a struggling burro, on the litters of South Sea Islanders, in the arms of medical corpsmen, and all bespoke the urgent need for plasma where soldiers and sailors were fighting and dying.

While attention and interest were centered on the production of blood substitutes for the treatment of traumatic shock as the main objective of the Blood Donor Service, thought was also directed to the possible medical value of the red blood cells that were being discarded in such great volume. A useful purpose was first found for a small amount of the so-called cellular residue for the production of peptone, a substance used in growing the bacteria from which sera and antitoxins required by the armed forces were produced.

Later, the technical staff of the Blood Donor Service devised a plan by which the red blood cells could be selected and suspended in solutions that preserved them. These red blood cell suspensions were used as transfusions in the treatment of anemia and other chronic conditions in which blood transfusions were of much benefit. A red blood cell transfusion service was organized in several of the blood donor centers situated near a processing laboratory, and from these centers the cells were supplied to military hospitals and used for clinical investigation in a few civilian hospitals. This service is fully described in the fourth and fifth publications in the references.

Although this service might never compare in magnitude with the Blood Donor Service for the collection of blood, it served to augment the valuable functions of dried plasma and serum albumin. Just as these substances had an invaluable place in treating the acute conditions characterized by traumatic shock on the battlefield, the red blood cell transfusions had their less dramatic but valuable place in the treatment of the chronic and prolonged results of serious wounds in those who were returned to military hospitals in this country. In many of these patients, blood regeneration was disturbed and great benefit derived from transfusions, which could be supplied freely with such a large reserve of red blood cells to call upon as that which the Blood Donor Service provided.

The success of the Blood Donor Service stands as a tribute to the devotion of the American people to the causes for which this war has been fought, and to those in our armed forces who have been fighting at the battle fronts. It serves also as an example of the ability of the Red Cross to carry out its charter obligations to "furnish volunteer aid to the sick and wounded of armies." The value of this particular project, already indicated by reports from the combat zones, probably will be realized even more fully when the final story of the war is written.

Of the scores of other Red Cross activities carried on in this country, and by several thousand workers attached to the armed forces overseas, there are four which deserve special mention here because of their direct relationship to the medical or medical-social aspects of the war.

These are the recruitment of nurses for the Army and Navy; social case work and recreation work in Army and Navy hospitals in this country and abroad and on hospital ships; the production of surgical dressings for the armed forces; and certain phases of the work of Red Cross Home Service, through which the Red Cross carried out its charter responsibility to "act in matters of voluntary relief and in accord with the military and naval authorities as a medium of communication between the people of the United States of America and their Army and Navy."

Red Cross Home Service was organized during the First World War. Then, and afterward, its primary function was to act as a link between the men in the armed forces and their families. Reduced to its simplest terms, servicemen who worried about their families got in touch with Red Cross Field Directors serving with the troops, who initiated requests for information which were fulfilled by workers in the local Red Cross chapters, assistance being provided where needed. The same system worked in reverse when the families at home wished to establish emergency contacts with relatives in the service.

Requests for information poured in from all sides—from families seeking information concerning their loved ones, from the men overseas regarding their families back home, and from officers requiring information about home conditions of their men. During 1918, 500,000 families with men in the armed forces received information, advice, financial help, or other assistance from the Red Cross. Never had the Red Cross been able to employ to better advantage its vast network of chapters and branches throughout the United States.

In 1944, Red Cross Home Service was a streamlined version of the 1918 organization, with hundreds of paid and volunteer workers handling thousands of cases a month. When the family needed advice about allowances or allotments or, in the case of a disabled ex-serviceman or the dependents of a deceased serviceman, when help was needed in filing claims for government benefits, or when financial assistance was needed pending the receipt of government benefits or any other requirement of this group, Home Service assisted in carrying out the obligations of the Red Cross. Little publicized, the nature of its work being confidential, it was one of the largest and most important of all Red Cross wartime activities. Here, truly, was the soldier's closest emergency link with home, and the value of this work as a morale-builder received the warm praise of commanding officers throughout the war zones.

The production of surgical dressings, another important wartime activity, was carried on by the women of America in Red Cross chapter workrooms throughout the country, and more than a billion surgical dressings were delivered to the armed services. In this work, which goes back to the Civil War, thousands of volunteer workers, many of them with sons overseas, sat quietly day after day, folding and packing the surgical dressings to staunch the flow of blood on some far-distant field.

In many respects, one of the most difficult assignments that the Red Cross undertook was the recruiting of nurses for the Army and Navy Nurse Corps at the request of the Surgeons General of the Army and Navy.

The complexity of this problem resulted from the limited number of nurses available and the great demand for their services in hundreds of hospitals and industrial plants in this country. The scarcity of nurses became so acute that at the request of the nursing profession, in July, 1943, the War Manpower Commission set up a system of procurement and assignment to determine the availability of nurses for military service or their essentiality for civilian service.

Despite these difficulties, the Red Cross, as of June 1, 1944, had recruited approximately 40,000 nurses for service with the Army Nurse Corps, and approximately 10,000 who accepted commissions in the Navy, and it continued to enroll additional nurses.

In a further effort to relieve the shortage of civilian nurses, the Red Cross, during the twenty-nine months ending May 31, 1944, trained and issued home nursing certificates to approximately 1,133,000 women; and during the three years ending June 1, 1944, issued approximately 137,000 Volunteer Nurse's Aide certificates.

These volunteer nurses' aides became familiar to patients in hundreds of hospitals throughout America, where their work was most useful. Recognizing their value, the Surgeon General of the Army called upon nurses' aides who had had at least 150 hours of service to accept full-time assignments as salaried civilian employees in Army hospitals in this country when requested by their Army Service Commands.

In Army and Naval hospitals at home and abroad and on hospital ships evacuating the injured, professional medical-social workers and recreation workers of the American National Red Cross rendered important services to the sick and wounded. The case workers assisted the patients in the solution of personal problems which might be retarding recovery, aided in their orientation to the hospital, obtained social history material for the medical officers, provided funds for convalescent or therapeutic furloughs when needed, secured reports on the welfare of the relatives of patients, and rendered numerous humble though important services, such as tracing lost clothing, providing, among other things, stationery, cigarettes, toothbrushes and razor blades for patients temporarily without these necessary articles.

The recreation workers conducted medically approved diversional activities in centrally located recreation halls and in the hospital wards, and provided a wide variety of games and equipment, including musical instruments. Motion pictures were shown in the recreation halls, and when appropriate, in wards. The recreation workers also helped the patients to organize special interest groups for book reviews, music appreciation, dancing classes, foreign language study and amateur dramatic production.

Those patients about to be discharged from military service helped to plan for their readjustment to civilian life by Red Cross case workers, who informed them of the resources through which they might obtain follow-up medical care, vocational rehabilitation, employment and financial assistance. Their privilege of applying for veterans' pensions was discussed, and they were aided in executing their applications. Patients who required further case work assistance after discharge were referred to the Home Service workers of the Red Cross chapters in their home communities.

It is through activities such as these that the Red Cross has performed its traditional function as an auxiliary of the armed forces.

REFERENCES

The following publications by members of the Technical Staff of the Red Cross Blood Donor Service describe and discuss many of the technical operations and problems of the Service:

1. Taylor, Earl S., Blood Procurement for the Army and Navy. Preliminary Report. *Journal of the American Medical Association,* Dec. 20, 1941, Vol. 117, pp. 2123–2129.

2. Taylor, Earl S., Procurement of Blood for the Armed Forces. *Journal of the American Medical Association,* Sept. 12, 1942, Vol. 120, pp. 119–123.

3. Heiss, Mary E., and Taylor, Earl S., Standards for the Protection of Blood Donors, *Hospitals,* Nov., 1943.

4. Taylor, Earl S., Thalhimer, William, and Cooksey, Warren B., The Organization of a Red Cross Blood Cell Transfusion Service. *Journal of the American Medical Association*, Apr. 1, 1944, Vol. 124, pp. 958–960.

5. Cooksey, Warren B., and Horwitz, William H., Use of Salvaged Red Cells. *Journal of the American Medical Association*, Apr. 1, 1944, Vol. 124, pp. 961–964.

6. Taylor, Earl S., and Heiss, Mary E., American Red Cross Blood Donor Service, *Journal of the American Medical Association*, Apr. 15, 1944, Vol. 124, pp. 1100–1103.

7. Boynton, Mary Heiss, and Taylor, Earl S., Complications Arising in Donors in a Mass Blood Procurement Project. In press.

HOW THE NATIONAL RESEARCH COUNCIL STREAMLINED MEDICAL RESEARCH FOR WAR

President Woodrow Wilson, during his incumbency, created a new quasi-governmental agency known as the National Research Council. During World War I, its activities were mobilized in aid of our armed forces. In the intervening period between World War I and World War II, it carried on projects of research in many fields, including particularly the field of medicine.

With the beginning of World War II, Dr. Lewis H. Weed became chairman of the Council's Division of Medical Sciences. Then followed a tremendous expansion to meet the requests of our Army and Navy medical departments for standardization of medical methods in diagnosis, prevention and treatment of disease. Daily new problems developed. Soon every great agency of our government, both those concerned particularly with the war and those which are permanent factors in our government, began calling on the Division of Medical Sciences for advice and authority. As the work expanded, Dr. Weed called to assist him, among others, Dr. George B. Darling, who had been president of the W. K. Kellogg Foundation in Battle Creek, Michigan. Dr. Darling holds the degree of doctor of public health from the University of Michigan.

When Dr. Darling accepted the position of Vice Chairman of the Division of Medical Sciences of the National Research Council, he familiarized himself with its many activities, and this is reflected in the record which follows of the many ways in which medical scientists, in some instances too old or too important in their civilian lives to enter the war, contributed their knowledge for the protection of the lives and health of the men and women in the armed forces, and of the nation in general.

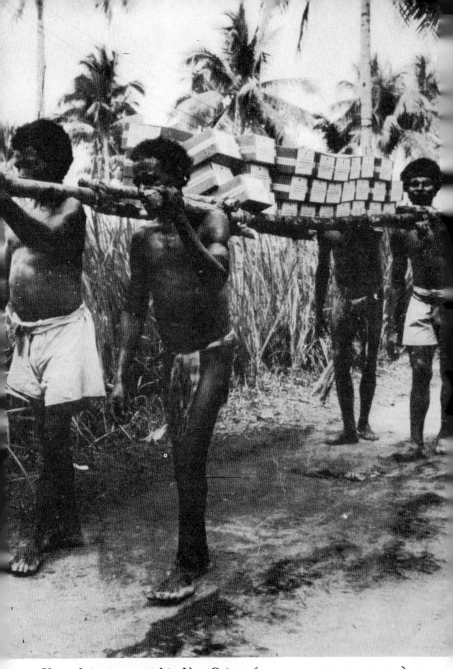

Plasma being transported in New Guinea. (RED CROSS PHOTO BY POAGUE)

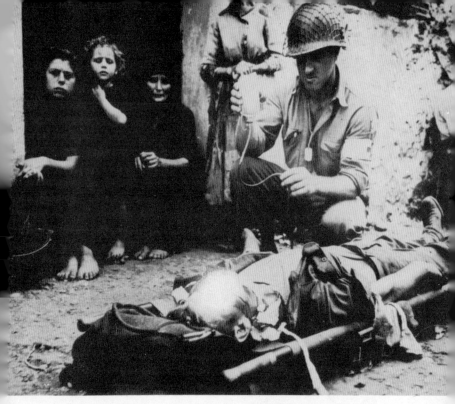

Plasma in use during Sicilian campaign. (U. S. ARMY SIGNAL CORPS PHOTO)

CHAPTER XVI

HOW THE NATIONAL RESEARCH COUNCIL STREAMLINED MEDICAL RESEARCH FOR WAR

By
GEORGE B. DARLING, M.D.
Vice Chairman of the Division of Medical Sciences,
National Research Council

THE IMMENSE SCALE on which World War II has been waged has multiplied the number and nature of medical problems far beyond previous experience. We have had to contend not only with natural enemies lurking in corners of the globe with which we have not ordinarily been concerned, but we have had to face entirely new problems created by the tremendous technological advances that have given us a new mastery in the air, on the land, and on and under the sea.

Many of these problems could be successfully attacked only by the complete cooperation of many groups through careful organization, including the mobilization of professional manpower for both military and civilian needs; the integration of training programs with general mobilization plans; the selection of essential medical and hospital supplies and equipment and their production; the development of special educational programs both for our own professionals and those of liberated nations. Of paramount importance has been the establishment of a mechanism to provide for the adequate marshaling of the scientific knowledge and experimental facilities of medicine so that decisions might really be made on the basis of the best contemporary knowledge and belief. That mobilization of medical mind-power is the subject of this chapter.

Such a program has two major phases: first, the coordination of knowledge already won (often in widely divergent fields) for application to the problem at hand, and second, the prosecution of new research to answer new problems or old problems that have suddenly assumed a new importance. Both are significant, but the pressures of war tend to accelerate the first at the expense of the second. Certainly the war accentuated the need for effective channels for the prompt exchange of hard-won knowledge from the points of discovery to the points of application.

A state of war introduces both positive and negative factors. Acceleration is undoubtedly enhanced by merging the entire nation's professional interests into one united effort. This motivation for rapid pooling of professional contributions counteracts the normal peacetime tendency toward individual effort. However, difficulties are multiplied by the dislocation of brain power and the restricted publication of research findings. The job is to take the greatest advantage of the positive factors and then neutralize, as far as possible, the negative.

War needs in the medical field included:

(1) A neutral forum for free discussion of common problems by military and civilian leaders.

(2) A mechanism for summarizing information, recommendations and the best contemporary thought of the entire profession, both in and out of uniform, for the guidance of military or governmental officers, when requested.

(3) An adequate organization for the planning, investigation, supervision and coordination of new investigative work.

(4) Sufficient funds to provide for all three.

To meet these needs, we have had the total resources of the nation in men, facilities and money. The problem was to organize the professional men efficiently, to inform them completely and promptly, and to finance them adequately.

The National Research Council recognized the necessity for making adequate provision for such programs early, and the Division of Medical Sciences, accepting its traditional responsibilities, offered its services to the armed forces in the first months of 1940. At the request of the Surgeon General of the Army, with the wholehearted concurrence of the Surgeons General of the Navy and the United States Public Health Service, two advisory committees on military medicine (chemotherapy and transfusions) were first established in May, 1940. Committees on Medicine,

Surgery and Information followed shortly thereafter. This was a logical development. The National Research Council had been created to advise the government during the previous world war as an outgrowth of the earlier National Academy of Sciences.

The National Academy of Sciences has an honorable history of important scientific contributions to the nation's war efforts since the early days of the Civil War, when one of its committees worked with the Navy on problems concerning the new "iron-clads." The original charter of the National Academy of Sciences, passed by Congress and approved by President Lincoln in 1863, provides that

. . . the Academy shall, whenever called upon by any department of the government, investigate, examine, experiment and report upon any subject of science or art, the actual expense of such investigations, examinations, experiments and reports to be paid from appropriations which may be made for the purpose, but the Academy shall receive no compensation whatever for any services to the government of the United States.

The National Research Council was organized in 1916 at the request of the President of the United States by the National Academy of Sciences under its Congressional charter, as a measure of national preparedness. The Council served the government in a cooperative capacity during the First World War as the Department of Science and Research of the Council of National Defense, and also as the Science and Research Division of the United States Signal Corps.

The duties of the National Research Council, as set forth in the Executive Order signed by Woodrow Wilson at the White House on May 11, 1918, were as follows:

1. In general, to stimulate research in the mathematical, physical and biological sciences, and in the application of these sciences to engineering, agriculture, medicine and other useful arts, with the object of increasing knowledge, of strengthening the national defense, and of contributing in other ways to the public welfare.

2. To survey the larger possibilities of science, to formulate comprehensive projects of research, and to develop effective means of utilizing the scientific and technical resources of the country for dealing with these projects.

3. To promote cooperation in research, at home and abroad, in order to secure concentration of effort, minimize duplication, and stimulate

progress; but in all cooperative undertakings to give encouragement to individual initiative, as fundamentally important to the advancement of science.

4. To serve as a means of bringing American and foreign investigators into active cooperation with the scientific and technical services of the War and Navy Departments and with those of the civil branches of the government.

5. To direct the attention of scientific and technical investigators to the present importance of military and industrial problems in connection with the war, and to aid in the solution of these problems by organizing specific researches.

6. To gather and collate scientific and technical information, at home and abroad, in cooperation with governmental and other agencies, and to render such information available to duly accredited persons.

This was as good an outline of responsibilities in 1944 as it had been in 1916.

The National Research Council is composed of nine major divisions, of which the Division of Medical Sciences is one. These divisions are arranged in two groups, one relating to the main branches of science and the other to foreign and educational relations. Each division has a governing body consisting of representatives from the leading national scientific societies in the field with which it is concerned and also certain members at large. The National Research Council thus constitutes a democratic organization acting for the great body of scientific men of the United States.

The record of the Division of Medical Sciences in the First World War and the national character of the organizations making up its membership indicated its choice as the agency for handling the scientific phases of the medical problem. The problem of funds for administrative overhead and the adequate financing of contracts for new investigative work remained.

In the history of World War II, we find no dearth of coordinating agencies. Many agencies at one time or another have been charged with broad and often overlapping responsibilities. The Health and Medical Committee of the Council of National Defense, established on September 19, 1940, was created, according to the Executive Order, to "advise the Council of National Defense regarding the health and medical aspects of National Defense and to coordinate health and medical activities affecting national defense." This committee, under the chairmanship of Dr. Irvin Abell, consisted of the Surgeons General of the Army, Navy and Public Health Service, and the Chairman of the Division of Medical Sciences of the National Research Council. Six subcommittees, representing large sectors of medical interests, were created on (1) medical education, (2) hospitals, (3) industrial medicine, (4) nursing, (5) Negro health, (6) dentistry. These committees made important contributions in their respective fields. Shortly after its organization, the Health and Medical Committee requested the National Research Council to establish committees on aviation medicine and neuropsychiatry.

On November 28, 1940, the Council of National Defense designated the Federal Security Administrator coordinator of "all health, medical, welfare, nutritional, recreational and other related fields of activity affecting the national defense." An initial fund of $250,000 was then made available by the Budget Bureau. Of this amount, the Division of Medical Sciences was allocated approximately $60,000 for the preparation of special reports, committee meetings, etc., and approximately $67,000 for support of research projects. Unfortunately, because of technical difficulties, payments on the research fund were not made until May, 1941.

Prior to these allocations, the Division of Medical Sciences had to depend on private organizations for support. In October, 1940, the sum of $10,000 was received from the Carnegie Corporation for the work of the committees advisory to the Surgeons General. The American College of Physicians appropriated $10,000 for the support of investigations on human plasma under the Committee on Medicine. The Committee on Neuropsychiatry was financed at first by a grant of $500 from an anonymous donor.

On June 28, 1941, President Roosevelt issued an Executive Order establishing the Office of Scientific Research and Development within the Office of Emergency Management. This order provided for Presidential appointment of a director who should be responsible for the coordination, direction and supervision of scientific and medical research pertaining to the national defense. Under the Office of Scientific Research and Development, the order specified that there should be two main committees: (1) the already existent National Defense Research Committee, and (2) a Committee on Medical Research. The Committee on Medical

Research was by Executive Order to consist of four civilians and representatives of the Secretary of War, Secretary of the Navy, and Administrator of the Federal Security Agency. This Committee was authorized to

. . . advise and assist the Director in the performance of his medical research duties with special reference to the mobilization of medical and scientific personnel of the nation. To this end it shall be the responsibility of the Committee to recommend to the Director the need for and character of contracts to be entered into with universities, hospitals and other agencies conducting medical research activities for research and development in the field of the medical sciences. Furthermore, the Committee shall from time to time, on request by the Director, make findings and submit recommendations with respect to the adequacy, progress and results of research on medical problems related to national defense.

In July the Committee on Medical Research was appointed, with Dr. A. N. Richards as Chairman and Dr. Lewis H. Weed (the Chairman of the Division of Medical Sciences of the National Research Council) as Vice Chairman. There were two other civilian members (Dr. A. R. Dochez and Dr. A. Baird Hastings) and representatives of the Army, the Navy and the United States Public Health Service (Colonel J. S. Simmons, Rear Admiral H. W. Smith and Dr. L. R. Thompson).

At an early meeting of the Committee on Medical Research, the relationship of the committees on military medicine of the Division of Medical Sciences to the new governmental agency was defined. The Committee on Medical Research recommended the appointment of the chairmen of the main military committees of the Division as special consultants in the various fields designated. Furthermore, the Committee on Medical Research recommended the drawing of a contract between the Office of Scientific Research and Development and the National Academy-National Research Council whereby the Division of Medical Sciences would arrange meetings of the various groups and submission of reports and recommendations regarding medical research problems. The sum of approximately $45,000 was made available by transfer of funds from the Federal Security Agency. Later, the Office of Scientific Research and Development entered into a further contract with the National Academy-National Research Council in the amount of $150,000, under the same general terms for the furnishing of committee reports, recommendations and other expenses incidental thereto. (This was continued annually, with gradual increases as the work expanded, so that through June, 1944, contracts of approximately $670,000 had been written with the Office of Scientific Research and Development.)

As the contract with the Office of Scientific Research and Development was on a reimbursable basis, the need for a revolving fund to finance expenditures became obvious early in the fall of 1941. The John and Mary R. Markle Foundation appropriated $60,000 to the National Research Council on November 5, 1941, to serve as a revolving fund for the divisional activities in military medicine.

The prompt and spontaneous action of the several private agencies mentioned was timely and invaluable. Without this support, the Division would have been unable to meet its opportunities and obligations. The nation is greatly in their debt.

A little late then, but still in time to be effective, the basic organization was completed, financed partly by public and partly by private funds, to meet the four immediate needs of doctors at war.

From the modest beginning in 1940, additional standing committees were organized as required until a total of fourteen main and forty-two subcommittees were established, with a total membership of 379. Effective liaison with the military services was essential. Beginning with Colonel C. C. Hillman and Commander C. S. Stevenson in 1940, a distinguished list of officers in the Army and Navy and United States Public Health Service served in this capacity. In 1944, Presidential appointments as liaison officers to the Division of Medical Sciences were held by Brigadier General J. S. Simmons and Colonel Roger G. Prentiss, Jr., of the Army, and Captain W. W. Hall and Captain E. H. Cushing of the Navy. In addition, some fifty officers received official designation as contact officers to various committees. These men were all specialists in their fields and spoke with authority on the technical conditions, requirements and needs of the different elements of their services. The results obtained were due in no small measure to the realistic manner in which they presented their problems and participated in the deliberations of the committees.

In the spring of 1944, there were the following committees on military medicine:

COMMITTEES ON MILITARY MEDICINE

(Including Present Chairmen)

Aviation Medicine (Eugene F. DuBois)
  Advisory Commission A (J. K. Lewis)
  Acceleration (Eugene M. Landis)
  Clothing (L. H. Newburgh)
  Decompression Sickness (John F. Fulton)
  Motion Sickness (Derek Denny-Brown)
  Oxygen and Anoxia (Detlev W. Bronk)
  Visual Problems (Detlev W. Bronk)
Chemotherapeutic and Other Agents (Chester S. Keefer)
Convalescence and Rehabilitation (Wm. S. Tillett)
Drugs and Medical Supplies (W. W. Palmer)
  Essential Drugs (Ernest E. Irons)
  Hospital and Surgical Supplies (Frederick A. Coller)
  Medical Food Requirements (Wm. D. Stroud)
  Pharmacy (Isaac Starr)
Industrial Medicine (Clarence D. Selby)
  Armored Vehicles (George M. Smith)
  Personal Relationships in Industry (Lydia G. Giberson)
Information (Morris Fishbein)
  Historical Records (John F. Fulton)
  Publicity (Morris Fishbein)
Medicine (O. H. Perry Pepper)
  Cardiovascular Diseases (Paul Dudley White)
  Clinical Investigation (J. H. Means)
  Infectious Diseases (Francis G. Blake)
  Medical Nutrition (J. S. McLester)
  Tropical Diseases (Henry E. Meleney)
  Tuberculosis (James Burns Amberson, Jr.)
  Venereal Diseases (J. E. Moore)
Neuropsychiatry (Winfred Overholser)
  Neurology (Foster Kennedy)
  Psychiatry (Arthur Ruggles)
Pathology (Howard T. Karsner)
Sanitary Engineering (Abel Wolman)
Shock and Transfusions (Walter B. Cannon)
  Blood Substitutes (Joseph T. Wearn)
  Shock (Alfred Blalock)
Surgery (Evarts A. Graham)
  Anesthesia (Ralph M. Waters)
  Infected Wounds and Burns (Allen O. Whipple)

Neurosurgery (Howard C. Naffziger)
Ophthalmology (Harry S. Gradle)
Orthopedic Surgery (George E. Bennett)
Otolaryngology (A. C. Furstenberg)
Physical Therapy (John S. Coulter)
Plastic and Maxillo-facial Surgery (Robert H. Ivy)
Radiology (A. C. Christie)
Thoracic Surgery (Evarts A. Graham)
Urology (Herman L. Kretschmer)
Vascular Injuries (John Homans)
Treatment of Gas Casualties (Milton G. Winternitz)

Board for the Coordination of Malarial Studies (Robert F. Loeb)
Panel on Clinical Testing (James A. Shannon)
Panel on Pharmacology (E. K. Marshall, Jr.)
Panel on Biochemistry (William Mansfield Clark)
Panel on Synthesis (Dr. Carl S. Marvel)

This marshaling of minds represents one of the most important functions of the Division. For either standing committees or *ad hoc* conference groups, professional men were needed with judgment, experience, imagination, energy, integrity and the ability to take an impersonal point of view in regard to the achievements and capacities of their colleagues. A proportional geographic representation was desirable to avoid provincialism. Certain tools were available to aid in selection, such as the Scientific Roster and the standard reference directories, but the extensive personal knowledge of the Chairman of the Division of the leaders in each field remained the most important factor. Upon him rested the responsibility of selecting the men best qualified to act as chairmen. They in turn could suggest their own committees.

Integration of this effort with that of other national organizations was obtained by the appointment of representatives to the appropriate National Research Council committees. These interlocking relationships were of tremendous importance in unifying the total professional effort. Coordination at the top was insured by the fact that the Chairman of the Division was also a member of the Health and Medical Committee of the Council of National Defense, Vice Chairman of the Committee on Medical Research of the OSRD, and Chairman of the Medical and Health Advisory Committee of the American Red Cross.

It should be mentioned that, with the exception of a small

administrative staff in Washington, all of the nearly four hundred men, specially selected from all over the nation because of competence in their particular fields, served on the various committees on military medicine without compensation except for the actual out-of-pocket expenses of travel to the meetings. They contributed their time and experience and judgment gladly as part of their contribution toward the total war effort.

Once the committees and members of the conferences had been selected, they were charged with three important functions:

(1) The informal exchange of experience made possible by bringing the men with similar problems and interests from the various armed services together with leaders from civil life.

(2) Formal recommendations drafted upon the request and for the guidance of the armed forces and governmental agencies.

(3) Review of contracts for investigative work to be carried out by universities, hospitals and other research organizations financed by contracts with the Office of Scientific Research and Development on recommendation of the Committee on Medical Research.

It will be noted that the committees were responsible for both professional and research advice. These two functions are interdependent. Professional problems indicated the direction research must take, and professional advice would be altered as achievements were reported.

When the committees had been selected, given their assignments, and adequately financed, there still remained the problem of keeping them informed as to both problems and discoveries in their field which had developed since the outbreak of the war.

It is sufficiently difficult to keep reasonably up to date on scientific developments in peacetime, but war complicates the problem greatly. Results normally reported in open literature are forced "underground" by the military requirements, so that much is classified as "secret," "confidential" or "restricted," and circulation is limited to individuals approved by appropriate security agencies. Obviously committee members and research investigators would soon find themselves behind the times unless special machinery were devised to keep them up to date. The Division of Medical Sciences, in cooperation with the Committee on Medical Research, consequently established a file of "classified" reports appropriately indexed, arranged for "clearance" of staff and committee members and research workers, and saw that these approved individuals received reports in their special fields.

The National Research Council was able to effect close liaison with the National Research Council of Canada, and prompt and unrestricted interchange of medical information went on between the two councils with considerable exchange of attendance at committee meetings. The relationship to the British Medical Research Council, which was established as a part of the Privy Council of Great Britain, could necessarily not be so close, but through liaison officers a good deal was accomplished. Informal contact was maintained with our other allies through their military medical representatives stationed in Washington.

Gradually new problems developed as the character of total war unfolded. The War Production Board found itself in need of professional advice as to the relative importance of various items of drugs, medical supplies and equipment; and in July, 1942, a contract was entered into between the National Research Council and the War Production Board to provide expert advice through similar committee procedures.

With the introduction of food rationing, the need for a medical committee that could advise as to the minimum dietary requirements, in excess of the ration allowances, of those suffering from particular diseases was recognized. In April, 1943, a contract was entered into with the War Food Administration to make arrangements for this medical service.

Later, as our international obligations toward liberated countries became clearer, the Division was asked first by the Office of Foreign Relief and Rehabilitation and later by the United Nations Relief and Rehabilitation Administration to prepare a list of basic drugs and supplies, laboratory manuals and education materials for use overseas. In 1944, it had been possible for the Division to meet these requests through various established committees.

Since the role of the Division of Medical Sciences of the National Research Council has been to make available to those charged with the prosecution of the war the best medical research minds and facilities of the nation, it is difficult to evaluate its exact contribution. Furthermore, a relatively high proportion of its activities still cannot be revealed. Scientific advances in medicine, perhaps for the first time in the history of man, have been equivalent to many military divisions.

The inoculating syringe and the insect repellent spray became secret weapons, providing our troops an important increased operating range. The stories of penicillin, of blood plasma, of DDT, and of the use of quinacrine (atabrine) in malaria, to name a few, are among the modern romances of medicine. Any one of these achievements would be worth many times the cost in time and money of the entire program. Other discoveries may ultimately prove to be equally important. Nor should the importance of so-called negative knowledge learned from experimental "failures" be lost sight of. Many lives were saved and the recovery of thousands of men hastened by a definite knowledge of what not to do, so that a high percentage of investigations which seemed to be non-productive to investigators and committee members concerned really contributed enormously to the total effort.

It may be worth while to review briefly the volume of work accomplished by the Council to indicate, at least to a degree, the extent of the effort involved.

Since long before Pearl Harbor, the Division of Medical Sciences held an average of thirteen committee meetings and four conferences a month. The attendance at these meetings averaged approximately thirty, of which perhaps a third were liaison officers from the armed services who brought the committees face to face with field problems. The importance of providing a forum, where members of all the various armed services and civilian leaders could pool their experiences and judgment, cannot be overemphasized. While its value was difficult to measure quantitatively, it can best be understood by trying to imagine what the situation would have been had this exchange not been possible.

As outlined above, the agenda of these meetings resulted largely from problems presented to the Council by representatives of the armed forces or other governmental agencies, but hundreds of requests for advice were handled by referring the problem directly to an individual or individuals whose advice would be most valuable.

A larger number of formal recommendations, averaging ten a month in the later war years, were transmitted to the Surgeons General of the Army, Navy and Public Health Service and other governmental agencies (such as the WPB, OPA, Veterans Administration, etc.) as a result of direct requests for advice. Usually these recommendations were eventually translated into service directives covering field, hospital and administrative procedures affecting the lives and welfare of millions of men in the armed forces.

One of the most important functions of the committees on military medicine was to initiate and supervise investigative work carried out largely in university laboratories and cooperating hospitals under governmental contract with the Office of Scientific Research and Development through the Committee on Medical Research. The official governmental responsibility for such contracts rested with the Director of OSRD, who acted on the recommendation of the CMR, which fortified its judgment with the advisory assistance of the NRC committees. In this connection, the committees and conferences acted as advisory bodies for a scientific program for which grants were made totaling well over $10,000,000 by the spring of 1944. The major fields of investigation included tropical diseases, insect repellents, infections of wounds and burns, penicillin, blood substitutes and general problems of shock, aviation medicine, nutrition, venereal diseases and neurosurgery. The committees judged projects submitted according to four main classifications: A, urgent; B, desirable; C, longterm project but desirable, or R, reject. They could recommend modifications of program, personnel, time or appropriation. Over the years, between 6 and 10 per cent of the proposals were denied.

In order that the committees on military medicine might be able to carry out their duties adequately, a number of direct services were provided by the Division's professional staff.

The volume of this work grew steadily until by the spring of 1944 the joint report section of the Division of Medical Sciences and CMR edited, mimeographed and mailed an average of 20,000 copies of 230 reports of committees and research investigations a month. Of these, 7,000 copies went to the Army and Navy (including the eight theaters of operations) and to liaison offices in England, Canada, Australia and New Zealand. A modest secretarial staff turned out this huge volume of work with phenomenal accuracy. Without it, medical opinion would have been hopelessly outdated when faced with its greatest problems.

The indexing unit received, indexed, carded and filed an average of 500 classified documents each month. In addition to the material from civilian and military sources in the United States, reports were received regularly from our allies in England, Australia, Canada and New Zealand, and occasionally from Russia and China. Classified documents were circulated daily to the professional personnel of the Division of Medical Sciences and the Committee on Medical Research. The files were consulted by civilian and military research specialists both from the United States and our allies. By the spring of 1944, the number of documents accessioned had exceeded 8,000. This material consisted of:

(1) Restricted publications of the armed forces (our own and our allies).

(2) Reports of results or of projected studies from the various investigative units of the armed services.

(3) Military intelligence reports bearing on medical problems.

(4) Reports from official representatives of NRC and CMR abroad.

(5) Reports from liaison officers of medical services of Allied governments.

(6) Reports from research councils of Allied countries.

(7) Progress and/or final reports of the investigators under contract with the Office of Scientific Research and Development through the Committee on Medical Research, National Defense Research Committee, and so forth.

(8) Minutes of National Research Council committees and conferences.

The opportunities for an office of information located in the midst of the medical intelligence center were recognized early. Starting as a service for the staff, the scope was first broadened by a grant of $17,000 from the Carnegie Corporation of New York and later by a grant of $75,000 for a period of years by the Johnson & Johnson Research Foundation. The Office of Medical Information integrated the "open" published material with the "classified" master index already mentioned. A daily news bulletin, prepared for the staff of the Division of Medical Sciences and the Committee on Medical Research, summarized items appearing in representative daily newspapers (including the London *Times*) and the more important medical publications, including the military.

Another function of this office was to distill the essence of important work reported in the committee minutes and the reports of research workers. A topical index listing recently accessioned documents of interest to the members of the committees was sent to them in advance of scheduled meetings. Special reports were prepared when it was necessary to summarize all the investigative results relating to a complex problem or to issue a definitive statement of research findings that indicated new treatment methods. A number of special monographs were released, including: "Burns" (March, 1943), "Blast" (June, 1943), "Anthiomaline Bibliography" (August, 1943) and "Antimalarial Drugs" (July, 1944).

As the process of liberation of countries formerly occupied by the enemy began, the Division of Medical Sciences was requested by OWI and UNRRA to prepare pamphlets on medical subjects to summarize the advances of the last few years for the physicians and medical workers in liberated countries.

The office is under the direction of the former Surgeon General of the United States Army, Major General James C. Magee, U.S.A. (Retired).

While most of the deliberations of the committees on military medicine found their greatest effectiveness in directives issued by the Army, Navy or other governmental services, some of their labors resulted in publications released under the imprint of the Council itself. The Manuals of Military Surgery, published by W. B. Saunders & Co., were particularly valuable in the early stages of the war, and played an important role in the education of new officers and medical students. The list included: I. "Plastic and Maxillo-facial Surgery"; II. "Ophthalmology and Otolaryngology"; III. "Abdominal and Genito-urinary Injuries"; IV. "Orthopedic Subjects"; V. "Burns, Shock, Wound Healing and Vascular Injuries"; VI. "Neurosurgery and Thoracic Surgery"; as well as the "Manual of Dermatology" and "Fundamentals of Anesthesia."

The "Bibliography on Aviation Medicine" served as a valuable reference work for investigators in the field of aviation medicine.

In addition, appropriate committees of the Division reviewed a number of technical manuals for the Army, beginning with revision of the War Department publications, MR 1-9, "Standards of Physical Examination," and TM 8-210, "Guides to Therapy for Medical Officers." The most recent to be revised were TM 8-233, "Methods for Pharmacy Technicians," and TM 8-227, "Methods for Laboratory Technicians."

Many important publications were prepared for release by other organizations, as for example, the technical manuals of the Office of Civilian Defense on the "Preservation and Transfusion of

Whole Blood" and "Citrated Human Blood Plasma," and the "Manual of Occupational Therapy" prepared with the Council on Physical Therapy of the American Medical Association and the American Occupational Therapy Association.

Reports that could be released on work sponsored by the committees appeared in the appropriate professional journals. As might have been expected, the *Journal of the American Medical Association, War Medicine* and the technical publications of the Army and Navy *(Bumed News; Naval Medical Bulletin; Hospital Corps Quarterly; Army News; Army Technical Bulletin)* carried the bulk of these papers. Many others were held up until such time as their publication would no longer be of value to the enemy.

It was not unnatural that in the early days of the development of the huge military forces of the United States many problems arose which could properly be expected to be handled by military testing laboratories. In fact, the work of the committees sometimes led to the establishment of such service laboratories, so that the committees practically put themselves out of a job. The Subcommittee on Armored Vehicles, of the Committee on Industrial Medicine, is a good example of this evolutionary development. The committee was instrumental in establishing the Armored Medical Research Laboratory at Fort Knox, Kentucky, and recommended the major personnel.

A similar history, varying in degree, could be cited for some of the Air Force Laboratories, the Climatic Food and Clothing Laboratories of the Quartermaster General, the Chemical Warfare Laboratory and some of the naval laboratories. Much of the work of these laboratories, of course, revolved around improvements and testing of mechanical equipment. However, as more experience was gained in mechanized warfare, the importance of adapting machinery to the men who operate it so as to obtain a maximum of efficiency with a minimum of fatigue became increasingly obvious.

While the exact role of the military laboratories still remained to be decided in 1944, it seemed likely that they would be principally concerned with practical problems. It appeared unlikely that such laboratories would be in a position to undertake "basic" research. Every military energy had to be devoted to winning the war. It proved to be difficult to staff adequately Army and Navy laboratories with competent professional teams and keep them together long enough to make significant contributions. It was seemingly inevitable that fundamental research had to be carried on in university and industrial research centers.

The range of problems in physiology faced by the Committee on Military Medicine defies description. Heat, cold, humidity, excessive dryness, altitude and pressure, all had to be counteracted or compensated for. The very mechanisms by which we increase man's ability to see and hear and travel in the air, on land, and on and in the sea increase proportionately the importance of the fundamental knowledge of the capabilities and limitations of the human eye and ear, hand and body, and reduce the time required for response to stimuli to fractions heretofore met only in laboratories.

Basic studies on normal human physiology assumed an importance unknown before. Even items that contributed to the comfort of the operator of the tank or airplane, which could be disregarded in the early days because of the relatively brief periods that men operated them, now became matters of military importance. It certainly was worse than useless for a man to fly for several hours, only to find himself unable to complete his mission or defend himself because of cramps or fatigue brought about by poor design. All the engineering and production skill poured into military landing craft were of no avail if the men who made up the assault teams were too seasick to fight effectively when they finally got ashore into combat. A gun might be perfect in itself, but ineffective if the fire control mechanism was so awkward that a man could operate it easily only for a short time. In complicated control mechanisms, the kinesthetic sense could be used to help the operator or confuse him, depending upon the degree to which the design was based upon knowledge of human physiology. Many of the committees dealt with these problems in a fundamental way.

The problem of clothing for a world-wide military force is a fascinating one. At one moment a flier may need protection against a temperature of 40 degrees below zero and as adequate protection against flak and gunfire as body armor can provide. The next moment he may need to escape rapidly with a parachute from a machine out of control. A few seconds later he may find himself facing a long exposure to sea water at near freezing temperatures, and will need something that will keep him warm, dry and afloat. Even the design of satisfactory uniforms for the celebrated G-I

Joes was a problem to stump the experts. In the Arctic, he had to be kept warm without sacrificing freedom of movement. In the tropics, he had to be kept as cool as possible and still be protected effectively against insects. His clothing had to withstand torrential downpours and high humidity, repel insects and protect him against the ever-present threat of chemical warfare—all this without having the protective agents interfere with one another, harm the wearer, or dissolve the uniform! A great deal of the time and of many committees was directed toward the physiological aspects of these puzzling problems, and much of value was accomplished.

Proper food for the fighting man is all-important. First there are the dietary needs of military men under normal conditions or conditions which are made to approximate normal by the hard-working and efficient mess officers and men. Then there are special rations, designed for combat conditions, landing operations, or other circumstances when transport difficulties or other factors prevent normal food service. Finally, there are true emergency rations and water supplies for fliers forced down in out-of-the-way spots, or fliers or sailors lost at sea. Other problems involved water replacement needs, salt requirements, vitamins and so forth. All these problems needed and received due consideration from the advisory committees.

Adequate examinations for entrance into the Army and Navy and for particular branches of these services were important in this specialized type of warfare as never before. Beginning with the standards for physical examination issued by the War Department as pamphlet MR 1-9, the committees made many important contributions in this field.

The neuropsychiatry committees concerned themselves with the whole gamut of problems from pre-military, through the military to the post-military stages. While a number of important contributions were made in the early days of the war, these had primarily to do with the weeding out of men unfit for the military machine. Probably the most significant findings will result from studies of men whose performance in battle can be compared with their history (including an adequate neuropsychiatric examination) prior to and at the time of entrance into the armed forces. Other interesting studies are being made comparing the relative effectiveness of batteries of psychological examinations with interviews by psychiatrists and various mechanical neurological tests.

Many, if not most, of the problems in this new field still await the investigators.

One of the first assignments given to the Division of Medical Sciences by the Army in the spring of 1940 was the investigation of the problem of shock and methods for its treatment. A great deal of investigative work has been sponsored by appropriate committees of the Division to explore this problem in the test tube, in animals and in man.

In January, 1941, the American Red Cross and the Research Council were asked by identical letters from the Surgeons General of the Army and Navy to assume responsibilities in regard to the procurement of human blood plasma for the armed forces. In this cooperative venture, the Red Cross undertook to recruit the donors for the blood, to provide all necessary collection equipment for the bleedings, to transport the citrated drawn blood to processing centers, to centrifuge the blood and to store the resultant plasma in refrigerated chambers. The Division of Medical Sciences was asked to supply the professional advice and professional supervision for the collection of blood. The project was started with an initial organization in New York City and was rapidly extended, as facilities for centrifuging and drying were developed, to the entire nation. The Army and Navy contracted for the drying of the plasma as furnished by the Red Cross and were furnished with the huge quantities required for cases of shock, hemorrhage and burns. The armed forces adopted both dried plasma and human albumin as the result of recommendations of appropriate committees of the Division.

The procurement program expanded to enormous proportions. By the spring of 1944, blood donor centers reported over 8,000,000 bleedings since February, 1942, with a current average of approximately 100,000 a week. Here again we have magnificent evidence of the response of a democracy to total war in the medical field. The number of individuals involved in this program, in one way or another, was incalculable. The armed services, scientific laboratories, a great service organization, and countless thousands of private citizens all participated. The psychological value of this program in uniting the home and fighting fronts was without parallel in the history of man.

As a result of the contracts developed by the Committee on Medical Research, the scientific achievements were of an equally high order. Practical methods for large-scale production had to be developed. New instruments had to be devised. Simple tests were developed for the safeguarding of donors by measurement of hemoglobin. The fractionation of blood involved scientific problems of great complexity. It may well be that the value of the by-products developed as a result of this research may ultimately equal the original contribution of the plasma program itself. To mention only one or two items, the control of measles by the use of immune globulin is a fascinating story. The development of thrombin and fibrin foam provides a hemostatic and adhesive agent that solves some of the most troublesome problems of surgery.

The extensive use of gasoline-powered vehicles on land and in the air made the subject of burns an extremely important one. Here it was as important to rule out things that should not be done as it was to evolve an effective therapy. New treatments were offered to the uninitiated each week. Much time was spent by the committee investigating the claims of new products, some of which were presented by well-intentioned but inexperienced individuals, whose desire to help far outran their competence or judgment. Unfortunately, this field is an easy one for individuals with interests in proprietary remedies to exploit. The amount of pressure brought to bear by private individuals in high places was fantastic. It should be recorded that because of the importance of the problem and the committe members' desire not to overlook any possibility, no matter how remote, preliminary animal tests were run on all remedies for which any evidence whatever could be brought forward. Their experience, however, calls attention to the need for some type of trial board which could arrange for the tests of new therapeutic procedures, set up the conditions under which these remedies would be accepted for testing, and approve the investigative protocols.

A great deal of emphasis has been placed upon neurosurgery, one of the major problems of military medicine. Orthopedic and plastic and maxillo-facial surgery also came in for their share of study. Surgical infections and their control with débridement, sulfa drugs, etc., were, of course, of major interest. Gas gangrene, which was relatively unimportant in the African campaign, became of greater interest when operations were resumed on the Continent of Europe. Much needed to be known (and still does) about the mechanisms of wound healing, and considerable investigative work was sponsored in this field. In spite of the fact that a great deal has been learned about shock, the final chapter had not been written by D-Day for the Normandy invasion.

The catalogue of diseases especially studied in relation to the war includes all the familiar ones and some not so familiar. Major emphasis, however, has been placed on two chemotherapeutic agents, penicillin and the sulfa compounds, and on the diseases of syphilis, gonorrhea, malaria and typhus.

The story of penicillin has become a classic, not only because of the remarkable properties of the product but also because of the great number and diverse nature of the agencies that cooperated to make it available to the greatest number in the shortest possible time. Discovered in 1929 by Fleming, its potentialities were first recognized by Florey in 1940. Some months before Pearl Harbor, Dr. Florey was brought to this country as a guest of the Rockefeller Foundation. He came at once to Washington, where he made contact with the officers of the Committee on Medical Research and the National Research Council. Dr. A. N. Richards, Chairman of the CMR, immediately became greatly interested in the total problem presented by penicillin and put Dr. Florey in touch with various commercial firms interested in proceeding with production at that time. Dr. Richards convinced these firms of the government's serious interest in penicillin, and the WPB that the necessary priorities should be given to producers.

From this modest and almost casual beginning, a program of tremendous proportions was developed. Dr. Robert D. Coghill, in charge of the Northern Regional Laboratory of the Fermentation Division of the United States Department of Agriculture at Peoria, Illinois, found strains of penicillium and culture methods which increased productiveness some fifty-fold within six months. Production was started in this country, and Dr. Keefer's Committee on Chemotherapeutic and Other Agents sponsored a series of experimental clinical trials. As pencillin became available, it was released to cooperating physicians for use on selected cases. Complete reports were required to be filed with the committee for evaluation. By this method the medical services of the country were mobilized to evaluate in a remarkably short period the effectiveness of a new therapeutic agent which it might otherwise have taken years to document. Recommendations were transmitted to the armed forces for the use of penicillin in an increasing list of diseases and conditions as fast as the experimental evidence warranted. On the recommendation of the Committee on Chemotherapeutic and Other Agents, the Committee on Medical Research of the Office of Scientific Research and Development authorized a gradually expanding program of clinical testing, and many university laboratories and individual clinical investigators were drawn into the picture.

The aid of the War Production Board was obtained to facilitate production in amounts sufficient for adequate clinical testing, and priorities for equipment were allocated. The Office of Production Research and Development of the WPB set up a study of production methods with the aid of production experts of pharmaceutical houses and (because of the nature of the process) distilling interests. Complicated legal obstacles were overcome in order to exchange knowledge won on production methods in one place with the workers in other industrial houses. A special agreement with the Department of Justice was required so that representatives of the private firms might meet to discuss common problems without being subject to prosecution under the antitrust and restriction of trade laws.

The romance of penicillin has certain parallels to the Curies' discovery of radium in so far as the infinitesimally small amounts of active substances derived from huge quantities of raw material are concerned, and a great deal of new equipment and supplies had to be allocated by the WPB to facilitate production. In June, 1943, allocations of penicillin were made by the WPB in conference with a committee in which the Army, Navy, United States Public Health Service and OSRD were represented. The entire supply was allocated to these four agencies until May 15, 1944.

The uses and limitations of penicillin are well known and have been extensively reported elsewhere. The list has not yet been completed. In the spring of 1944, production in this country, at least, had climbed to the point where limited quantities could be made available to civilian hospitals as distribution centers for private cases. Up to that time the OSRD had made available over a million and a half dollars for the purchase of penicillin, and until then no civilian patient for whom it was used had to pay for it—or could pay for it.

The experimental work goes forward with great energy. Production methods have been rapidly simplified. Other molds and fungi are being investigated in the hope of finding an even more active substance, or one that will be effective in conditions that are not helped by penicillin. The chemists are hard at work at synthesis. Nevertheless, the achievements to date have been tremendous. All those who have had a part in it can take pride in the accomplishment. The discoverer, the developer, the laboratory workers, the production specialists, the physicians who did the clinical testing, the business men, the lawyers, the governmental agencies and the research councils all contributed their share to a magnificent program.

A great deal of work was done on the venereal diseases in assaying prophylactic methods and the development of intensive treatments. The studies on the use of penicillin springing from the pioneer work of Dr. J. F. Mahoney of the United States Public Health Service, for example, resulted in recommendations to the armed forces which revamped military treatment methods and promised eventually to revolutionize civilian practice as well.

The importance of malaria is well known. The need for a well-integrated program of basic research for the prevention and treatment of this disease required close coordination of Army, Navy, Public Health Service and civilian workers. In the fall of 1943, at the suggestion of the Chairman of the Division of Medical Sciences, a Board for the Coordination of Malarial Studies was created as an outgrowth of an earlier committee of the Division. This Board, with officially designated representatives from the Army, Navy, United States Public Health Service, OSRD and NRC, was appointed with full responsibility and power and given complete autonomy. The Board took over the over-all strategy for the fight against this disease. The attacks in special fields were carried on by panels on Clinical Testing, Pharmacology, Biochemistry, and Synthesis of Antimalarials.

The early work of the committee of the Division related largely to the development of the most effective use of quinacrine. Much work needed to be done to determine proper dosage levels, establish the limitations of the drug, and perfect plans for adequate "malaria discipline" for the troops. This had been so well done by the spring of 1944 that despite earlier untoward experiences, particularly among British troops in Africa (which were adequately explained by later work), quinacrine proved so effective as a malarial suppressive in the field that the announcement of the chemical synthesis of quinine in May, 1944, was only of academic interest and had no military importance. Quinacrine was doing a better job than quinine.

The coordination of the work of the synthetic chemists in the production of the chemical compounds tested for antimalarial activity presented interesting organizational complications. Contributions of great theoretical importance to our knowledge of the life cycle of the human malarial organisms have been made by studying the developmental forms of the malarial infections in chickens. This provided leads as to the specific action of the drugs on different stages of the organism. Methods based on the measurements of fluorescence by electronic photo-fluorometers have been devised for the determination of quinine and quinacrine in the blood plasma, which have contributed greatly to a rational development of dosage regimes.

Although quinacrine is more effective than quinine, its action is similar in that it suppresses but does not prevent or cure most forms of malaria. The Board is trying to find a new drug that will be better than either. By the spring of 1944, more than 8,000 chemical compounds had been tested for antimalarial activity, and the work is being pressed forward with increased energy. The solution is only a question of time, and there are already some indications that this may not be too far in the future.

The work on tuberculosis is a good example of the interrelation of medical research with that of allied specialties. The important contribution to x-ray technique made possible by the adaptation of the photo-electronic cell to exposure meters and exposure control apparatus is well known, as is the small 5×8 film made possible by the development of a new lens for direct photography of the fluoroscopic image.

The development of effective insecticides and insect repellents was of tremendous importance to the military effort. Investigations of an empirical nature, conducted over a period of two years, succeeded in establishing the usefulness of certain insect repellents and insecticides against a number of important flying and crawling insects. The most noteworthy contribution was the discovery of DDT for use in the insecticidal field, yet substantial progress was made also in the search for efficient insect repellents. The impressive performance of the United States of America Typhus

Commission in controlling the Naples outbreak of typhus in the winter of 1943–1944 is only one of the examples that can be cited as to the effectiveness of this program. The importance of these discoveries to the war in the Pacific can well be imagined. This is another triumph of coordinated research. Applications to civilian life have awaited only adequate production.

Much of the most important work of the committees on military medicine cannot be reported at this writing for security reasons. Some of this work was in the nature of defense against agents that might be used by the enemy, but which fortunately had not been utilized by mid-1944. Others dealt with industrial and military aspects of secret weapons.

The Committee on the Treatment of Gas Casualties is an excellent example of this type of service. Methods of treatment, manuals and directives were prepared not only for the protection of the soldier and civilian who might be subjected to chemical warfare agents, but also for the protection of the industrial worker, should production of these materials be found necessary. The advantages of integration of work of this type in the over-all program of the committees on military medicine were illustrated by the development of new forms of therapy for other conditions (particularly poisoning occasionally associated with the therapeutic use of heavy metals) which were suggested by findings of the Committee on the Treatment of Gas Casualties.

A world-wide war calls for the conservation of medical supplies and equipment. Plans are needed to insure the production of essential items and to prevent their dissipation in ineffective or unimportant programs. For this reason the National Research Council was asked in March, 1942, to set up a Committee on Drugs and Medical Supplies to advise the War Production Board, and a contract was written to meet the costs of this service.

The committee gave invaluable aid in determining the relative priority ratings for supplies and equipment. The committee also advised on distribution problems. Requests ran the gamut from large items of expensive hospital equipment to the simplest prescriptions.

As the war progressed, the committee was often called upon to revise the system of priorities for the use of drugs or equipment in which shortages developed because of the necessary diversion of raw supplies or intermediary products to new emergency needs. Production problems included those brought on by the vital need for penicillin, the conservation and development of antimalarial drugs, vitamins, the use of rubber in items ranging from hospital equipment to baby pants, elastic girdles and foundation garments! As production patterns became established, the work changed from decisions on national problems to advice for international relief organizations, such as the UNRRA, the Civil Affairs Division of the Army, the American Red Cross, etc.

The Office of Price Administration ran into many problems of a medical nature in determining the allocation of food supplies, not only for the general population, but for various groups suffering from particular diseases that had, or were thought to have, special nutritional needs. The OPA asked the NRC for advice, and the Subcommittee on Medical Food Requirements was set up in the Division of Medical Sciences under a contract written with the Food Distribution Administration. The minimum requirements for the nutritional needs of infants, children and adults were established, and agreement was reached in regard to the special dietary needs of those suffering from diseases in which dietary supplements or modifications were required.

At the request of the OPA, the committee recommended a panel of medical consultants specially trained in the nutritional field to act as advisers to local ration boards throughout the United States. Suitable recommendations were speedily transmitted and were subsequently published in the *Journal of the American Medical Association*. However, the corresponding directives to the local boards were not issued until much later, when the volume of troublesome decisions and applications for additional rations had reached proportions that made the wisdom of the original recommendations clearly apparent.

The two committees of the Division of Medical Sciences on nutritional problems worked closely with the Food and Nutrition Board of the Division of Biology and Agriculture of the National Research Council. The committees also cooperated in advising the Offices of the Surgeons General and the Quartermaster General in the development of standard and emergency rations previously mentioned.

Close collaboration with UNRRA and its organizational precursor, OFRRA, began in the planning stages and included not only the question of drugs and medical supplies but the general field of medical care and preventive medicine for the liberated countries. The Committee compiled lists of drugs to be distributed, established the lists of equipment for the first replacement laboratories, and set up manuals for the use of the drugs and for the laboratory procedures. All these were then reviewed by representatives of the European nations concerned, and arrangements completed with the American Medical Association for their translation into appropriate foreign languages. It was expected that the Division of Medical Sciences would have a correspondingly increasing role to play in this connection as the program of UNRRA developed.

When the British Red Cross appealed for a thousand physicians for service with the Royal Army Medical Corps or the Emergency Medical Service of Great Britain, the American Red Cross, which acted as the recruiting agency, requested an evaluation of the personal and professional qualifications of the applicants from the NRC.

In the early days of mobilization, the personnel divisions of the offices of the Surgeons General requested evaluations of medical men throughout the country to assist in making the proper assignments to big positions. Many of the committees gave valuable assistance. These evaluations were transmitted also to the roster of physicians compiled by the American Medical Association, and were made available to the Procurement and Assignment Service of the Office of Defense Health and Welfare.

Following a suggestion of the Office of the Surgeon General of the Army, lectures in tropical medicine were sponsored in medical schools throughout the United States. Staff members from many medical schools took short courses in tropical medicine, either at the Army Medical Center at the Walter Reed Hospital or at Tulane University. An appropriation of $50,000 was made by the John and Mary R. Markle Foundation on June 25, 1942, to make this service possible. In addition to this major appropriation, the Division of Medical Sciences administered another grant of $3,000 from the same source to enable the Office of the Surgeon General of the Army to distribute educational material on tropical medicine to medical schools.

At the request of the Army Air Forces, a series of postgraduate lectures on pathology was arranged in many of the larger Air

Force Hospitals. A Division committee selected the lecturers, who contributed their time. Their expenses were paid and discussion material was sent from the American Registry of Pathology (under the auspices of the NRC) in the Army Medical Museum under a grant of $5,500 from the Josiah Macy Foundation.

The committees of the Division also cooperated with the Macy Foundation's program for the distribution of reprints of important new articles to members of the armed forces.

In the fall of 1943, the Division was asked to advise the Archivist of the United States on the question as to which of the medical records of the armed services and other governmental agencies should be preserved for research purposes. Through the interest and assistance of the Markle Foundation, funds were obtained for a study of representative samples of records and a committee was established to review the situation. It eventually became clear that all records with any potential research value would have to be preserved indefinitely because of administrative requirements. but a number of suggestions were offered to make their utilization by research workers more effective.

The Committee on Sanitary Engineering played an important part in the procurement of engineer officers in this specialty as an agency of the War Manpower Commission. The armed forces were assisted in obtaining the men best adapted for military service, and at the same time key personnel were reserved when required for important civilian needs. The Committee sponsored a number of studies of far-reaching significance, including the safeguarding of water supplies, cross-connections on piers and docks and the mushrooming war plants, sewage treatment systems, milk supplies for the Army, and many other projects of similar importance.

The Committee on Information reviewed the reports of committees and investigators and arranged for publication in the most appropriate journals of such reports as could receive general distribution in the "open" category. The Committee was instrumental in setting up an advisory group in the Office of the Surgeon General of the Army to facilitate news releases on items of general interest to the public. The Committee succeeded in obtaining the appointment of a general reclassification board for reconsideration of classified documents so that releases of important scientific contributions could be made as soon as the military situation permitted. The Subcommittee on Historical Records developed a plan for the medical history of the war which has been carefully integrated with the histories of the various services.

The Committee on Convalescence and Rehabilitation, in co-operation with a number of the other committees on military medicine, developed a far-reaching program to bridge the gap between the war and postwar periods for individuals who were casualties as a result of military action, disease or accident. Important lessons have been learned which should be of great significance to the medical management of the convalescent patient in civilian practice, particularly in respect to the importance of reducing the average period of complete bed rest, the mobilization of limbs, and adequate nutrition. Some of those findings will not only greatly expedite the recovery of the individual and contribute markedly to his morale, but will also effect tremendous savings in hospital management and medical care. This committee, together with the Committee on Industrial Medicine, is also studying, in considerable detail, industrial plans for more effective return and rehabilitation of men physically or mentally handicapped as a result of the war.

This brief and necessarily sketchy survey of the activities of the Division of Medical Sciences of the National Research Council will at least indicate the scope and, to some extent, the importance of the programs with which it has been deeply concerned. A really definitive statement cannot be published until the war is won. However, we can consider with profit some of the lessons that our war experience has taught us.

The lessons learned in meeting these tremendous problems in military medicine have both military and civilian implications for the future.

It is obvious to all that an efficient military machine will be required for a great many years to come. It would be calamitous if this program, which has functioned so well on the whole, should not be used to derive the greatest possible benefit from our military medical experience.

Experience has shown the need for detailed plans for the mobilization of the scientific resources of the country in the medical field around three major elements: (1) research laboratories and facilities; (2) the production of supplies and equipment; and (3) the best utilization of scientific mind-power.

Research needs a carefully integrated policy as to the role to be played by the various service laboratories and how these are to be related to civilian laboratories.

Funds must be made available so that research work required in the nation's interest can be carried out under contract in civilian research centers. Our experience in this war will provide a good starting point for such a program.

The organization of civilian research facilities should take into consideration the increasingly important role played by the research divisions of industrial organizations. Necessary legislation to obtain immediate pooling of information should be promulgated. Such legislation should protect individual and corporation rights in new developments and provide adequate incentives (utilizing both professional recognition and the profit motive in a manner compatible with our American philosophy of individual enterprise) without sacrificing the controls that have been found necessary to prevent monopolies, price-fixing and other abuses of economic power. We should not be faced again with the need for emergency legislation because the solution of a scientific problem requires the contravention of the letter, if not the spirit, of the law. We can ill afford to let totalitarian forms of government possess an organizational advantage, particularly when organization is supposed to be one of our fortes. American ingenuity can solve these problems within our own economic pattern.

Methods of production control based on the relative importance of medical needs should be developed for future "M-Days" and revised as circumstances dictate. Many of the present provisions for the production of supplies and equipment, rationing, etc., need little modification for their effectiveness in the future. However, experience has shown the tremendous importance of intimate collaboration of the various scientific disciplines, including medicine, *before* final models and plans are accepted and production methods are frozen. Improvements in design of incalculable importance to the fighting man have been made again and again in this war as a result of the study of the physiological performance of man in relation to his new machines, and again and again it has been found that these changes, important as they may be, cannot be made because they would upset production schedules. Here, too, is overwhelming evidence of the importance of continuation of the committees on military medicine. If these committees could have held meetings in the years *prior* to this war as part of the regular machinery for national defense, there can be no doubt that thousands of lives would have been saved and the war materially shortened.

Plans for the mobilization of scientific mind- and manpower are desperately needed. Only a nation rich in scientific resources of men and machines could afford the severe dislocations and inefficient use of technical personnel that have been the rule in this war. It is a truism, of course, that war is always wasteful and that we must expect a terrific loss of time and energy, even with the most favorable organization. But there is no need to aggravate this by thoughtless action resulting from the lack of a plan or of time to make one. The relation of scientific workers to selective service should be clearly defined. Adequate provision for training should be made, and matters of policy, such as whether scientific workers should be in uniform or wear civilian clothes, receive citations for important contributions, etc., should be worked out in time of peace if they are to be effective in time of war.

The opportunities afforded by the Division through its committees on military medicine for the exchange of experience between officers in the various services should be made use of to evaluate technics employed in the war. The practice of including the best civilian minds available in these discussions has proved its value. Ways and means should be found to make this a continuing rather than an emergency service. The problems of equipment, supplies, treatment methods, nomenclature, record forms and training manuals are all fruitful fields for further work.

While the Council has no coordinating responsibilities, nevertheless a great deal of unification has been made possible when the various services have asked the same technical committee to review their manuals. In this way, many inconsistencies of policy and method have been avoided. This simple technic could have been used to greater advantage had its potentialities been recognized earlier in the war, when the manuals and directives were first being prepared. There is no reason why the Council's committees could not serve the armed forces in this way in the years of peace. When problems and resources are identical, the procedures in the various services should be comparable. They should vary only because of special circumstances or because of the traditional language of the branch concerned. Needless differences of policy and technic unnecessarily confuse the relationships of the various branches of the armed forces with local and State public health agencies.

The question of publication or suppression of medical papers on research work and therapy needs close examination and a clearly defined policy for the future. The experience in this war should be evaluated to determine whether the holding of scientific developments in a restricted category has resulted, or could possibly have resulted, in any military advantage to our forces sufficient to compensate for the retardation of further scientific discoveries as a result of suppression. Many medical men, both civilian or military, have been critical of our haphazard policies in World War II. Not only from the traditional obligation of the physician to heal rather than to destroy, but from the very practical military consideration that as our forces advance, disease and even environmental hazards of the liberated or captured peoples become our responsibility, a good case can be made for treating everything but the most exceptional research findings in an "open" category. If such diseases or conditions have not been controlled or corrected by the enemy, we must treat them. On the other hand, if it were agreed in advance that all investigations in certain fields were to be restricted, adequate machinery could be established to insure circulation of such reports among those who need them in getting on with the war. Any policy is better than none—or several.

The importance of having an organization like the National Research Council in each country with which we are allied has been well demonstrated. Without such an organization, effective liaison is out of the question. It is, in fact, impossible to exchange restricted information with another country unless it has a similar mechanism. By the same token, a common policy on publication and restriction of medical papers must obviously be adopted by all cooperating nations. In the medical field our problems are so vast, our ignorance so great, and scientific minds so few that we can ill afford to disregard the opportunities offered by international collaboration.

These are only a few of the examples that might be given to

illustrate why the contributions of the committees on military medicine of the Division of Medical Sciences of the National Research Council, valuable as they have been during this war, would have been many times more valuable had they been carried out in the years prior to the outbreak of hostilities. It is obvious that the work will always be intensified in war and that many problems either do not develop or do not seem acute until the conflict is on, but there are enough of these to consider without also having to do basic planning under such conditions.

It has been apparent to everyone who has had a small part to play in the cooperative work involved in meeting military problems that humanity would be greatly served if only a fraction of this time and energy could be given to medical problems in time of peace. It is a curious commentary on life that in the midst of the holocaust we reach heights of service to our fellow men that we find difficult to achieve without the emotional stimulus of a nation at war. Nevertheless, it is hard to believe that we cannot find a way to harness at least some of the factors of this cooperative activity even in the midst of the distractions of peace.

The National Research Council has served successfully as a clearing house for the armed forces. There is every reason to suppose that the Council might also serve other agencies in a similar capacity. If ways and means could be found to provide traveling expenses, cost of meetings, and a modest amount for administration, committees for the coordination and appraisal of research work could serve civilian as well as military needs.

There are four major organizational groups for which service of this nature would be invaluable: (1) local, State and Federal government agencies; (2) universities; (3) foundations; and (4) industrial groups, represented either by trade institutes or by individual corporations. Executives in all these groups are continually faced with decisions that require an evaluation of the latest and best available knowledge. The question comes up again and again as to whether they should investigate a particular problem themselves or whether work is already in process elsewhere. Committees or boards of review to advise as to the promise, usefulness and need of proposed investigations would be extremely useful. This is exactly the kind of service the committees on military medicine are now performing for the armed services and the OSRD. A large number of foundations support research work in the medical field.

It is conceivable that they might find it worth while to support such review committees for the authority the Council could provide, and to avoid duplication of effort and obtain a pooling of results. Industry presents special problems, but the value of having as complete a knowledge as possible both of projects under way and of the people qualified to undertake special types of investigation is obvious.

It might be found desirable to amplify somewhat the formal membership of the medical division of the National Research Council. The possibility of organizing government, university, industrial and foundation groups on some type of representative basis might be considered. It should be possible, as a result of wartime experience, to make the division more representative of the really research-minded groups in the country, and at the same time to increase its sensitivity to problems and effectiveness in dealing with them. The theoretical ideal would be for the division to function as a national problem-solving agency in the research field, bringing men with the problems into contact with others with abilities and facilities and, if necessary, to the attention of potential financial sponsors.

The problem of providing machinery for adequate laboratory, experimental animal, and clinical trials of new therapeutic procedures and drugs has been emphasized by the war. Experience, both with reputable individuals having a worth-while idea and with others interested in promoting a profitable if valueless remedy, indicates the importance of such a service. This problem will probably have to be attacked eventually either by the A.M.A. or by some government agency. However, should this be long delayed, the Council might help by issuing a statement as to the evidence required before such a trial should be considered, and perhaps even develop basic protocols for the evaluation of the more common types of therapy.

The National Research Council has an honorable history in guiding fellowship programs. This is obviously not a wartime activity, but experience has shown the wisdom of considering advanced fellowships on a national and sometimes on an international basis. Many organizations which now have their own fellowship programs could be more effectively served and the fellows themselves more adequately guided if their programs could be planned by men with a wide knowledge of the experimental field, the individuals who work in it, and the problems that need to be solved. Perhaps the Council could extend its present program on request to provide service to foundations, professional societies and other organizations interested in fellowships. A clearing house would certainly be of great value. It is not hard to imagine a situation where far too many scholarships might become available in certain fields while other important fields were entirely neglected. With the government itself entering the field, the need for coordination of official and private effort certainly becomes apparent. The postgraduate training programs under consideration for returning medical officers emphasize the desirability of such a center. After all, our training facilities are limited, and careful planning is necessary if the various programs are not to overlap. Leadership in this field is needed which the National Research Council could provide.

Experience in keeping the committees on military medicine informed calls attention to the great need for a coordinated abstract service covering the major scientific fields. A plan might be developed by which the National Research Council could sponsor, and its divisional committees supervise, a complete series. The journals of original publication could require abstracts of all their authors, to be edited and forwarded with the journals to the abstracting service. Both the value to the nation and the cost of the service suggest that funds should be provided by the Federal government. Foreign language editions exchanged between various national research councils would greatly accelerate the development of science, and incidentally would be a tremendous factor in developing international good will and understanding at the professional level. Think what it would mean if we had foreign language editions to bring the liberated countries of Europe up to date on the scientific developments that took place during their enslavement. But first we need English editions. The return on the investment would be tremendous.

One other implication (of the many that might still be cited) should be mentioned. It will be interesting to watch the effect of the new discoveries on the character of medical practice. The trend in recent years has been increasingly toward specialization. The scientists are hard at work reducing the amount and kind of this specialization once more. With each specific therapy or diagnostic aid, the general practitioner grows in stature and the importance of the specialist declines. Moreover, the costs of medical care are reduced. Losses due to delayed diagnosis and treatment are avoided, convalescence shortened, and the average patient greatly benefited.

Great advances in technical knowledge and in methods of organization to increase the effectiveness of this knowledge in reducing human suffering and loss of life have been made during the war. Let us make the most of the gains for which so great a price has been paid.

INDEX

Fleet Marine Force, 224
Fleming, 14, 383
Flies, 133
Flight Nurse, 276, 299
  Surgeons, 112, 209, 220, 275-9, 299
Floor space, 144
Florey, 14, 383
Florida, 83
Fluorograph, 258
Flying clothing, 210, 286
"Focke-Wulf" jitters, 290
Food, 144, 153, 208, 380
  and Nutrition Board, 388
  Distribution Administration, 388
  experts, 92
Foreign languages, 97, 397
  School Graduates, 100
Fort Benning, Ga., 276, 299
    Parachute School, 276
  George Wright, Wash., 317
  Hancock, 338
  Knox, Ky., 378
  Pierce, Fla., 21
Fowler, Lt. Col. L. H., 105
Fox, Lt. Col. J. C., 105
Fractures, 197, 227
Frament, Paul Stanley, 234
France, 3, 16, 21, 59, 109, 257, 337-41
French physical standards, 9
Freon bomb, 17
  -pyrethrum bomb, 123, 169
Frostbite, 144, 210, 286
Fulton, Dr. John F., 370
Fumes, 231
Functional disorders of expressive movements, 54
"Fundamentals of Anesthesia," 377
Furstenberg, Dr. A. C., 371

Gage, Lt. Col. I. M., 105
  Lt. Col. M., 106
"Gallon Club," 351
Gamma globin, 19, 157
Garrison ration, 145
Gas, 111
  casualties, 217, 371, 387
  gangrene, 151, 382
Gasolines, 265
  high-octane, 265
Gastro-Enterology, 104
Gastro-intestinal diseases, 151, 153
  syndrome, 54
Gelatin, 15
General hospitals, 93, 102, 113, 116, 120, 187-8, 192, 196, 199, 200-3, 215
  surgery, 104, 182
Geneva Convention, 298
  Treaty of, 339
Genitalia defects, 40, 51-2
  wounds, 245

Genito-urinary diseases, 10
George Washington University Medical School, 136
Georgia, 83, 273
German physical standards, 9
Germany, 59, 109, 196, 211
Giberson, Lydia G., 370
Gilbert Islands, 226
Gillespie, Dr. R. D., 50
Girth of Registrants, 42
Glandular therapy, 14
Glenolden, Pa., 343
Gliders, 215
Global epidemiology, 136
Goethals, Col. T. R., 105
Gonococcus, 14
Gonorrhea, 40, 49, 51-2, 123, 143, 160-1, 256-7, 383
  intensive treatment of, 256
Goyas, 167
Gorman, William Louis, 234
Governors, 32
Gradle, Dr. Harry S., 371
Graduated Mild Exercises, 305
Graham, Dr. Evarts A., 370
Gramicidin, 14
Grant, Major Gen. David N. W., 12, 275-301
Granuloma inguinale, 160
Graw, Brig. Gen. Malcolm C., 209-10, 284
Great Britain, 21, 200, 204, 207, 212, 257
Great Lakes, Ill., 21
Greece, 257
Griffith, Dr. Charles Marion, 320-35
Group examinations, 34, 48
Guadalcanal, 68, 183, 232-9, 337
Guam, 20
Guantanamo Bay, 224
"Guides to Therapy for Medical Officers," 377
Guillotine amputation, 117-19, 242
Gums, 231
  defects, 40, 51-2
Gunshot wounds, 241-2
Guy, Lt. Col. C., 106
Gymnastics, 26
Gynecology, 104

Half-tracks, 211
Hall, Capt. W. W., 369
Hardy, John Ellis, 236
Harper Hospital, Detroit, 105
Hartford, 16
Harvard School of Public Health, 136
  University, Cambridge, Mass., 105-6
Hashinger, Lt. Col. E. H., 107
Hastings, Dr. A. Baird, 368
Havre, Mont., 239
Hawaii, 225, 255, 322

Nutrition, 11, 14, 141-7, 168, 180, 222
  Division, 144
  experts, 92
Nutritional problems, 224

Oakland, Cal., 229
Obstetrics, 104
Occupational health, 141
  reconditioning, 25
Office for Emergency Management, 61
  of Chief Surgeon, 216
      Administrative division, 216
      Dental division, 216
      Gas Casualties division, 216
      Historical division, 216
      Hospitalization division, 216
      Medical records division, 216
      Nursing division, 216
      Operations division, 216
      Personnel division, 216
      Preventive medicine division,
        216
      Professional services division,
        216-17
      Rehabilitation division, 216
      Supply division, 216
      Veterinary division, 216
  Civilian Defense, 269-70
      Hospital Section, 270
      Medical Division, 269
  Defense Health and Welfare Serv-
    ices, 36, 61, 63, 389
  Emergency Management, 367
  Foreign Relief and Rehabilitation,
    272, 373, 388
  Price Administration, 374, 388
  Production, Research and Develop-
    ment, 384
  Scientific Research and Develop-
    ment, 5, 7, 123, 154, 167, 170,
    367-9, 371-2, 375-6, 384-5
  War Information, 377
Officer Candidate Schools, 113
  Procurement, 220
Ohio, 83, 264
  plan, 34
Oiling, 19
Oklahoma, 83, 252
  State University, Oklahoma City, 106
Onchorcerciasis, 266
Operation with carpenter's tools, 133
Operations, 216
Operational fatigue, 288, 291
Ophthalmologic surgery, 188
Ophthalmology, 104
  Committee on, 371
"Ophthalmology and Otolaryngology,"
  377
Optical defects, 10
Optometrists, 92

Oral hygiene, 223
Oran, 297
Order of Carlos J. Finlay, 136
Oregon, 83, 255
"Organization and Operation American
  Red Cross Blood Donor Service," 347,
  349
Orient, 16
Orlando, Fla., 168
Orthopedic committee, 118
  shops, 118
  "subjects," 377
  surgery, 18, 104, 111, 182
      Committee on, 371
Osteomyelitis, 118-19
Otolaryngology, 104
  Committee on, 371
Overholser, Dr. Winfred, 35, 370
Overseas Hospital Ration, 145
Overweight, 40, 51, 53
Oximeter, 124
Oxygen, 298
  equipment, 284
  mask, 210
Oxygenation equipment, 224

Pacific Ocean, 21, 218
Palmer, Dr. W. W., 370
Panama, 275
Pan-American Highway, 269
  Sanitary Bureau, 142, 272
Pappataci fever, 164
Papua, 297
Paraffin, 17
Parasites, 40, 51, 53
Parasitologists, 79
Paratroop battalion surgeons, 112
Paratroopers, 144
Paratyphoid fever A, 151
      B, 151
Paresis, 15
Parker, Thaddeus, 235
Parran, Surgeon Gen., Thomas, 16, 38,
  247-73
Parsons, Lt. Col. Wm. B., 105
Pathology, 104
  Committee on, 370
"Patient Load of Physicians in Private
  Practice," 80
Paton, Major D. M., 106
Patterson, Com. J. K., 239
Paullin, Dr. James, 63
Pawling, N. Y., 317
Pearl Harbor, 12-13, 16, 45-7, 49, 58, 103,
  220, 225, 230, 270, 294, 338, 374, 383
Pediatrics, 104
Peiping (China) Union Medical College,
  336

414

415

WAVES, 72, 222, 230
Wayne University, Detroit, 105
Wearn, Dr. Joseph T., 370
Weed, Dr. Lewis H., 362, 368
Weight, Selectees, American, 8
    British, 9
    Canada, 8
    French, 9
    German, 9
    Japanese, 9
    registrants, 42-3
    rejections, 41
    Russian, 9
Welch, Lt. Col. John M., 93
Wells, Capt. C. Raymond, 36
Wentworth, Col. E., 105
Wessellhoeft, Jr., Second Lt. Robert, 12
West Suburban Hospital, Oak Park, Ill., 106
    Virginia, 84, 252
Western Pennsylvania Hospital, Pittsburgh, 106
Westinghouse Co., 17
Weston, Lt. Col. F. L., 106
Whipple, Dr. Allen O., 370
White House, 218, 365
    Paul Dudley, 370
Whole blood, 130, 246
    transfusions, 190, 213, 227
Wiggers, Prof, Carl J., 340
Williams, Lt. Col. J. P., 106
Wilson, Woodrow, 365
Winans, Lt. Col. H. M., 107

Winternitz, Dr. Milton G., 371
Wisconsin, 84
Wolman, Dr. Abel, 370
Woman physicians, committee on, 65, 77
Women, 26
Women's Medical Assn., 95
    Army Corps, 326
    Reserve, 222
    Reserve of the Coast Guard, 326
    Navy and Marine Corps, 326

Work load of physicians, 81
Workers in industry, 26
World War I, 3-4, 8, 19, 70, 102, 140, 143, 151, 153, 155, 157-8, 161, 169, 172, 174, 181, 187, 208, 230, 257, 259, 275, 280, 320-2, 324, 326, 331, 340, 357, 362, 365-6
    II, 3-4, 8, 14, 17, 26, 59, 139, 143, 151-2, 155, 157-8, 161, 165, 167, 172, 219, 230, 280, 297, 320-1, 324-6, 331, 334, 362-3, 366, 394
Wounds, 18, 180, 230, 233, 240, 375
    abdominal, 174, 179, 189, 233, 238, 240, 243
    bladder, 245
    chest, 174, 179, 189, 233, 238, 240, 243-4
    face, 240
    genitalia, 245
    head, 134, 179, 233, 238, 240, 242
    incidence, 177
    intestinal, 244-5
    mouth, 242
    neck, 243
    scalp, 242
    spinal, 245
    traumatic, 190, 240
Wright Field, Ohio, 283, 298
Wuchereria bancrofti, 20, 164
Wyoming, 84, 157

X-ray, 116, 143, 202, 213, 217, 258, 386
    mobile units, 258
    specialists, 76
    technicians, 92, 114

Yale University Medical School, New Haven, Conn., 105, 253
Yaws, 20
Yellow fever, 20, 133, 151, 161-2, 166, 169, 207
    vaccine, 266
"Your Body in Flight," 284
Yudin, Dr., 15

Zippers, 22